ASPERGER SYNDROME OR HIGH-FUNCTIONING AUTISM?

CURRENT ISSUES IN AUTISM

Series Editors: Eric Schopler and Gary B. Mesibov

University of North Carolina
Chapel Hill, North Carolina

ASPERGER SYNDROME OR HIGH-FUNCTIONING AUTISM?

Edited by

Eric Schopler and
Gary B. Mesibov

University of North Carolina
Chapel Hill, North Carolina

and

Linda J. Kunce

Illinois Wesleyan University
Bloomington, Illinois

PLENUM PRESS • NEW YORK AND LONDON

Library of Congress Cataloging-in-Publication Data

On file

ISBN 0-306-45746-6

© 1998 Plenum Press, New York
A Division of Plenum Publishing Corporation
233 Spring Street, New York, N.Y. 10013

http://www.plenum.com

10 9 8 7 6 5 4 3 2 1

Contributors

MARK ALLEN, Laboratory for Research on the Neuroscience of Autism, Children's Hospital and Health Center, La Jolla, California 92037

DARIEN BROOKS, Wilmington, North Carolina 28412

MYRA BETH BUNDY, Department of Psychology, Eastern Kentucky University, Richmond, Kentucky 40475

ERIC COURCHESNE, Laboratory for Research on the Neuroscience of Autism, Children's Hospital and Health Center, and Department of Neurosciences, University of California at San Diego, La Jolla, California 92093

STEPHAN EHLERS, Department of Child and Adolescent Psychiatry, Annedals Clinics, S-413 45 Göteborg, Sweden

MICHAELA ENE, California School of Professional Psychology—San Diego, San Diego, California 92121

CHRISTOPHER GILLBERG, Department of Child and Adolescent Psychiatry, Annedals Clinics, S-413 45 Göteborg, Sweden

CAROL A. GRAY, Jenison Public Schools, Jenison, Michigan 49428

ELLEN HANSON, California School of Professional Psychology—San Diego, San Diego, California 92121

STEPHEN R. HOOPER, Department of Psychiatry and The Clinical Center for the Study of Development and Learning, University of North Carolina School of Medicine, Chapel Hill, North Carolina 27599-7255

AMI KLIN, Child Study Center, Yale University School of Medicine, New Haven, Connecticut 06520

LINDA KUNCE, Illinois Wesleyan University, Bloomington, Illinois 61702-2900

ALAN LINCOLN, Laboratory for Research on the Neuroscience of Autism, Children's Hospital and Health Center, La Jolla, and School of Professional Psychology—San Diego, San Diego, California 92121

VAN BRUCE MacDONALD, Denver, Colorado 80210

CHRISTOPHER J. McDOUGLE, Section of Child and Adolescent Psychiatry, Department of Psychiatry, Indiana University School of Medicine, Indianopolis, Indiana 46202

THOMAS A. McKEAN, Columbus, Ohio 43229

GARY B. MESIBOV, Division TEACCH, Department of Psychiatry, University of North Carolina at Chapel Hill, Chapel Hill, North Carolina 27599-7180

SALLY OZONOFF, Department of Psychology, University of Utah, Salt Lake City, Utah 84112

JEFFREY B. PIGOTT, Raleigh, North Carolina 27607

JOHN C. POMEROY, Department of Psychiatry and Behavioral Science, State University of New York at Stony Brook, Stony Brook, New York 11794-8790

ERIC SCHOPLER, Division TEACCH, Department of Psychiatry, University of North Carolina at Chapel Hill, Chapel Hill, North Carolina 27599-7180

DAVE SPICER, Asheville, North Carolina 28805

PETER SZATMARI, Department of Psychiatry, McMaster University, Hamilton, Ontario L8N 3Z5, Canada

DIANE TWACHTMAN-CULLEN, Autism and Developmental Disabilities Consultation Center, Cromwell, Connecticut 06416

FRED R. VOLKMAR, Child Study Center, Yale University School of Medicine, New Haven, Connecticut 06520

LORNA WING, National Autistic Society Centre for Social and Communication Disorders, Bromley, Kent BR2 9HT, United Kingdom

SULA WOLFF, Formerly of the Royal Hospital for Sick Children and the Department of Psychiatry, University of Edinburgh, Edinburgh EH9 1RL, Scotland, United Kingdom

Preface

This volume, like the other nine in the *Current Issues in Autism* series, grew from an annual TEACCH Conference. The book, however, is more than simply a compilation of conference proceedings. It is, instead, built around the conference participants whose work on high-functioning autism and Asperger syndrome (AS) has achieved national and international recognition. Each of these experts was asked to develop a chapter around their presentations, and other authorities on these topics were also asked to contribute. Although we were unable to include everyone who has contributed to this important area of inquiry, the volume represents our best effort to organize the most current knowledge and state-of-the-art practices involving high-functioning people with autism and AS.

Although the precise relationship between high-functioning autism and AS is still under discussion, this book is relevant to those interested in both of these overlapping areas. Each author has expressed a personal view about how high-functioning autism and AS might relate, and readers will find the most current thinking about the debate. Although this volume does not include every facet of research and practice in high-functioning autism and AS, it is a comprehensive and useful integration of the state of the art and should be of great interest to teachers, parents, and researchers.

ERIC SCHOPLER
GARY B. MESIBOV

Acknowledgments

As with all of the volumes in this autism series, this book would not have been completed without the help of many dedicated people. First, we are grateful to Helen Garrison, who organized the conference that was the impetus for this book. Each year our TEACCH conferences continue to grow, but Helen always meets the extra demands with grace and skill. Superb secretarial assistance has been available from Jill Cagle and J. P. Barfield. Molly Compton has added her assistance in reading and editing each of the manuscripts and organizing the review and editing process. Not only are we fortunate in having such skilled people working with us, but their good cheer and cooperative spirit make these projects much more pleasant and efficient.

As with all of our activities, these books would not be possible without our many superb TEACCH colleagues, too numerous to name. Their clinical insights and skills, so willingly shared with us, have been our entree into this topic. Their many observations are seen throughout the book and have greatly enhanced our understanding of the important issues.

We especially appreciate the contributions of the many families we see throughout the year. Their willingness to share their struggles and insights consistently inspire all of our clinical and scholarly efforts.

Finally, the School of Medicine at the University of North Carolina at Chapel Hill, and especially the Department of Psychiatry, have provided the kind of environment that cultivates and nurtures our activities. The University of North Carolina at Chapel Hill's emphasis on scholarly research and public service encourages us to blend our scholarly work and clinical practice into a book of this kind. We are also most grateful to the members of the North Carolina General Assembly, who continue to support services, scholarly research, and training aimed at understanding and ameliorating the effects of autism and related developmental disorders.

ERIC SCHOPLER
GARY B. MESIBOV

Contents

Chapter 6

ASPERGER SYNDROME AND NONVERBAL LEARNING
DISABILITIES   107

Fred R. Volkmar and Ami Klin

Chapter 7

SCHIZOID PERSONALITY IN CHILDHOOD: THE LINKS WITH
ASPERGER SYNDROME, SCHIZOPHRENIA SPECTRUM
DISORDERS, AND ELECTIVE MUTISM   123

Sula Wolff

Part III: Neuropsychological Issues

Chapter 8

NEUROBIOLOGY OF ASPERGER SYNDROME: SEVEN CASE
STUDIES AND QUANTITATIVE MAGNETIC RESONANCE
IMAGING FINDINGS   145

Alan Lincoln, Eric Courchesne, Mark Allen, Ellen Hanson, and
Michaela Ene

Part IV: Treatment Issues

Chapter 9

SOCIAL STORIES AND COMIC STRIP CONVERSATIONS WITH
STUDENTS WITH ASPERGER SYNDROME AND
HIGH-FUNCTIONING AUTISM   167

Carol A. Gray

Part V: Related Conditions

Chapter 13

REPETITIVE THOUGHTS AND BEHAVIOR IN PERVASIVE
DEVELOPMENTAL DISORDERS: PHENOMENOLOGY AND
PHARMACOTHERAPY   293

Christopher J. McDougle

Chapter 14

LEARNING CHARACTERISTICS OF INDIVIDUALS WITH
ASPERGER SYNDROME   317

Stephen R. Hooper and Myra Beth Bundy

Part VI: Personal Essays

Chapter 15

A PERSONAL ACCOUNT OF AUTISM   345

Thomas A. McKean

Chapter 16

AN ESSAY OF FAITH, PERSERVERANCE, AND HARD WORK   357

Jeffrey B. Pigott

Chapter 17

HOW FATE TAUGHT ME THE VIOLIN   363

Darien Brooks

Chapter 18

HOW THE DIAGNOSIS OF ASPERGER'S HAS INFLUENCED MY
LIFE   367

Van Bruce MacDonald

Chapter 19

AUTISTIC AND UNDIAGNOSED: MY CAUTIONARY TALE   377

Dave Spicer

Part VII: Conclusion

Chapter 20

PREMATURE POPULARIZATION OF ASPERGER SYNDROME   385

Eric Schopler

1

Overview

Introduction

ERIC SCHOPLER and GARY B. MESIBOV

In the 5 years since we edited *High-Functioning Individuals with Autism* (Schopler & Mesibov, 1992), an increasing tide of referrals has come to TEACCH. A majority of these carry a possible diagnosis of Asperger syndrome (AS) or Asperger disorder (AD). With our TEACCH faculty and staff engaging in training and consultation in other regions of the United States and distant countries, they have brought back reports of increasing referrals in this same direction. Increase in prevalence is also confirmed by research data (Honda, Shimizu, Misumi, Niimi, & Ohashi, 1996).

With the publication of *High-Functioning Individuals with Autism*, we had assumed that no significant clinical distinction existed between high-functioning autism (HFA) and AS. However, because of the growing number of studies using subjects diagnosed with AS, we thought it important to edit a volume in our *Current Issues in Autism* series focusing on AS and how it compares with HFA. For this purpose we assembled a distinguished panel to author chapters on various aspects of AS, including its history, diagnosis, related conditions, and treatment. We also invited a few essays from individuals qualified to report on what the designation of AS means to them from the inside out.

We were unable to include contributions from all of the major researchers who have published their work on this diagnostic label, but we have been assured that virtually all such investigators are at least included in the references of this volume. Our respective chapter authors have presented interesting snapshots of

ERIC SCHOPLER and GARY B. MESIBOV • Division TEACCH, Department of Psychiatry, University of North Carolina at Chapel Hill, Chapel Hill, North Carolina 27599-7180.

Asperger Syndrome or High-Functioning Autism?, edited by Schopler *et al.* Plenum Press, New York, 1998.

an aspect of AS in which they have had a special interest. We refer to these chapters as photographs because the issues defining AS are still in motion, and will no doubt provide a different set of snapshots during the next decade. This volume is intended to provide a status report on research and interventions with this population. The AS diagnosis also raises important issues in the classification of mental disorders. Is there a distinction between AS and HFA? If the answer is no, what are the consequences for both research and treatment? The controversy over the existence of AS as a disorder raises broader questions about the labeling process in general.

In an attempt to provide our readers with a better understanding of the labeling process, we have requested that all contributors discuss their view as to whether a distinction between AS and HFA exists or whether these are different labels for essentially the same condition. For most issues informing new social policies in the United States, our politicians are proposing planks of a platform "to form a bridge to the twenty-first century." This volume is offered as a modest plank in the neuro-microcosmic issue of our understanding of HFA and AS in the next century.

For an overview of this fascinating disorder, Lorna Wing presents the history of AS, including similar individuals in historical and fictional accounts predating Asperger's own publication. Wing provides clues about its resurgence after four decades of relative dormancy. No one is better qualified to do so, as her paper on AS (Wing, 1981) is credited by many with inspiring this renewed interest. Although Asperger did not publish a list of essential diagnostic criteria, he did describe many different characteristics of these children. Wing lists eight points that he emphasized. It will be useful for the reader to bear these in mind because they differ from the AS "criteria" designated by Gillberg and Gillberg (1989) and Szatmari, Bartolucci, and Bremner (1989). Even on features of social and language problems, each of these groups suggests interesting differences.

John Pomeroy presents a model for subtyping the Pervasive Developmental Disorders (PDD). After a selective review of the literature, he focuses on a study addressing the validity of PDD subtypes. Pomeroy's data suggest that it is justifiable to define three subtypes of PDD without mental retardation. The subtypes include an autistic group with higher verbal than performance skills, a language-impaired group, which did not show any of the unique strengths typically seen in high-functioning individuals with autism, and a non-language-impaired PDD group with higher verbal than performance skills. Pomeroy's study suggests that there are distinctive, noncontinuous subgroups among the high-functioning group and several of these subtypes might be distinct from AS as well. The study also suggests that these subtypes might be further delineated through empirical research. Ongoing efforts to identify subtypes of HFA seem promising.

Readers will have their overview of AS and HFA further expanded by the documentation of five research distinctions in the Szatmari chapter. He finds that

AS can be distinguished from PDD and from autism, but not from HFA. The reader is led through an intriguing research trek to learn about the possibilities of diagnostic distinctions between AS and other disorders including schizoid, schizotypal, schizophrenia, semantic and pragmatic language disorders, obsessive-compulsive disorders, and social phobias. He concludes that a differential diagnosis of AS is premature, that no clear distinction between HFA and AS has yet been established, but that the rate of improvement in language may offer the distinction between AS with more rapid improvement and HFA with slower improvement.

Gillberg and Ehlers provide a valuable compilation of the published literature on AS. They have found at least 140 English-language articles were published in the 14 years since Wing's 1981 inspirational paper, with more than two-thirds of these appearing in the last 5 years, and only 4 prior to 1980. This chapter both establishes the onset of the AS resurgence and it also offers a remarkable demonstration of the confusion produced in the process.

Although Asperger himself published no AS criteria, Gillberg and Gillberg (1989) developed their own, distinguished from those of Szatmari and colleagues (1989) and other researchers who prioritized their own favorite criteria be they clumsiness, impaired executive function, or pedantic speech. To give the discussion an additional spin, this chapter helps the reader to understand how the research criteria of ICD-10 (WHO, 1993) differ from the clinical criteria of DSM IV (APA, 1994). This leaves us pondering how research progress on AS will proceed if the clinical population studied meets different criteria than those studied in formal research. It is a small wonder that the chapter is written as if AS is established, yet the authors conclude that it is not possible to distinguish AS from HFA.

Volkmar and Klin join the previously cited authors in acknowledging that the state of confusion over the AS label is not confined to the overlaps between AS and autism. The confusion is generously extended to other diagnostic concepts such as schizoid personality disorders, semantic–pragmatic disorder, developmental learning disability of the right hemisphere, and so on.

The material on AS in this chapter is based on the DSM-IV field trial, which was a primary factor bringing AS into official existence. Its use in DSM-IV is, of course, no assurance that the various field trial participants used the same AS definition for their count. They were expected to base it on the ICD-10 research definition, stipulating no clinically significant delay in language or cognitive development. The possibility of circular reasoning plaguing other AS studies is acknowledged by the authors. Nevertheless, the authors optimistically conclude that autism and HFA can be clearly distinguishable whereas AS and nonverbal learning disability (NLD) cannot be distinguished. These demonstrations include deficits in tactile perceptions, psychomotor coordination, visual-spatial organization, nonverbal problem solving, and well-developed rote verbal memory. For example, AS students and people with NLD have difficulty in adapting to new situations, and they were also poor in language perceptions and prosody. Although Volkmar and Klin do not claim to resolve the confusion over the AS diagnosis, the connections they suggest between AS and NLD hold the promise for diagnostic grouping that will be meaningful regardless of how the AS controversy plays out.

Sula Wolff has been interested in schizoid personality of childhood for over 30 years. In this chapter she concurs with the authors of other chapters that diagnostic confusion over the AS classifications abounds; she argues for additional labels of overlap, adding schizophrenia spectrum and elective mutism, benign psychosis, ego disturbance, borderline states, circumscribed interest patterns, right hemisphere deficits, and multiplex developmental disorders. It is a small wonder that she reports that children with AS and with symptoms of schizoid personality resemble, and also differ from, each other. Both groups show abnormalities of social reciprocity, circumscribed and repetitive interests, and communication. The differences are that social differences showed in school with peers for schizoid personality disorders rather than at home, special interests were more sophisticated than for the autistic, and communication problems were more subtle. Because Wolff suspects a common genetic process for these related labels, differences between them could be indicative of differences in their socializing conditions rather than in their disabilities.

A focus on neurological factors is provided in the Lincoln *et al.* chapter. These authors offer a preliminary report on seven cases of AS studied with magnetic resonance imaging (MRI) procedures. They observed intriguing structural characteristics. Four of the seven cases had relatively small neocerebellar vernal lobules VI and VII compared with normal controls. They suggest that these AS cases show some degree of cerebellar hypoplasia and that this is similar to what they have reported for cases of autism. Larger samples are needed, however, to see if these brain measures hold up across the two diagnostic labels, or whether distinguishing differences will be found.

The reader may wonder whether a meaningful intervention can be formulated for a diagnostic category with uncertain status like AS. However, we are inclined to agree with Volkmar and Klin that the qualitative distinctions reported between characteristics of AS and HFA are more closely tied to research than to treatment.

Carol Gray's chapter offers an interesting guided tour through her intervention using social stories and comic strip conversations. Social stories offer individualized lessons on social situations "obvious" to most, but confusing to individuals diagnosed with either HFA or AS. The stories include orientation as to where, when, who, what, and why. The topic and context are presented from the students' perspective. The likelihood of a literal interpretation needs to be considered.

Comic strip conversations are another forum for developing group conversations using pictures and conversation balloons. Gray admits that some students are not interested in these, some even refuse to participate, but many find them most helpful. Outcome studies have not yet been completed, but the social story comic strip technique has evoked considerable interest as a most promising educational tool. There is no distinction in its application between AS and HFA.

The Twachtman-Cullen chapter offers a most useful insight into how language and communication in individuals with AS or HFA deviate from the general population. This chapter is not a review of the formal aspects of language but is rather a focus on language as communication and social interaction. This is the area in which both researchers and individuals with the AS/HFA impairment experience the most difficulty. The pragmatics of language or the various uses of it include functions such as requesting, criticizing, asking, discussing opinions, expressing complex thoughts, feelings, and emotions, speculating, negotiating, deceiving, imploring, and understanding others. These are examples of communication difficulties for AS and HFA.

Body language, including gestures, facial expression, eye gaze, and voice intonation and stress, all constitute often underrated aspects of communication. Research is cited showing that only 7% of the emotional meaning of a message is based on words, while the other 93% is expressed through body language. Along with their communication difficulties, individuals with AS and HFA tend to be literal and have trouble making inferences and interpreting metaphors. Given these problems of communication, it follows that such individuals have trouble managing conversational topics and processing facts and factual information. Twachtman-Cullen's clear review of the communication problems is not translated into interventions in this chapter, but it does leave the reader with a better understanding of individuals confined by the communication problems of HFA and AS.

Kunce and Mesibov describe educational approaches to teaching students with HFA and AS in the classroom. They describe the principles and strategies of structured teaching, a central component of the TEACCH Program since its inception, and demonstrate how it can be utilized in the design of educational interventions for students with HFA and AS. Teachers, parents, and practitioners will find these classroom applications especially interesting and useful. Although structured teaching is the focal point, intervention strategies based on a variety of effective treatment approaches are described and demonstrated. Historically, Division TEACCH was associated with separate classrooms for students with autism, and this chapter shows how the techniques have been expanded to include a wide range of interventions representing a full continuum of services.

Sally Ozonoff's chapter guides us through the definition, assessment, and intervention of executive function deficits. The large majority of past studies have found deficiencies in executive functions for individuals in the autism spectrum. Executive function is a broad, multifaceted concept and its dysfunction is found in many conditions outside the autism spectrum. Nevertheless, to remediate this disorder it is first necessary to identify its individual expression. Ozonoff provides a most useful review of available neuropsychological tests, behavioral observations, and interventions with parents and teachers. Interventions emphasized involve cognitive and behavioral approaches including self-management techniques, monitoring their own behavior, and cognitive structures that can be implemented through classroom modifications.

McDougle's chapter offers intriguing distinctions between the obsessive-compulsive behaviors among the pervasive developmental disorders. Comparing obsessive-compulsive disorder (OCD) with repetitive thoughts and behaviors in PDD, he documents some clinically significant differences. He reports that obsessions best describe OCD including aggressive, sexual, or religious thoughts not usually found with autism. On the other hand, autism is characterized by compulsions usually seen in observable behaviors. Likewise, individuals with OCD are aware of and can articulate internal thoughts, an awareness found less frequently in autism. This distinction might be accounted for by differences in IQ. Serotonin uptake inhibitors, among other drugs, have been demonstrated to be effective in double-blind studies with adult OCD patients, and may also be effective for PDD. However, they may be better tolerated by adolescents and adults than by children.

Hooper and Bundy review the various studies that have examined the learning characteristics of individuals with AS. In 9 of these 20 studies, AS subjects were compared with HFA subjects. The authors conclude that there are subtle differences in learning characteristics between AS and HFA. AS will show higher verbal than nonverbal abilities, and also higher scores on theory of mind tasks, relative to HFA. Hooper and Bundy underscore observations made in the Volkmar and Klin chapter that the implications for assessment and treatment may be more similar for nonverbal learning disabilities and AS than for AS and HFA. The question of the distinction between AS and HFA is also still far from resolved for these authors.

Next we have some personal essays from high-functioning people with autism/AS who describe their experiences and perceptions in compelling first-hand accounts. This articulate group recounts their early experiences, coping strategies, personal defeats, and major triumphs. No book on this topic would be complete without hearing from the clients themselves. Readers will enjoy these wonderful opportunities to enhance their own understanding and insights.

In the final chapter of this volume, Schopler provides a provocative synthesis of why most of the chapter authors felt that a clear distinction between AS and HFA has not yet been established. He discusses the ease with which such a distinction could be defined, by consensus, but suggests possible consequences, primarily dysfunctional. For him the preponderant evidence indicates that the currently assumed diagnostic status for AS produces unnecessary, counterproductive confusion and is premature.

REFERENCES

American Psychiatric Association. (1994). *Diagnostic and statistical manual of mental disorders* (4th ed.). Washington, DC: Author.

Gillberg, I. C., & Gillberg, C. (1989). Asperger syndrome—some epidemiological considerations: A research note. *Journal of Child Psychology and Psychiatry, 30,* 631–638.

Honda, H., Shimizu, Y., Misumi, K., Niimi, M., & Ohashi, Y. (1996). Cumulative incidence and prevalence of childhood autism in children in Japan. *British Journal of Psychiatry, 169,* 228–235.

Schopler, E., & Mesibov, G.B. (Eds.) (1992). *High-functioning individuals with autism.* New York: Plenum Press.

Szatmari, P., Bartolucci, G., & Bremner, R. (1989). Asperger's syndrome and autism: Comparisons on early history and outcome. *Developmental Medicine and Child Neurology, 31,* 709–720.

Wing, L. (1981). Asperger's syndrome: A clinical account. *Psychological Medicine, 11,* 115–129.

World Health Organization. (1993). *International classification of diseases: Tenth revision.* Chapter V. Mental and behavioral disorders (including disorders of psychological development): Diagnostic criteria for research. Geneva: Author.

2

The History of Asperger Syndrome

LORNA WING

In physical medicine, the identification of recurring patterns of signs or symptoms suggesting a common pathology and etiology has led to major advances in prevention and treatment of a range of conditions. The "specific disease" model is appropriate and useful in some but not all disorders. A major theme in the history of psychiatry is the ongoing struggle to identify discrete patterns among the variety of symptoms and signs of emotional, cognitive, and behavioral disturbances in order to facilitate research into causes and treatments. The identification of syndromes among the developmental disorders affecting behavior is particularly difficult. Overt behavioral abnormalities in such conditions are the outcome of impairments of psychological functions, resulting from abnormalities of brain functions, caused by biochemical and/or structural neuropathology, produced by the original etiology. Added to this are the effects of individual differences in brain organization, changes with increasing age, individual personality, and environmental influences. Recognizing patterns within this bewildering complexity is akin to classifying clouds.

Attempts to identify syndromes among disorders of psychological development can be based on overt behavior, developmental history, psychological functions, brain pathology, etiology, or a mixture of these different levels of discourse. This can lead to the same conditions being defined on different types of criteria by different workers and not recognized as the same. Variation in selection criteria can also give rise to suggested "syndromes" that overlap but

LORNA WING • National Autistic Society Centre for Social and Communication Disorders, Bromley, Kent BR2 9111, United Kingdom.

Asperger Syndrome or High-Functioning Autism?, edited by Schopler *et al.* Plenum Press, New York, 1998.

are not identical. Definitions can be made narrow and specific or placed within a broader spectrum.

The above discussion is of particular relevance to the history and present status of the concept of Asperger syndrome. In this chapter, Asperger's original account of his syndrome will be outlined, followed by examples of characters in legends and literature who resembled Asperger's descriptions. The guises in which the syndrome appeared in the psychiatric literature before Asperger published his first paper on the subject will be discussed. The minimal recognition of Asperger's work in the English language literature during the period 1944 to 1980 will be compared with the situation in continental Europe during this time and with the escalation of interest from the early 1980s to the present day. The relationship of the syndrome to other developmental disorders and psychiatric conditions and its current classification in the standard diagnostic systems will be examined. The concept of a spectrum of autistic disorders will be explained. Finally, the contribution made by Asperger's work in this field will be evaluated.

ASPERGER'S DESCRIPTION OF HIS SYNDROME

Asperger was an Austrian pediatrician specializing in remedial pedagogy. He wrote his first paper on what has come to be known as his syndrome in 1944, in a German journal of psychiatry and neurology (Asperger, 1944, translated by Frith, 1991). He chose the label *autistic psychopathy* using the latter word in the technical sense of an abnormality of personality. Because the term *psychopath* has come to be equated with antisocial behavior, the neutral term *Asperger syndrome* is now in common use. Asperger outlined the clinical picture, gave some lengthy case histories, and discussed his views on the nature of this unusual pattern of behavior. He described many facets of the behavior of children with his syndrome but did not give a list of essential diagnostic criteria. However, he particularly emphasized the following points:

1. The children were socially odd, naive, inappropriate, emotionally detached from others.
2. They were markedly egocentric and highly sensitive to any perceived criticism, while being oblivious of other people's feelings.
3. They had good grammar and extensive vocabularies. Their speech was fluent but long-winded, literal and pedantic, used for monologues and not for reciprocal conversations.
4. They had poor nonverbal communication and monotonous or peculiar vocal intonation.
5. They had circumscribed interests in specific subjects, including collecting objects or facts connected with these interests.

6. Although most of the affected children had intelligence in the borderline, normal, or superior range on tests, they had difficulty in learning
   conventional schoolwork. However, they were capable of producing
   remarkably original ideas and had skills connected with their special
   interests.
7. Motor coordination and organization of movement was generally poor,
   although some could perform well in areas of special interest to them,
   such as playing a musical instrument.
8. The children conspicuously lacked common sense.

In addition to the above, Asperger also mentioned stereotyped play, odd
responses to sensory stimuli, including oversensitivity to sound, fascination with
spinning objects, stereotyped body movements, aggression, destructiveness, and
restlessness. These all often occur in Kanner's autism, a point that will be
enlarged on later. As in Kanner's autism, there was a marked excess of males
among those with Asperger syndrome.

Asperger summed up the children's problems in his hypothesis that they
failed to assimilate the automatic routines of everyday life (such as motor skills,
basic academic skills, and social conventions) but followed their own spontaneous interests regardless of any environmental constraints. He emphasized that
the traits were lifelong, though the most able achieved success in adult life,
sometimes of a high order, by finding a niche in which they could use their special
interests and associated talents. He remarked that the parents had not usually
noticed any abnormality in the children before the age of 3 years and sometimes
not until they started school.

THE SYNDROME IN LEGENDS AND FICTION

This constellation of features has, presumably, always existed among
human beings. Uta Frith (1989) explored this theme with insight and humor in
relation to the wider spectrum of autistic conditions. Some of her examples
undoubtedly fit Asperger's description. Among the legends of the early followers
of St. Francis of Assisi were some concerning Brother Juniper. He was honest
and humble but exhibited startling social naiveté and literal interpretation of the
rules of his order, including, on several occasions, giving away his own clothes.
He had to be constantly watched by the other brothers, who evidently regarded
him with a mixture of admiration, affection, amusement, and bewildered exas-
peration.

Uta Frith also pointed out how individuals with the traits described by
Asperger appear in fiction. One example she gives is that of Sherlock Holmes.
The author, Sir Arthur Conan Doyle, sprinkled clues throughout the series of
Sherlock Holmes stories that indicate many Asperger-like traits. In the first

chapter of the first book, Dr. Watson comments on the surprising gaps in Holmes's general knowledge in contrast to his remarkable collection of facts about abstruse subjects, such as the 140 varieties of tobacco ash. There is also an older brother, Mycroft Holmes, appearing in one or two stories, who has even more of the syndrome than Sherlock himself. Grove (1988) suggested that the Charles Dickens's character, Barnaby Rudge, was autistic. A good case can be made that he has characteristics of Asperger syndrome. He is naive and inappropriate in his social relations and has fluent speech, though the content is odd. His greatest love is for Grip, his pet raven. Some people with Asperger syndrome are closely attached to animals, unlike those with autism, who tend to be indifferent to them. Asperger emphasized that the quality of single-mindedness and detachment from competing demands is essential for success in the arts and sciences. The eccentric artist and absent-minded professor are long-accepted stereotypes that are familiar in comedy but are based on reality.

THE SYNDROME IN PSYCHIATRIC LITERATURE BEFORE 1944

In the psychiatric literature published before Asperger's first paper on his syndrome, there are descriptions and discussions of personality traits that overlap with those found in Asperger syndrome. Among Kretschmer's (1925) case histories of people with "schizothymic" personality disorder, one or two seem very similar to the Asperger picture. One young man, for example, had no friends at school, was odd and awkward in social interaction, had difficulty with speaking, never took part in rough games, was oversensitive, and was unhappy when away from home. Together with his sister, he invented a detailed imaginary world. Definitions of schizothymic or schizoid personality included lack of empathy, single-mindedness, odd communication, social isolation, and oversensitivity.

Some accounts of individuals who pursue their own interests with ruthless indifference to other people's feelings and needs suggest similarities to Asperger syndrome. Schneider (1923) termed them *affectionless psychopaths*, also known as *cold callous psychopaths*. It is possible that, among those given this diagnosis, there are included some of the very small proportion of people with Asperger syndrome who commit crimes, especially those who harm others in pursuit of their special interests (Asperger, 1944; Baron-Cohen, 1988; Mawson, Grounds, & Tantam, 1985; Wing, 1981).

The problem with early writings on these personality disorders is that the descriptions were couched in imprecise general terms, almost all were concerned with adults, and little or no information was given on development in infancy and childhood. It seems likely that the way these labels were used included some people with Asperger syndrome but also embraced a wider range of clinical pictures. Sula Wolff (1995) refers to one early paper, by Ssucharewa (1926), that was concerned with children. This Russian author described a group of boys with a pattern of behavior she called *schizoid personality of childhood*. Her description suggests an overlap with Asperger syndrome.

Another source of case histories that strike a chord is found in writings on the so-called "savant syndrome." Treffert (1989) reviewed the historical accounts, starting with Langdon Down's lecture on the subject in 1887. As Treffert pointed out, whereas many savants are severely mentally retarded apart from their special skills and best fit a diagnosis of typical autism, some have intelligence in the normal range and have many similarities to Asperger syndrome.

The most striking coincidence in the literature was the publication, in 1943, of Leo Kanner's first paper on the syndrome he named *early infantile autism*. Both Kanner and Asperger, independently of each other, followed Bleuler in using the words *autism* and *autistic* to capture the lack of social instinct in the children they described. Later, Asperger (1979) referred to Kanner's work, but, as far as the present author can ascertain, Kanner never mentioned Asperger's papers. The clinical pictures drawn by Kanner and Asperger overlap to a large extent, despite some differences. Asperger (1979) noted the many similarities between his and Kanner's group but tended to feel that the conditions were different. In his first paper, Kanner considered that his syndrome was unique and separate from all other childhood conditions.

THE SYNDROME IN PSYCHIATRIC LITERATURE AFTER 1944

Kanner and Asperger wrote their first papers on their respective syndromes during the Second World War. Kanner published in English in an American journal. His work became known in English-speaking and other countries. The numbers of publications on autism by other authors grew slowly at first, but with increasing rapidity from the 1960s onwards. In 1971 the first issue was published of the *Journal of Autism and Childhood Schizophrenia* devoted to autism and related topics, which, for its first 3 years, was edited by Kanner. Eric Schopler became the editor in March 1974. From June 1979 onwards, the title was changed to the *Journal of Autism and Developmental Disorders*.

Asperger, on the other hand, wrote in German, in a German language journal and for many years was little heard of in the United Kingdom or the United States. However, during the 1950s, through the 1970s his work became known in clinical psychiatry in German- and Dutch-speaking countries and in Russia. The syndrome was described in occasional papers in various journals and in at least one textbook of psychiatry, published in the Netherlands (Prick & Van Der Waals, 1965). Some writers considered that Kanner and Asperger syndromes were different entities while others regarded them as overlapping manifestations of the same condition. For example, Lutz, in Switzerland, considered they had much in common and he referred to Van Krevelen's report of three pairs of siblings, in each of which one had Kanner and the other had Asperger syndrome (Lutz, 1964). Paradoxically, Van Krevelen (1971) argued that the syndromes were different (see below). As far as is known to the present author, during this period there was no systematic research on the syndrome. It appears that there was little or no knowledge of Asperger's work in French-speaking countries. The present author has no information concerning interest in Asperger syndrome in Eastern Europe or Asia, apart from Russia.

In 1962, the Dutch workers, Van Krevelen and Kuipers, published a paper in English on Asperger syndrome because they considered that Asperger's work was insufficiently known in English-speaking countries. Van Krevelen wrote in English again in 1971, in the first issue of the *Journal of Autism and Childhood Schizophrenia*. In this paper he contrasted Kanner and Asperger syndromes, concluding that they were different but noting how both could occur in members of the same families. He listed a number of reasons for regarding the syndromes as different; for example, a child with early infantile autism walks early and talks late, if at all, whereas the converse is true for Asperger syndrome; in autism, speech, if present, is not used to communicate, whereas the child with Asperger syndrome tries to communicate but in a one-sided way. The problem with Van Krevelen's formulation is that many, perhaps the majority of, individuals manifest a mixture of the characteristics that he thought differentiated the syndromes. In his final point, that early infantile autism is a "psychotic process," whereas Asperger syndrome is a "personality trait," he uses terms that, in effect, have no useful meaning. He suggested that an autistic child had the genes for Asperger syndrome but became autistic because of some perinatal organic brain damage.

In 1970, a book by Bosch was translated into English. It was originally written in German and published in 1962. This was mainly concerned with an abstruse but fascinating discussion of the nature of language disturbances in autistic conditions. Bosch also compared Kanner and Asperger syndromes and suggested that there was a close relationship between the two conditions. In 1974, the Russian psychiatrists, Isaev and Kagan, wrote in English about "autistic psychopathy." A paper by Mnukhin and Isaev on the probable organic nature of some forms of "autistic or schizoid psychopathy" was translated from the Russian and published in English in 1975. In a book on autism published in 1976, the present author referred briefly to Asperger syndrome and raised the question of its relationship with Kanner's autism but without reaching any conclusion (Wing, 1976a, b).

At the beginning of the 1980s, the present author (Wing, 1981) published a paper discussing the clinical features, course, differential diagnosis, and management of Asperger syndrome, based on Asperger's own account and on 35 subjects, ranging in age from 5 to 35 years, seen and diagnosed by the author. The purpose was to present the hypothesis that the so-called syndrome was a variant of autism, although the author gave the arguments for and against this view. Following this paper, interest in Asperger syndrome began to grow, possibly because Wing emphasized its relevance for adult psychiatry. Tantam

(1986, 1988), in his study of adults with Asperger syndrome, found that the diagnostic features present in childhood continued into adult life. Interest was heightened with the publication of the book on autism and Asperger syndrome edited by Frith (1991) in which she included her translation into English of Asperger's original paper, making this accessible to English-speaking workers. As can be seen from the other chapters in this volume, the literature in this field has steadily expanded and now includes work on etiology, neuropathology, diagnosis, differential diagnosis, education, and other ways of helping.

Wing (1981) discussed the epidemiology of Asperger syndrome. A study in the Camberwell area of London, England, carried out in the years 1972–1976 (Wing & Gould, 1979) identified only about 2 in 10,000 children with the behavioral features described by Asperger. The problem was that the children included in this study were all receiving some form of special education, so the rate suggested was a gross underestimate. Ehlers and Gillberg (1993) published an epidemiological study of children aged 7–16 years attending mainstream schools in Gothenburg, Sweden. They calculated a rate of 71 per 10,000 for all children with social impairment and IQ of 70 or more, of whom half (36 per 10,000) had the diagnostic criteria for Asperger syndrome used by the authors that were based on Asperger's own account.

ASPERGER SYNDROME BY OTHER NAMES

Parallel with the development of the literature on Asperger syndrome, some papers have appeared that focus on one particular clinical feature that can be found in the syndrome. The authors do not mention Asperger's work but the descriptions of the general behavior of the individuals concerned strongly suggest that they had the full syndrome.

One of the most fascinating examples is Luria's (1965/1969) account of the "mnemonist" who had an extraordinarily vivid and accurate visual memory. He earned his living with his memory act in the music halls but was an odd, socially isolated individual. The details that can be gleaned from Luria's book suggest he may have had the features of Asperger syndrome.

Robinson and Vitale (1954) wrote about children with circumscribed interest patterns and gave three case histories that were closely similar to Asperger's descriptions of his children. Leo Kanner was one of the discussants of this paper and his comments were also published. The authors and Kanner mentioned the similarities with autism and "childhood schizophrenia" but Asperger's work appeared to be unknown to them. Adams (1973), in a book on "obsessive" children, described some with clinical pictures resembling Asperger syndrome but without any reference to his publications.

Some writers have concentrated on impairments of the semantic and pragmatic aspects of language (Blank, Gessner, & Esposito, 1979; McTear,

1985). Impairments of the pragmatics of language are, by definition, an essential feature of Asperger syndrome. Rapin and Allen (1983) hypothesized the existence of a "semantic–pragmatic syndrome without autism." In this "syndrome," the structural aspects of language are unimpaired but there are marked problems in using language in social and interpersonal contexts. Lister Brook and Bowler (1992) discussed this hypothesis and examined 10 publications on this subject appearing from 1979 to 1989. They found that, where details were given, the children were described as impaired in social interaction and communication and rigid and repetitive in their play. Lister Brook and Bowler concluded that the semantic–pragmatic syndrome was part of the autistic spectrum. Where descriptions of the pattern of behavior are given, it is clear that at least some of the children could be diagnosed as having Asperger syndrome.

Rourke and his colleagues (Rourke, 1982; Rourke, Young, Strang, & Russel, 1986) studied children with deficiencies in arithmetical skills combined with average or above-average language, reading, and spelling skills. They were found to be markedly impaired in visuospatial organizational abilities and tended to be clumsy. Rourke et al. described the characteristics of these children. These included seriously deficient social skills, having few if any friends, unable to join in other children's play, being seen as "different" by others, learning through rote memory, unable to cope with change, sensitive to imagined slights, and having poor self-esteem. They had particular problems in reading nonverbal social cues such as gestures and facial expressions. Their handwriting and organization of schoolwork were poor. These features are familiar in the context of Asperger syndrome. Rourke and his colleagues hypothesized central processing deficiencies particularly in the right hemisphere. They did not make comparisons with Asperger syndrome. It is interesting that, among the children with the pattern described by Rourke et al., there was a slight preponderance of females. Weintraub and Mesulam (1982) described a similar clinical picture, including avoidance of eye contact and lack of gestures and prosody, which they also attributed to a right-hemisphere dysfunction.

Sula Wolff has made a long-term study of children whom she diagnosed as having "schizoid personality disorder of childhood." As she discusses in her book (Wolff, 1995), there is a marked overlap with Asperger syndrome (see Chapter 7, this volume).

ASSOCIATION WITH OTHER DEVELOPMENTAL AND PSYCHIATRIC DISORDERS

Gillberg, Rasmussen, Carlström, Svenson, and Waldenström (1982) described a group of children with disorders of attention, motor control, and perception, which they first classified as "minimal brain dysfunction" and later referred to using the acronym "DAMP syndrome." Follow-up showed that of 14 children with this syndrome, 8 had autistic-type traits, 3 of whom had Asperger syndrome and 4 had some of the criteria for this syndrome (Gillberg, 1992; Gillberg & Gillberg, 1989).

Studies of adults have shown that superimposed psychiatric illnesses can complicate Asperger syndrome. Most of the adults described by Wing (1981) and more than one third of those described by Tantam (1991) had such conditions. However, most of the individuals seen by these authors had been referred to adult psychiatric services and so were more likely to have had psychiatric illnesses than other people with Asperger syndrome who were not referred. The exact size of the risk has not been calculated in an epidemiological study. Affective disorders, especially depression, appear to be particularly common but any variety of illness can occur. Gillberg (1992) noted the co-occurrence of autism and anorexia nervosa.

There is an overlap of Asperger syndrome with Tourette's syndrome (Kerbeshian & Burd, 1986) and obsessive-compulsive disorder (Wing, 1996). A small proportion of adolescents and adults with autistic spectrum disorders, including Asperger syndrome, develop catatonic features of varying degrees of severity (Wing, 1981, 1996). Taking a retrospective view, it seems likely that some people in the old mental hospitals diagnosed as having "catatonic schizo-phrenia" had Asperger syndrome with catatonia developing in adolescence. Some individuals develop symptoms of obsessive-compulsive disorder, such as repetitive hand-washing, dressing rituals, or repetitive thoughts. They gradually become slower in completing actions because of their rituals and then begin to show catatonic features such as freezing in postures, inability to cross thresholds, and echopraxia. A few decline into stupor.

The interrelationships of autism, Asperger syndrome, obsessive-compulsive disorder, Tourette's syndrome and catatonia are of considerable interest from the point of view of the neuropathology of all of these conditions.

THE CLASSIFICATION OF ASPERGER SYNDROME

The debate concerning the status of Asperger syndrome as a separate entity is still ongoing. The most intense discussions concern the relationship with Kanner's autism and other autisticlike disorders and with the schizoid personality disorder of childhood as described by Wolff (1995).

Asperger syndrome appeared for the first time in the latest versions of the *International Classification of Diseases,* 10th edition (ICD-10) (WHO, 1993) and the *Diagnostic and Statistical Manual of Mental Disorders,* 4th edition (DSM-IV) (APA, 1994). It is included with autistic disorders under the general heading of "Pervasive Developmental Disorders." The criteria in both systems demand development of language, self-care skills, adaptive behavior, and curiosity about the environment consistent with normal development up to 3 years of age. The other criteria are qualitative abnormalities in reciprocal social interaction, and circumscribed interests and repetitive, stereotyped patterns of activities, both defined in the same ways as for the criteria used for autism. This definition has moved away from Asperger's description, which emphasized the children's particular style of communication and social interaction. Also, Asperger did not describe normal early development of skills other than speech. In his first paper he made the statement "From the second year of life we find already the characteristic features...," even though he noted that the parents usually did not recognize the problems until later (Frith's 1991 translation of Asperger's paper, p. 67). Asperger also wrote that his syndrome could occur "in the less able, even in children with severe mental retardation" (pp. 58–59).

The term *schizoid personality* occurs in the section entitled "Personality Disorders" in DSM-IV and "Disorders of Adult Personality and Behaviour" in ICD-10. In neither of these classification systems is schizoid personality disorder of childhood mentioned. The definitions of the adult disorder are presented as a set of descriptions of current features. These include emotional detachment, consistent choice of solitary activities, taking pleasure in few if any activities, excessive preoccupation with fantasy and introspection, no close friendships, and marked insensitivity to social norms and conventions. There is no mention of the course of development in childhood.

Although these international classification systems have given official existence to Asperger syndrome, they are of little help in solving the issues of the overlap with autism and Wolff's "schizoid" children. The arguments concerning the similarities and differences between Asperger syndrome and various other conditions are pursued in other chapters in this book. Here the more general questions of the meaning of diagnosis and specificity in this field will be discussed.

IS ASPERGER SYNDROME A SPECIFIC ENTITY?

The strongest reason for regarding a condition as specific is if the original cause is known and is different from that of other conditions. This cannot be claimed for Asperger syndrome as yet because the cause is unknown. There is much clinical evidence for inherited factors in Asperger syndrome but also for its association within families with other autistic spectrum disorders (Bolton *et al.*, 1994; Bowman, 1988; Burgoine & Wing, 1983; Gillberg, 1991; Van Krevelen, 1971). Many different kinds of specific genetic, metabolic, and infectious conditions have been reported in association with autistic spectrum disorders, including Asperger syndrome (Gillberg, 1992; Gillberg & Coleman, 1992). Although the degree of association varies from minor to major, none invariably results in an autistic disorder, and none is associated with any one specific subgroup of the autistic spectrum.

A second possibility is that the syndrome has a specific type of neuropathology. The neurological basis of Asperger syndrome is being investigated and, at the time of writing, no conclusions have been reached.

Third, a consistent and unique pattern of psychological dysfunction would justify regarding the cluster of features described by Asperger as a specific syndrome. Results of psychological testing are variable. The most usual finding is that verbal scores are higher than performance scores and marks are lost because of inability to work fast on timed items. Some, however, do better on performance tasks, while others achieve roughly the same scores on both types of measures. Although profiles on subtests are, in the majority, patchy, there are some individuals whose profiles are fairly even. Differences between Asperger syndrome and high-functioning autism were found by Klin, Volkmar, Sparrow, Cicchetti, and Rourke (1995), who included in their criteria for Asperger syndrome the absence of significant delay in language or cognitive development and delayed motor milestones and the presence of clumsiness. However, the differences found by Klin et al. were based on the numbers of individuals in each group showing deficiencies in various aspects of nonverbal learning. Significant differences were found in 9 of 22 items, but, for all items, some individuals in one or both groups had test results that were more frequent in the other group. Considering the criteria used for subgrouping, it is perhaps not surprising that the significant items included clumsiness (worse in the Asperger group) and verbal output and articulation (better in the Asperger group). Ozonoff, Rogers, and Pennington (1991) showed better performance on "theory of mind" tests and verbal memory in children with Asperger syndrome compared with high-functioning autism. However, the criteria for diagnosing Asperger syndrome included no general language retardation at the time of the study. It is possible that language level is related to performance on theory of mind tests.

Fourth, a syndrome could be defined as a separate entity if it was manifested as a specific clinical picture, including course over time. There is no doubt that it is possible to select individuals who are typical representatives of Kanner's autism and Asperger syndrome and who show the very marked contrasts in behavior pattern, the former being aloof, mostly silent, and absorbed in stereotyped routines such as making long lines of objects and the latter being naively inappropriate in social interaction, delivering nonstop monologues on abstract interests, such as meteorology or the characteristics of varieties of crustaceans. The problem is that the most marked contrasts are seen when the testable verbal intelligence of the child with autism is low and that of the child with Asperger syndrome is high. The closer the IQs converge, the more similar are the clinical pictures. Another difficulty in separating the groups is that there are many individuals who have a mixture of features of Kanner's autism and Asperger syndrome. It is quite common to find some who fit Kanner's description in early childhood, including delayed language, who change with age until they precisely fit Asperger's descriptions. The course and prognosis are closely related to level of ability, not to the clinical syndrome (Wing, 1988, 1991).

Finally, a specific response to a unique method of intervention would justify regarding a syndrome as a specific entity. So far, no medication has been proved to be effective in treating the social and communication impairments underlying autism, Asperger syndrome, or mixed pictures. Drugs sometimes help to alleviate associated symptoms such as anxiety or depression, or behavior such as aggression, but the same medications are equally variable in their effects in all of the above clinical patterns. The educational approaches that are helpful are based on structured, organized, predictable programs with emphasis on concrete, visual modes of presentation of information and instructions, whether the diagnosis is autism or Asperger syndrome. Differences in program content are related to the intellectual ability and severity of social impairment of the individuals concerned and not to the syndrome (Jordan & Powell, 1995).

THE HYPOTHESIS OF THE AUTISTIC SPECTRUM

How can some sense be made of an extremely wide spectrum of disorders in which those at the "mildest" end of the scale appear, superficially at least, completely different from those who are most severely affected?

The first point to be made is that exposure, through epidemiological studies and clinical work, to the whole unselected range of social and communication disorders gives a different view from that of research workers who see only individuals selected on specific criteria for experimental studies. From the former perspective, Wing and Gould (1979) concluded that children with Kanner's autism, Asperger syndrome, and other clinical pictures with autistic features have in common a triad of impairments affecting social interaction, communication, and imagination, accompanied by a narrow, rigid, repetitive pattern of activities. They developed the hypothesis of a continuum or spectrum of autistic disorders held together by this triad (Wing, 1988).

There are also many other features that are often but not invariably associated with the triad, such as language delay and deviance, odd responses to sensory stimuli, clumsiness and peculiarities of posture and movement, and disorders of eating, drinking, and sleeping. Epilepsy is common among people with the triad and the possibility of superimposed psychiatric illnesses has already been mentioned. Each of the elements of the triad and the accompanying repetitive pattern of activities can be manifested in a wide range of ways, some of them very subtle indeed. The picture is further complicated by the variation in overall level of ability from profound retardation to superior levels of cognitive skill on testing.

Because the numbers of clinical features and the severity and manner in which each is shown can vary widely among individuals with the triad, the range of possible clinical pictures is enormous. Certain patterns, such as those described by Kanner and Asperger, can be recognized. The problem is that, among the whole range of people with the triad, these subgroups make up under one half (Ehlers & Gillberg, 1993; Wing & Gould, 1979) and considerably less if the most strict criteria for Kanner and Asperger syndromes are rigidly applied. In clinical work, it is evident that any pattern can occur, though some combinations are somewhat more likely than others.

Why should autistic spectrum disorders be considered as a group if the causes and clinical pictures are so diverse? The reason is that the autistic social impairment, in whatever form it is manifested, has major effects on development, learning, behavior and adaptation to all aspects of life that are different from those of any disability in which social interaction is preserved. It may be that the most fruitful line of research is to analyze the nature of autistic social impairment and to try to identify the psychological dysfunctions and the neuropathology underlying that aspect of the autistic spectrum.

Gillberg (1992) extended the theme of a spectrum of disorders by suggesting that autistic conditions are a subgroup among a broader group of disorders of empathy that include not only autism, Asperger syndrome, and Wolff's schizoid personality disorder of childhood but also overlap with obsessive-compulsive disorder, the DAMP syndrome, Tourette's syndrome, paranoid disorder, and anorexia nervosa. There is a case to be made for including schizophrenia as a disorder associated with impairment of the empathic skills appearing in adolescence or adult life (Frith, 1992).

In the view of the present author, Asperger syndrome and high-functioning autism are not distinct conditions. There is no evidence that Kanner, Asperger, or anyone else has as yet succeeded in identifying a separate syndrome. If lists of several features contrasting Asperger syndrome and autism are compiled, as in Van Krevelen (1971), many individuals have items from both. If a list of features of Asperger syndrome is compiled without reference to autism, as in Ehlers and Gillberg (1993), virtually all of the items can also be found in clinical descriptions of high functioning adolescents and adults originally diagnosed as autistic, including those of Kanner (1973). If Asperger syndrome and autism are separated on the basis of one aspect of the clinical picture, such as speech and cognitive development, as in ICD-10 (WHO, 1993), other major features are found in both groups.

The most useful method of grouping for clinical purposes is to ignore the eponymous syndromes, to diagnose an autistic spectrum disorder when it is present and to subgroup on quality of social interaction and level of ability in verbal and nonverbal skills. Wing and Gould (1979) identified three types of social interaction, namely, "aloof and indifferent," "passively accepting," and "active but odd" social approaches (Borden & Ollendick, 1994; Gillberg, 1992;

O'Brien, 1996). A fourth can be added for the most able adolescents and adults, namely, "stilted and overformal" (Wing, 1996). Information on the quality of social interaction and level of verbal and nonverbal skills is considerably more useful in practice as a guide to an individual's needs at any one time than a diagnosis of typical autism, Asperger syndrome, or "autistic features." Any additional conditions, such as epilepsy, and any known causes have to be described separately. It should always be remembered that the clinical picture, and therefore the individual's needs, can change over time.

The search for identifiable syndromes can be pursued by research workers. Clinical practice requires more down-to-earth, here-and-now methods of classifying and conveying information.

EVALUATION OF ASPERGER'S CONTRIBUTION

What advantages have accrued from recognizing Asperger's work? In the author's clinical experience in the United Kingdom, drawing attention to Asperger's descriptions of the group of children he studied has made professionals and the general public aware of the range of the autistic spectrum. Parents who are unable to accept a diagnosis of autism because their child has grammatical speech and makes positive, though one-sided social approaches are more willing to consider Asperger syndrome as a possibility even when informed that it is related to autism. Psychiatrists concerned with mental illness in adults, who previously knew of autism only as a disorder of childhood, are becoming aware that autistic conditions, such as Asperger described, can present as psychiatric disorders in adult life. It has increased understanding of a group of people whose disabilities cause them much suffering and which have often resulted in ridicule and rejection rather than sympathy and help. If Asperger's work had not become known and *autism* had remained as the only term used in the field, it is possible that interest in social impairment in all of its manifestations would not have developed in the way that it has or, at least, would have grown much more slowly. This might have been the case because of the semantic constraints imposed by Kanner's descriptions of his autistic syndrome and his belief in its uniqueness.

Schopler (1985, 1996) pointed out the problems caused by the use of the term *Asperger syndrome*, particularly the confusion over its relationship with high-functioning autism. The disadvantages of the idea of Asperger syndrome are also semantic, arising from the different ways the concept is interpreted. By the same token, there would have been similar diagnostic problems if the only label for children with autistic disorders and average or high IQs were high-functioning autism. Some workers are mainly interested in discrete categories. They look for defining criteria and exclude individuals who do not precisely fit, leaving them and their families without any explanation or help for their difficulties. Others are inclined to see everything as part of a seamless continuum but this can also deny access to useful information and treatment. A more constructive approach is to recognize similarities across the autistic spectrum while searching for useful ways to subdivide for particular purposes, reserving judgment on all of the categories that have so far been suggested. These semantic problems apply equally to other labels under the heading of "Pervasive Developmental Disorders" in DSM-IV or ICD-10, particularly "atypical autism," "childhood disintegrative disorder," and (in ICD-10 only) "overactive disorder associated with mental retardation and stereotyped movements," which have considerably less value in clinical practice than "Asperger syndrome."

Separate from the arguments about diagnostic groups, Asperger's accounts of the children he worked with should be read for his remarkable insights into the details of their patterns of disabilities, their special skills, and the way they experience the world and other people. He was also very perceptive in his suggestions on how to interact with, educate, and help the children. His ideas are as relevant now as when they were written.

The history of Asperger syndrome is similar to many other disorders in psychiatry. At first, the condition is an unrecognized part of a vague general group of conditions. Then one clinical observer, because of some special experience, recognizes what seems to be a group of individuals with a cluster of features in common. At this stage, some suggested syndromes fall by the wayside. Those that survive are the ones that evoke a feeling of recognition among other workers. Eventually, there is general acceptance, the final accolade being inclusion in the ICD and DSM systems. However, there are always arguments about the true status of any condition for which the criteria are mainly behavioral. In the case of Asperger syndrome, its recognition has resulted in its placement among developmental disorders in general and autistic spectrum disorders in particular. It may well be proved to have no independent existence but this does not detract from Asperger's achievement in discerning something very special in the children he described.

The abilities involved in reciprocal social interaction are subtle and intangible but of immense importance in human life. It is fitting that they should at last be considered to be an appropriate subject for scientific research.

REFERENCES

Adams, P. L. (1973). *Obsessive children: A sociopsychiatric study*. London: Butterworths.
American Psychiatric Association. (1994). *Diagnostic and statistical manual of mental disorders* (4th ed.). Washington, DC: Author.
Asperger, H. (1944). Die "autistischen Psychopathen" im Kindesalter. *Archive für Psychiatrie und Nervenkrankheiten, 117*, 76–136.
Asperger, H. (1979). Problems of infantile autism. *Communication, 13*, 45–52.
Asperger, H. (1991). 'Autistic psychopathy' in childhood (U. Frith, Trans.). In U.Frith (Ed.), *Autism and Asperger syndrome* (pp. 37–92). Cambridge: Cambridge University Press.

Baron-Cohen, S. (1988). An assessment of violence in a young man with Asperger's syndrome. *Journal of Child Psychology and Psychiatry, 29,* 351–360.

Blank, M., Gessner, M., & Esposito, A. (1979). Language without communication: A case study. *Journal of Child Language, 6,* 329–352.

Bolton, P., MacDonald, H., Pickles, A., Rios, P., Goode, S., Crowson, M., Bailey, A., & Rutter, M. (1994). A case–control family history study of autism. *Journal of Child Psychology and Psychiatry, 35,* 877–900.

Borden, M., & Ollendick, T. (1994). An examination of the validity of social subtypes in autism. *Journal of Autism and Developmental Disorders, 24,* 23–38.

Bosch, G. (1970). *Infantile autism.* Berlin: Springer-Verlag.

Bowman, E. P. (1988) Asperger's syndrome and autism: The case for a connection. *British Journal of Psychiatry, 152,* 377–382.

Burgoine, E., & Wing, L. (1983). Identical triplets with Asperger's syndrome. *British Journal of Psychiatry, 143,* 261–265.

Ehlers, S., & Gillberg, C. (1993). The epidemiology of Asperger syndrome. A total population study. *Journal of Child Psychology and Psychiatry, 34,* 1327–1350.

Frith, C. D. (1992). *The cognitive neuropsychology of schizophrenia.* Hillsdale, NJ: Erlbaum.

Frith, U. (1989). *Autism: Explaining the enigma.* Oxford: Blackwell.

Frith, U. (Ed.). (1991). *Autism and Asperger syndrome.* Cambridge: Cambridge University Press.

Gillberg, C. (1991). Clinical and neurobiological aspects of Asperger syndrome in six family studies. In U.Frith (Ed.), *Autism and Asperger syndrome* (pp. 122–146). Cambridge: Cambridge University Press.

Gillberg, C. (1992). The Emanuel Miller Memorial Lecture 1991. Autism and autistic-like conditions: Subclasses among disorders of empathy. *Journal of Child Psychology and Psychiatry, 33,* 813–842.

Gillberg, C., & Coleman, M. (1992). *The biology of the autistic syndromes.* London: Mac Keith Press.

Gillberg, C., Rasmussen, P., Carlström, G., Svenson, B., & Waldenström, E. (1982). Perceptual, motor and attentional deficits in six-year-old children. *Journal of Child Psychology and Psychiatry, 23,* 131–144.

Gillberg, I. C., & Gillberg, C. (1989). Asperger syndrome—some epidemiological considerations: A research note. *Journal of Child Psychology and Psychiatry, 30,* 631–638.

Grove, T. (1988). Barnaby Rudge — a case study in autism. *Communication, 22,* 12–16.

Isaev, D. N., & Kagan, V. E. (1974). Autistic syndromes in children and adolescents. *Acta Paedopsychiatrica, 40,* 182–190.

Jordan, R., & Powell, S. (1995) *Understanding and teaching children with autism.* New York: Wiley.

Kanner, L. (1943). Autistic disturbances of affective contact. *Nervous Child, 2,* 217–250.

Kanner, L. (1973). How far can autistic children go in matters of social adaptation? In *Childhood psychosis: Initial studies and new insights* (pp. 189–213). Washington: Winston/Wiley.

Kerbeshian, J., & Burd, L. (1986). Asperger's syndrome and Tourette syndrome. *British Journal of Psychiatry, 148,* 731–735.

Klin, A., Volkmar, F. R, Sparrow, S. S., Cicchetti, D. V., & Rourke, B. P. (1995). Validity and neuropsychological characterization of Asperger syndrome: Convergence with nonverbal learning disabilities syndrome. *Journal of Child Psychology and Psychiatry, 36,* 1127–1140.

Kretschmer, E. (1925). *Physique and character.* London: Kegan Paul, Trench, Trübner.

Lister Brook, S., & Bowler, D. (1992). Autism by another name? Semantic and pragmatic impairments in children. *Journal of Autism and Developmental Disorders, 22,* 61–82.

Luria, A. R. (1969). *The mind of a mnemonist* (L.Solotaroff, Trans.). New York: Avon Books. (Original work published 1965).

Lutz, J. (1964). *Kinderpsychiatrie.* Stuttgart: Rotappel-Verlag.

Mawson, D., Grounds, A., & Tantam, D. (1985). Violence and Asperger's syndrome: A case study. *British Journal of Psychiatry, 147,* 566–569.

McTear, M. (1985). Pragmatic disorders: A case study of conversational disability. *British Journal of Disorders of Communication*, 20, 129–142.

Mnukhin, S. S., & Isaev, D. N. (1975). On the organic nature of some forms of schizoid or autistic psychopathy. *Journal of Autism and Childhood Schizophrenia*, 5, 99–108.

O'Brien, S. (1996). The validity and reliability of the Wing Subgroups questionnaire. *Journal of Autism and Developmental Disorders*, 26, 321–336.

Ozonoff, S., Rogers, S. J., & Pennington, B. F (1991). Asperger's syndrome: Evidence of an empirical distinction from high functioning autism. *Journal of Child Psychology and Psychiatry*, 32, 1107–1122.

Prick, J. G. G., & Van Der Waals, H. G. (Eds.). (1965). *Nederlands Handboek van de Psychiatrie*. Arnhem: Van Loghum Slaterus.

Rapin, I., & Allen, D. (1983). Developmental language disorders: Nosologic considerations. In U. Kirk (Ed.), *Neuropsychology of language, reading and spelling* (pp. 155–183). London: Academic Press.

Robinson, J. F., & Vitale, L. J. (1954). Children with circumscribed interest patterns. *American Journal of Orthopsychiatry*, 24, 755–766.

Rourke, B. P. (1982). Central processing deficiencies in children: Towards a developmental neuropsychological model. *Journal of Clinical Neuropsychology*, 4, 1–18.

Rourke, B. P., Young, G. C., Strang, J. D., & Russell, D. L. (1986). Adult outcome of central processing deficiencies in childhood. In I. Grant & K.M. Adams (Eds.), *Neuropsychological assessment of neuropsychiatric disorders* (pp. 244–267). London: Oxford University Press.

Schneider, K. (1923). *Psychopathic personalities*. Vienna: Deuticke.

Schopler, E. (1985). Editorial. Convergence of learning disability, higher-level autism and Asperger's syndrome. *Journal of Autism and Developmental Disorders*, 15, 359–360.

Schopler, E. (1996). Are autism and Asperger syndrome different labels or different disabilities? *Journal of Autism and Developmental Disorders*, 26, 109–110.

Ssucharewa, G. E. (1926). Die schizoiden psychopathien im kindesalter. *Monatschrift für Psychiatrie und Neurologie*, 60, 235–261.

Tantam, D. (1986). *Eccentricity and autism*. Ph.D. thesis, University of London (unpublished).

Tantam, D. (1988). Lifelong eccentricity and social isolation: I. Psychiatric, social and forensic aspects. *British Journal of Psychiatry*, 153, 777–782.

Tantam, D. (1991). Asperger syndrome in adulthood. In U. Frith (Ed.), *Autism and Asperger syndrome* (pp. 147–183). Cambridge: Cambridge University Press.

Treffert, D. (1989). *Extraordinary people*. New York. Bantam.

Van Krevelen, D. A. (1971). Early infantile autism and autistic psychopathy. *Journal of Autism and Childhood Schizophrenia*, 1, 82–86.

Van Krevelen, D. A., & Kuipers, C. (1962) The psychopathology of autistic psychopathy. *Acta Paedopsychiatrica*, 29, 22–31.

Weintraub, S., & Mesulam, M. M. (1982). Developmental learning disabilities of the right hemisphere. *Archives of Neurology*, 40, 463–468.

Wing, L. (1976a). Diagnosis, clinical description and prognosis. In L. Wing (Ed.), *Early childhood autism* (2nd ed.) (pp. 15–64). Oxford: Pergamon.

Wing, L. (1976b). Epidemiology and theories of aetiology. In L. Wing (Ed.), *Early childhood autism* (2nd ed.) (pp. 65–92). Oxford: Pergamon.

Wing, L. (1981). Asperger's syndrome: A clinical account. *Psychological Medicine*, 11, 115 129.

Wing, L. (1988). The continuum of autistic characteristics. In E. Schopler & G. Mesibov (Eds.), *Diagnosis and Assessment in Autism* (pp. 91–110). New York: Plenum Press.

Wing, L. (1991). The relationship between Asperger's syndrome and Kanner's autism. In U.Frith (Ed.), *Autism and Asperger syndrome* (pp. 93–121). Cambridge: Cambridge University Press.

Wing, L. (1996). *The autistic spectrum: A guide for parents and professionals*. London: Constable.

Wing, L., & Gould, J. (1979). Severe impairments of social interaction and associated abnormalities in children: Epidemiology and classification. *Journal of Autism and Developmental Disorders*, *9*, 11–29.

Wolff, S. (1995). *Loners: The life path of unusual children*. London: Routledge.

World Health Organization (1993). *The ICD-10 classification of mental and behavioural disorders. Diagnostic criteria for research*. Geneva: Author.

3

Subtyping Pervasive Developmental Disorder

Issues of Validity and Implications for Child Psychiatric Diagnosis

JOHN C. POMEROY

INTRODUCTION

The use of the diagnostic term *pervasive developmental disorders* (PDD), as well as the value and purpose of subtyping the PDD has been a controversial issue. Such subtyping has been particularly relevant to disorders that are considered to be in the higher-functioning range of PDD. This chapter presents the author's own development of thought on this topic, and is divided into four main sections. The first is a selective review of opinion regarding the diagnosis of children with severe social withdrawal prior to the initial efforts of the American Psychiatric Association (1980, 1987) to provide diagnostic criteria for this clinical spectrum. Focusing on some of the findings from a study addressing the validity of PDD subtypes, the second section considers the prevailing diagnostic system (APA, 1994). The third section discusses research findings and clinical examples that support or contradict the presently accepted subtyping. The chapter concludes with a brief review of the present state of knowledge with some consideration of the ongoing research questions and how this can enhance clinical practice for

JOHN C. POMEROY • Department of Psychiatry and Behavioral Science, State University of New York at Stony Brook, Stony Brook, New York 11794-8790.

Asperger Syndrome or High-Functioning Autism?, edited by Schopler *et al.* Plenum Press, New York, 1998.

those assessing and treating young people with severe developmental/psychiatric disorders.

My introduction to this topic originated, not from a perspective of observing the outcome of individuals with a diagnosis of autism, but from study of a broad range of severe childhood psychopathology observed in child psychiatric clinical settings. Others have also noted that developmental and behavioral characteristics of PDD and high-functioning autism (HFA) overlap with a diverse group of disorders. These have included specific learning disorders (e.g., Shea & Mesibov, 1985), lateralized lesions of brain cortex (Weintraub & Mesulam, 1983; Voeller, 1986), and other putative psychiatric syndromes such as *schizoid* (e.g., Cull, Chick, & Wolff, 1984), *schizotypal* (Nagy & Szatmari, 1986), and *borderline* (see Petti & Vela, 1990) *disorders*. There has even been a reevaluation of the distinction between childhood-onset schizophrenia and PDD (Watkins, Asarnow, & Tanguay, 1988). Thus, at the risk of seeming idiosyncratic, this chapter, which addresses the validation of PDD subtypes, begins with a discussion of child psychiatric disorders that may, initially, seem unrelated to autism or autistic-like conditions. This perspective is important because mental health workers who evaluate and treat emotionally disturbed children are becoming increasingly aware of the impact on clinical practice of a broader concept of the PPD.

BEFORE DSM-III

Clinical Issues

As I began my training in child psychiatry in the late 1970s, I was intrigued by the apparent similarities between the disorders that a small number of children presented and the diagnostic concept of a schizophrenic spectrum (e.g., Kety, Rosenthal, Wender, & Schulsinger, 1968; Heston, 1970). One of my first child psychiatric patients typified such diagnostic issues:

A. was a 13-year-old boy who had a preoccupation with London at the time I first met him. (Ironically, I had recently emigrated from the United Kingdom.) His preoccupation would take the form of talking about London excessively but also perseveratively drawing pictures of well-known buildings (e.g., Tower Bridge). Although this interest should have provided a natural link to me, forming a personal relationship with A. was difficult.

A. was an adopted child living with professional parents and an older sister, who was a biological child of the adoptive parents. A. had been noted to be a "peculiar child" since his early years. There had been delays in his development of motor coordination, speech, and comprehension. Although using some words from 18 months of age, he could not form sentences until 4 years of age and at

5 years he was still noted to have very poor comprehension despite intellectual testing that suggested an average ability.

He was able to "hide" many of his unusual thoughts and behavior from people outside the family, but his parents reported that he had progressed through a number of different preoccupations (e.g., reptiles, the Bible, clocks, Disney characters), would destroy property that he felt had a slight imperfection or someone had moved from an appointed position; had become increasingly isolated; compulsively moved furniture around the room; kept all of the clocks in the house at a different time; and became easily frustrated and angered by inconsistency (e.g., if Bible stories presented on television were altered from the original biblical text). Along with social difficulties and these compulsive qualities, A. had evidence of academic learning disabilities and a marked deterioration in his functioning from 9 years of age. At that time, his level of destruction, because of perceived imperfections, increased (e.g., taking a sledge-hammer to his bicycle, killing his pet parakeet, destroying a grandfather clock). He became very angry with his family, accusing them of not wanting or liking him. He also became critical and irrationally fearful of certain peers.

On interview he was a tall, clumsy, tense boy who made no eye contact or true social rapport. His affect was incongruous with bursts of unprovoked laughter. His speech was rapid, monotonous, mechanical, but spontaneous. He was also repetitive and became more disorganized as attempts were made to explore his thought processes. At first he was only willing to admit to daydream-ing, but over a period of time he described experiencing auditory hallucinations (which included derogatory voices speaking about him), as well as ideas of reference (i.e., feeling people were looking at and talking about him); persecu-tory feelings; possible thought alienation (i.e., people could read, or interfere with, his thoughts); and ideas of destruction being associated with his compul-sive behavior. Physical examination and laboratory investigation revealed only a gait abnormality and subtle neurological deficits (e.g., abnormal reflexes) in his right lower limb.

Although A.'s clinical picture and, to some extent, his ongoing pattern of illness suggested a schizophrenic disorder, the lifelong pattern of rigid compul-sive behavior, socialization problems, delays in development of speech, and severe comprehension difficulties were more reflective of the unfolding of an abnormal developmental process. Some of these latter features were reminiscent of accounts of autistic children, but there had been a clear emphasis in then-cur-rent empirical research (e.g., Kolvin, Ounsted, Humphrey, & McNay, 1971) to justify a demarcation between the "psychoses of childhood" occurring before 3 years (i.e., *infantile autism*) and the later-onset disorders (usually after 5 years) which were thought, in most cases, to be an early manifestation of a schizo-phrenic illness. Differences in phenomenology, developmental history, family history, intellectual functioning, associated medical factors, and course of illness were all supportive of this dichotomy.

However, my early clinical experience, and review of the relevant emerging literature, made it apparent that such simple diagnostic separation did not adequately explain all of the disorders that children presented in which there were varied combinations of social deficits, compulsive and rigid behavior, and schizoid or schizophrenic-like symptoms.

Concepts of a Schizoid Disorder of Childhood

In an effort to explain inconsistencies in the research findings that addressed a presumed genetic causation of schizophrenia, workers, such as Heston (1970), proposed, and provided evidence from family studies, that some relatives, of individuals who have schizophrenia, inherit "schizoid" characteristics, rather than florid schizophrenia. These characteristics, considered part of a schizophrenic spectrum disorder, included rigidity of thinking, blunting of affect, anhedonia, exquisite sensitivity, suspiciousness, relative poverty of ideas, and micropsychotic episodes. The concept of a *schizoid disorder*, occurring more commonly in young boys and preceding the onset of dementia praecox, had been described by Kraepelin in 1907 (see Wolff & Chick, 1980), but Bleuler and, later, Kretschmer, who both provided broader clinical descriptions, felt that schizoid characteristics were part of an adult personality type that was not necessarily a disorder or disease.

Sula Wolff first presented her description of schizoid children in 1964. When work by Asperger became more well known, it was apparent, and was later discussed (e.g., Wing, 1984), that there were marked similarities between the descriptions of Wolff and those of Asperger, who had written his M.D. thesis on the disorder that he termed *autistic psychopathy* (Van Krevelen, 1971; Wing, 1981a; see Table 3-1). Following increased appreciation of the disorders described by Wolff and Asperger, it was also noted that other psychiatrists had previously observed similar clinical characteristics among obsessive children (Adams, 1973), young adults with soft neurological signs (Quitkin & Klein, 1969), and children of mothers who have schizophrenia (Mednick, 1970; Mednick & Schulsinger, 1970). As early as 1954, Robinson and Vitale had described three children with circumscribed interest patterns (e.g., chemistry, nuclear fission, corporate finance, bus routes) as well as solitariness, nonconforming attitude, and difficulty in emotional relationships. Furthermore, a less florid schizoid disorder had also been described (Childers, 1931; Jenkins & Glickman, 1946), in which communication and thought abnormalities were not so apparent but marked social avoidance , not related to an anxiety disorder, was the major deficit. This latter description constituted the diagnostic characteristics of *schizoid disorder of childhood*, which was present in DSM-III (APA, 1980), but not the later revisions of this diagnostic manual.

It was, perhaps, surprising that Wolff and Asperger both asserted that the childhood disorders they described represented personality types that continued

Table 3-1. Clinical Characteristics of Autistic Psychopathy and Schizoid Disorder of Childhood

	Autistic psychopathy (described by Asperger)	Schizoid disorder of childhood (described by Wolff)
Demographic characteristics	200 boys seen over a 10-year period All boys but similar relatives (including females)	3–4% of referrals to child psychiatry clinics Predominantly male
Onset	Starts after second year of life	Does not exhibit full features of autism before 3 years of age
Social behavior	Impairment of social adaptation (e.g., lack of empathy, maliciousness) Abnormality of gaze, poverty of expression and gesture, egocentric, lack of humor	Emotional detachment or solitariness Lack of empathy for others' feelings, callousness
Cognitive	Unusual thought and intelligence despite learning problems, internal distraction	Normal intelligence but educational difficulties
Language	Often talking before walking	Often has metaphorical use of language and marked lack of guardedness
Thought processes	Sensitivity, idiosyncratic interests and attachments	Sensitivity with suspiciousness and sometimes paranoid ideation Rigidity — at times assuming obsessional proportion, including long-lasting circumscribed interests
Outcome	Not a precursor to schizophrenia	Adults diagnosed as having a schizoid disorder on follow-up

into adulthood and did not precede the onset of schizophrenia. Assuming that schizoid disorder was part of a schizophrenic spectrum, it would have been reasonable to conclude that such early evidence of schizoid characteristics would be associated with a significantly increased risk to manifest schizophrenic psychosis in later life. As of 1980, the relationship between these "personality disorders" and descriptions of children with prepubertal onset of schizophrenic-like or obsessive-compulsive disorders remained unknown, but the previously cited clinical reports suggested some similarities. DSM-III (APA, 1980) did not satisfactorily address these diagnostic issues, and neither the literature nor my own efforts to isolate clinical cases of schizoid disorder for description could delineate a well-defined clinical group. Therefore, I embarked on a study to assess the use of empirical classification techniques to improve understanding of the nosology of schizoid and schizophrenic spectrum disorders among children with severe social withdrawal and/or obsessive-compulsive symptomatology and/or psychotic symptoms (Pomeroy, 1984). The findings from this study became, somewhat unexpectedly, relevant to the concept of a PDD spectrum.

Retrospective (Archive) Study of a Schizophrenia Spectrum in Childhood

This study applied cluster-analytic techniques to clinical data obtained from the records of all individuals under the age of 15 seen at the University of Iowa between 1930 and 1981, who had diagnoses that might include disorders within the spectrum to be considered. Children were included in the study if they had clear evidence in their records of (1) hallucinations and/or delusions, or (2) abnormal socialization (i.e., asocial or severely withdrawn, but not merely related to shyness or anxiety), or (3) obsessional ideation or compulsive behavior. Excluded were cases in which the child fulfilled diagnostic criteria for infantile autism (Rutter, 1971; APA, 1980) based on evaluations made before 5 years of age, plus any individual whose symptomatology was secondary to overt brain damage (e.g., open head injury). Thus, it was felt that children who were selected for the study would represent the broad descriptions of schizoid disorder in childhood, and included psychotic and obsessional children.

A total of 88 records were ultimately selected and reviewed. The methodology and procedures of the study will not be presented but are available to interested readers. The cluster analysis produced 11 clusters, which were considered tentative diagnostic groupings for closer examination. Eight of the clusters were predominantly of children whose disorders began in early years (under 5 years old). The other 3 clusters of children, whose disorders had begun in late childhood or early adolescence, were distinctive because of lack of reports of any significant developmental abnormalities and the relatively acute onset, in the peripubertal years, of symptoms that are commonly associated with major psychiatric disorders. These disorders separated into children with either florid psychotic illness or classical obsessional disorder (see Table 3-2 for brief clinical characteristics of the individual clusters).

The clusters of early onset disorders showed a separation (based on a correlation matrix) into two broader groupings. Unexpectedly, given the initial research goals, autism and autistic-like characteristics and development were a dominant feature of many of these early onset disorders. One of the broad groups was best characterized as an autistic spectrum. The shared clinical features of these clusters were speech abnormalities; lower intelligence; developmental histories revealing at least some characteristics of autistic disorder; short attention span; and a low incidence of anxiety and affective symptoms.

Three main clusters emerged within this group. The first (Cluster 1 in the study) was considered an autistic group, although (by study design) the subjects had not received an autistic diagnosis, at least before 5 years of age. Their IQ scores were mostly below 85. Many of the subjects could, in retrospect, have been considered more classically autistic. Cluster 5 was called an *autistic spectrum disorder* and included children with speech and language abnormalities

Table 3-2. Pilot Study: Brief Descriptive Characteristics of Individual Clusters

Autistic spectrum (34 subjects)
Shared features: Lower IQ; early onset; autistic-like history and speech abnormalities; short attention span; minimal anxiety and affective symptoms.

Cluster 1	Cluster 5	Cluster 3	Cluster 10[a]
IQ < 85	IQ higher than	Less severe motor or	Only two children with
Autistic features (in	Cluster 1, and	speech abnormalities	evidence of probable
speech, socialization,	• Less evidence of	Later hyperactivity, tics,	higher-functioning
and rigid behaviors)	motor problems	ritualism with	autism not detected
Motor problems	• Similar autistic	aggression, paranoia,	until adolescence
Toileting problems	features, except less	and phobias	
Temper tantrums	ritualistic	Most developed	
Self-harm	• Inappropriate and/or	hallucinations and	
	labile affect	delusions	

Schizoid Spectrum (25 subjects)
Shared features: Clinically resembled descriptions of schizoid children. Early and mid-childhood onset. Lower incidence of speech abnormalities, autistic characteristics and psychotic symptoms.

Clusters 6 & 7	Cluster 9	Cluster 8[a]
Clusters differed only in area	Predominantly male	Small group of children with
of cognitive functioning	Average IQ	early onset obsessional
(Cluster 6 — lower IQ, more	Chronically asocial	disorder
concrete thought processes)	Humorless, concrete	Differ from Cluster 2 in having
Predominantly male	Anxiety symptoms	lower IQ, hyperactivity,
Low average IQ	Low self-esteem	poor attention, early rituals,
Unusual social behavior	Often depressed and present	some autistic qualities
Significant motor problems	to clinic following unusual	Chronically asocial, humorless,
Behavior problems and	outburst of aggression	maneristic
anxiety symptoms		Obsessions and compulsions
Flat affect, thought disorder,		associated with somatic
omnipotence		complaints

Late-onset disorder (23 subjects)
Shared features: Disorder starting in late childhood or early adolescence. Few had any developmental abnormalities. Diagnosable as either obsessional disorder or psychotic illness.

Cluster 2	Cluster 4	Cluster 11
High IQ but social difficulties	Illness starts after age 10	Schizoid or withdrawn in
Anxiety symptoms	Recent deterioration	early years
Depressive features	Symptoms include perplexity,	High IQ
Obsessive personality	inappropriate affect, thought	Presented with catatonia —
characteristics as well as	disorder, hallucinations,	• stupor
true obsessions and	paranoia, sexual	• mutism
compulsions	preoccupations, poor reality	• mannerisms
Usually relate well and have	testing	and some affective symptoms
episodic illness	50% had affective symptoms	
	suggestive of mania and/or	
	depression	

[a]These clusters were small groups of uncertain significance and are therefore not included in the discussions of results.

limited to the autistic group but they tended to have higher intellectual functioning, few characteristics of developmental motor abnormalities and less "autistic" behavior. Cluster 3 was felt to be a childhood (or atypical) psychosis as children had some early autistic-like characteristics but later development of excess motor movements (overactivity, mannerisms, tics), aggression, paranoia, anxiety, and, in most, psychotic symptoms (i.e., hallucinations and/or delusions).

The second grouping of early onset disorders—the schizoid spectrum—was characterized by severe and chronic social difficulties and withdrawal but significantly less marked speech abnormalities and autistic-like histories. Three major clusters also emerged in this grouping. The first (Cluster 9) was characterized by children with chronic social withdrawal; concrete thought processes despite average to above-average intelligence; depression; anxiety; flattened affect; who often presented to the psychiatrist after a sudden outburst of severe aggression or hostility (e.g., two of these children murdered a parent in an impulsive gesture). Given the lack of evidence of developmental abnormalities in the first cluster (9), these clinical cases appeared more representative of schizoid disorder of childhood as defined in DSM-III (and, possibly, by Wolff). The other two clusters were very similar in many respects. The children in these clusters (6 and 7) had evidence of clumsiness, excess motor movements, and ritualistic behavior, but differences between the clusters were seen in level of intellectual functioning, flexibility of thought processes, and affective symptomatology. Retrospectively, it was apparent that these two clusters resembled descriptions by Asperger, and many of their reported clinical characteristics, with the notable exception of speech, resembled behaviors seen in some higher-functioning children with autistic or autistic-like disorders (i.e., PDD). Table 3-3 outlines more clinical and demographic data showing some group differences that provided further justification to consider these statistically derived entities as potential diagnostic groupings.

There are significant problems regarding the use of such powerful mathematical techniques in clinical diagnostic studies (see Paykel, 1981), but findings that I considered relevant to the active debate initiated by the introduction of PDD in DSM-III (APA, 1980) were:

1. Developmental deviations typically associated with the PDD (and/or autism) were seen in a somewhat wider range of severe emotional and behavioral disorders of childhood than had previously been considered for a diagnosis of autism.
2. Beyond the classical picture of autism (and excluding children with psychosis) there existed developmental disorders in which children had varying pieces of the autistic profile, of which two main subtypes were apparent:

    a. Language-impaired nonautistic PDD (autism spectrum). These children had autistic-like disorders but seemed less severely impaired and had relatively normal development of motor skills.

Table 3-3. Archival Study: Comparison between Clusters of Early Onset Disorders (Prepubertal) on a Number of Demographic and Clinical Features

	Cluster no.				
	1	5	6 & 7	9	3
Tentative diagnosis	Autistic disorder	Autism spectrum	Asperger syndrome	Schizoid disorder	Atypical or childhood psychosis
Male:female	11:6	5:2	14:0	7:1	8:2
Mean age at first professional intervention in years	4.9	5.9	6.9	11.75	5.9
(range)	(1–13)	(2–9)	(3–12)	(6–14)	(2–10)
Mean IQ	70.6	83.2	90.6	106.6	81.2
(range)	(40–89)	(68–90)	(56–126)	(100–117)	(62–117)
VIQ–PIQ split (> 10 points–Wechsler scale)					
V < P	3	3	1	4	2
V > P	1	0	8	1	0
Special education (percentage)	70	71.4	21.4	0	60
DSM-III autism characteristics (before 36 months) given as percentage passing criteria					
Pervasive lack of responsiveness	95	86	69	62.5	30
Gross deficits in language development	96	100	23	0	50
Peculiar speech	72.5	85	31	0	30
Bizarre environmental responses	82	86	72	25	40
Psychiatric symptomatology (percentage of subjects recorded as having such symptoms)					
Paranoia	11.6	14	21.6	12.5	80
Thought disorder	17.6	14	7	0	40
Poor reality testing	0	43	28.5	0	90
Hallucinations	0	0	0	0	50
Delusional ideation	6	43	29	0	60
Depressed affect	0	0	7	75	10
Panic attacks	0	0	0	37.5	0
School refusal	0	0	0	25	0
Phobic symptoms	23.5	14	28.5	25	70
Separation anxiety	0	0	36	25	20
Somatic anxiety	0	0	7	37.5	10

   b. Non-language-impaired nonautistic PDD. These children had clinical pictures that resembled some accounts of schizoid disorder but also exhibited ritualistic behavior and social deficits more typical of a PDD, without significant deficits in acquisition of speech. They also showed marked abnormalities in development of motor skills, plus an intellectual profile that tended to differ from autistic subjects in that there is often a verbal–performance IQ score discrepancy (higher verbal than performance scores) in a direction opposite that observed in classical autism. This group was later considered to be comparable to Asperger's description of autistic psychopathy.

The study also raised issues of some relevance to diagnostic issues within a broader spectrum. For example, there was evidence for the existence of a schizoid disorder of childhood, which differentiated from Asperger disorder on the basis of less deviant developmental history. Also, psychosis in childhood (prepubertal) was commonly preceded by developmental abnormalities that included speech disorders, and autistic-like characteristics. Although these broader issues of classification of prepubertal childhood psychosis and the validity of a schizoid personality in some children continue to be explored, the apparent clinical rarity of these disorders adds to the paucity of useful data on their appropriate diagnostic placement. The major research emphasis has, therefore, been toward the subtyping of PDD, which has led to the present compromise as delineated in DSM-IV (APA, 1994).

VALIDATING PDD SUBTYPES

The introduction of subtypes of PDD into the most recent diagnostic manuals for psychiatry does not represent a universally agreed consensus, nor was it the consequence of a body of research supporting their diagnostic validity. In fact, prior to the publication of ICD-10 (WHO, 1992) and DSM-IV (APA, 1994), most researchers had presented evidence to refute significant differences between HFA and PDD-NOS, most particularly Asperger disorder (e.g., Gillberg, 1989; Szatmari, Tuff, Finlayson, & Bartolucci, 1990; Kerbeshian, Burd, & Fisher, 1990). However, my colleagues and I (Pomeroy, Friedman, & Stephens, 1991) have argued that possible reasons for failing to find such differences were related to study designs that compared preselected children and young adults of varying age and range of ability, often using inconsistent criteria of uncertain validity for subgroup selection. In addition, diagnostic decisions were commonly based on retrospective assessment of developmental histories from old clinical records.

The archive study had somewhat less tendentious origins, as it began with no prior assumptions regarding diagnoses, and, fortuitously, included a broader range of higher-functioning children than is generally included in studies of autism spectrum disorders. This may explain why other applications of empirical classification procedures to subcategorize PDD, among younger or more cognitively impaired children (e.g., Sherman, Shapiro, & Glassman, 1983; Fein, Waterhouse, Lucci, & Snyder, 1985; Siegel, Anders, Ciaranello, Bienenstock, & Kraemer, 1986; Rescorla, 1988; Sevin et al., 1995) have not provided such clear differentiation. Wing (1981b) categorically stated that she found mathematical techniques unhelpful in separating groups in her epidemiological study of severely socially impaired children (Wing & Gould, 1979), although she did make a clinical subtyping of three groups based on the quality of social interaction. The only comparable analysis to my own, in which less severely impaired children were studied, was performed by Szatmari's group (Szatmari et al., 1990), who also found a pattern of three subtypes that resembled my observations, but they rejected their validity as distinct clinical groups (see Pomeroy, Friedman, & Stephens, 1990). A more recent cluster-analytic study (Eaves, Ho, & Eaves, 1994) using data from 166 children with a broad range of PDD did produce three subtypes that resemble those I have described, after a cluster of autistic children with moderate to severe mental handicap were excluded.

The archival work provided an impetus for a number of studies, of which the Stony Brook PDD study was devised, about 7 years before publication of DSM-IV (APA, 1994), to address diagnostic subgrouping among the PDD (Pomeroy, Stephens, Fennig, & Friedman, 1994; Fennig, Pomeroy, Stephens, Fennig, & Friedman, 1994).

The Stony Brook PDD Study

Introduction

Two observations from the archival study seemed relevant for examination of subtyping PDD. The first was that within the spectrum of PDD (excluding children with psychosis and/or mental retardation) there were potentially three major groups of disorders, namely, a classical autistic disorder as originally described by Kanner in 1943, an autistic-like disorder with speech and language deviation but less evidence of motor abnormalities or rigid behavior, and, a disorder, as had been described by Asperger, in which speech was well preserved but severe social difficulties and rigid behaviors predominated.

The second observation was that these disorders might be differentiated by distinct patterns of abnormal development and cognitive profile. More specifically, two models of differentiation might be of importance, one neuroanatomical and the other neuropsychological. In the former we might consider that language and motor skills are representative to some degree of dominant and nondominant cortical brain activity, respectively, whereas intellectual ability may be a function of both hemispheres or an independent variable. Thus, based on the archive study's findings it could be proposed that infantile autism is the product of damage or dysfunction in certain parts of both hemispheres in early development, associated more commonly with lower intellectual functioning. In children with more pronounced dominant hemisphere dysfunction, better intellect, but poor abstract thinking, a disorder that is clinically related to autism is apparent, but with no motor handicaps, as well as less ritualistic and manneristic behavior. Children with nondominant hemisphere dysfunction develop syndromes more compatible with the disorder described by Asperger. It was realized that this would probably prove to be too simple a concept, but the issue of lateralizing features among these disorders was an impetus to the research goals and design.

In many ways the neuropsychological issues mirrored these same lateralizing themes. Although our data were limited, there seemed to be evidence for a difference between the putative PDD subtypes suggesting that, at least comparing psychological profiles of autistic and Asperger subjects, we would expect to see distinctly different patterns of verbally mediated and visuospatial skills. Tanguay's theories (1984) had also influenced the study design. He argued that critical periods existed for development of different brain systems and if lines of development fail to occur at expected times uneven skills will become apparent, leading to psychopathology. He pointed out how patterns of strengths and weaknesses in the neuropsychologically derived concepts of holistic thinking (nonverbal integration of visual, kinesthetic, tactile, and auditory stimuli) and sequential thinking (coding and decoding of meaning in terms of relationship of elements within a sequence) lead to different clinical pictures. The models he discussed were in keeping with the observations of the pilot study if language and motor functioning were considered clinical correlates of sequential and holistic skills, respectively.

It should be noted that Tanguay's views and such models of differentiation have been considered idiosyncratic (e.g., Rutter & Schopler, 1987), and many have argued that these differentiations are artificial, stating that these disorders exist along a continuum and are merely variations of HFA disorders (e.g., Gillberg, 1989; Gillberg & Gillberg, 1989; Wing, 1991; Tantam, 1991). Studies that begin with categorical assumptions (such as cluster-analytic studies) cannot adequately address theories of a continuum but the prevailing data would suggest that at least two, rather than one, continuua have to be considered. One of these is in the direction of speech and language impairment and the other in a direction of motor impairment. Figure 3-1 shows the possible relationships (continuum or diagnostic overlap) for the diagnostic groups delineated in the archival study. It attempts to address the four different variables — IQ, motor skills, language skills, and age of onset — that seemed of most significance in differentiating the clusters. It is of note that with increasing IQ the diagnostic variation and the differentiation between groups tended to become more apparent. However, clinical examples from the study could be cited that genuinely crossed "diagnostic" boundaries supporting the idea that continuua were more relevant than discrete categories, or that the proposed diagnostic groups were not adequate to categorize all of the varied types of clinical presentation.

Based on these considerations it was decided that to address the validity of subcategorization of PDD a study should be a prospective evaluation of a broad range of higher-functioning children with PDD symptoms, within a

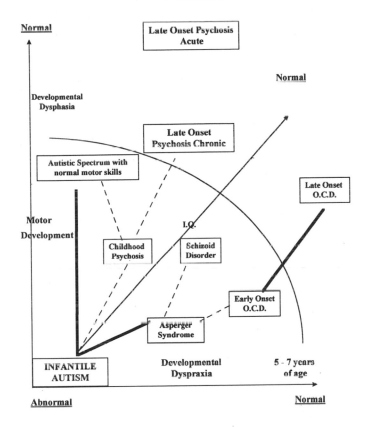

Fig. 3-1. Archival study: hypothetical diagnostic classification and relationships between the diagnostic groups.

discrete age and IQ range, and at a developmental stage when there was adequate verbal and cognitive skills to assess hypothesized group differences.

Method

Subjects

Eighty-nine children evaluated at the Child Psychiatric Clinic at University Hospital, Stony Brook, were recruited into an intensive evaluation study between the years 1987 and 1993. The recruited children had to be between the ages of 5 and 12 years, have a testable intelligence above 70 (on an individually administered IQ test), and be verbal. Three diagnostic groups were recruited:

1. Children who met the above selection criteria and had been given a clinical diagnosis of PDD. That is, they met DSM-IIIR (APA, 1987) diagnostic criteria for autistic disorder or PPD-NOS (43 subjects). Because there had been no specific criteria delineated for PDD-NOS, the study set the following minimal criteria for inclusion.* All children were required to have evidence of marked and chronic social withdrawal or inappropriateness prior to the age of 36 months, accompanied by at least one of the following features:

   a. Abnormal speech (e.g., echolalia, lack of prosody, lack of conversational speech)
   b. Unusual environmental responses or repetitive, rigid thought or behavioral patterns
   c. Unusual emotional reactions (e.g., sudden excessive anxiety; constricted or inappropiate affect)

2. Children who had a Developmental Receptive and Expressive Language Disorder (at least 1-year receptive language delay) but did not meet criteria for PDD (18 subjects). To expand the size of this group some subjects were recruited, by advertisement, from local special education settings.
3. Children with a disruptive behavior disorder (e.g., ADHD, conduct disorder) with no evidence of developmental disorder, based on a review of clinical data (27 subjects).

The latter two groups were matched as closely as possible for sex, age, and range of verbal and cognitive skills as the PDD group.

Measures

General Procedure. The research group consisted of a psychologist, speech pathologist, developmental pediatrician and child psychiatrist. Each child received: (1) a battery of neuropsychological tests; (2) a physical examination for minor physical anomalies, soft neurological signs, and major neurological

---

* Criteria were based on the only available DSM definition of characteristics of nonautistic PDD — childhood onset PDD (APA, 1980). Although this diagnosis has been invalidated because of the age criteria, the clinical criteria remain appropiate and are in keeping with the recently developed DSM-IV criteria for PDD-NOS.

abnormality; (3) videotaped interview; (4) speech and language evaluation; and (5) parent-completed diagnostic inventories and interviews. In addition, the first 30 PDD children recruited had chromosomal studies to detect fragile X syndrome (all of which were negative); a number of children had an assessment of blood platelet serotonin receptors; and most children had a neurophysiological assessment, initially using the "Neurometrics" Quantified EEG procedure and, later, assessing auditory brainstem evoked potentials only. Because the study spanned a long time period, some changes in assessment procedures occurred, but do not influence the findings presented in this chapter, which focuses on neuropsychological measures and clinical characteristics.

Neuropsychology. At the outset of this study a decision was made to use the Kaufman Assessment Battery for Children (K-ABC; Kaufman, O'Neil, Avant, & Long, 1987) as the major measure of general cognitive ability, for two reasons. The first was that the tests that constitute the K-ABC had been devised with a goal of addressing the neuropsychological measures that Tanguay (1984) had proposed were the underlying variants that could define different types of severe child psychopathology, namely, sequential and holistic (or simultaneous) skills. Second, children in special education settings receive routine psychological testing. Most of the children in the study would have received regular assessments on a Wechsler IQ measure (WISC-R in all of our subjects), and these data would therefore be available to us and could be presented for comparison, with the limitation that it was not measured in our standardized research setting. If WISC-R results were not available, most children in the study received this measure also.

Other neuropsychological tests included evaluation of visuomotor skills (VMI and Bender Gestalt tests), laterality tasks (Perdue Pegboard, Finger Tapping Test, Laterality Test), and one presumed measure of frontal lobe function (Trailmaking Test).

Subcategorizing the PDD Groups

Although we did not wish to establish preconceived diagnostic assumptions, it was decided for initial comparison studies to differentiate in a simple fashion between children who had classical autistic characteristics and those children who had nonautistic disorders (PDD-NOS). This was achieved by blind review of 32 items (see Appendix) from the semistructured diagnostic parent interview, which had originally been devised by Szatmari's group for their studies of Asperger disorder and HFA (Szatmari et al., 1990). The 32 items from the questionnaire were selected for their ability to adequately describe developmental abnormalities present before school age, which are typical of autistic disorder, in social (6 items), language (8 items), adaptive behavior and play (5 items) skills, as well as characteristics of schizotypal disorder (4 items) and psychosis (9 items) to ensure that children with symptoms of major psychosis had been excluded from the PDD groupings. The children were then placed in one of three categories.

1. Classical or Kanner's autistic disorder — these children had shown deficits in socialization, communication, and adaptive behavior sufficient to pass standard criteria for an autistic disorder. (Parents in this group endorsed 12 or more of the 19 autistic items from the parent interview, whereas in all other cases parents endorsed less than 10 of these items.) Thus, another group of PDD subjects who did not pass criteria for autism was created (PDD-NOS). Based on a review of their history of language development, this group was further subcategorized into two clinical groups:

2. Language-impaired PDD, if they had a history of significant delay in language development (e.g., no speech at 2 years, not forming sentences or lack of reciprocal speech at 3 years).

3. Non-language-impaired PDD (i.e., no significant delay in language development).

Although these diagnostic divisions did not use standard criteria, it would be reasonable to consider that Group B children would most likely receive a diagnosis, currently, of atypical autism and Group C children would be considered to have Asperger disorder (WHO, 1992; APA, 1994). The three PDD subgroups along with the language-impaired and behavior disorder (control) children, created five contrasting clinical groups.

Results

Some of the demographic and basic cognitive and language measures of the five groups are shown in Table 3-4.* Few females were identified for the PDD group and, therefore, the two contrasting groups were of similar sex ratio. The only age difference was that the non-language-impaired PDD group (PDD/NL) was older (by about 1 year) than most of the other groups, probably reflecting the later age of presentation that has been commonly reported for Asperger syndrome. Simple measures of language skills (i.e., receptive and expressive one-word vocabulary measures) reveal interesting group differences. The most severely language-impaired group was the language-impaired PDD group (PDD/L), showing a mean deficit of 2 years in receptive and 0.9 year in expressive vocabulary. More striking

*All significant measures presented in this study (in Tables 3-4 and 3-5) use Tukey's Studentized Range Test for significance applied to ANOVA for the five clinical groups.

Table 3-4. Stony Brook PDD Study: Descriptive Data of Comparison Groups

	Autistic	PDD/L	Language impaired (LI)	PDD/NL	Control
Number of subjects	13	16	18	15	27
Age in years	7.6 ± 1.2	8.2 ± 1.7	7.6 ± 1.9	8.6 ± 3.0^d	7.8 ± 2.1
Male:female	11:2	15:1	14:4	15:0	25:2
Wechsler Full Scale IQ (mean)	92 ± 21.1	81.3 ± 21.9	85.0 ± 13.1	105.1 ± 23.3	102.5 ± 14.7
Kaufman MPC (IQ equivalent-mean)	95.6 ± 17.5	84.5 ± 19.8	84.8 ± 15.6	94.8 ± 17.4	105 ± 19.7
Mean language difference (age skill level — chronological age)					
Peabody Picture Vocabulary Test (receptive)	−1.2	−2.0^c	−1.4	+4.3^a	+0.4
Expressive One Word Vocabulary Test	+0.4	−0.9^c	−0.4^c	+2.7^b	+1.3

^{a}Significantly ($p < .05$) greater than autistic, PDD/L, and LI groups.
^{b}Significantly ($p < .05$) greater than PDD/L group.
^{c}Significantly ($p < .05$) lower than control group.
^{d}Significantly ($p < .05$) greater than autistic group.

is the very superior vocabulary skills of the PDD/NL group showing mean skills of greater than 4 years above the normal age-related ability, in receptive vocabulary, and nearly 3 years greater for expressive vocabulary. That this reflected different underlying cognitive patterns for these clinical groups was apparent when neuropsychological measures were examined.

Autistic Group. Although this group, which may be considered a high-functioning autistic group, was selected on relatively simple diagnostic measures, the cognitive profile is striking for its similarity to other reports of high-functioning autistic individuals (see the excellent review by Rumsey, 1992). The mean IQ is well within the average range, but, as a group, there is a lower verbal than performance IQ score on the WISC-R. Furthermore, the very low abilities on many verbally mediated tasks (e.g., Vocabulary, Comprehension) were in contrast to their average to above-average ability in performance tasks such as Block Design and Object Assembly.

The patterns on the K-ABC are less dramatic, but again in keeping with previous studies. The autistic group as a mean fall well within the average range on the global scales of the K-ABC and do not show a significant difference between the sequential and simultaneous scales of this measure. The most dramatic pattern on the K-ABC that distinguished the autistic group was apparent on the Achievement scale. Here, we observed the superior ability of the autistic subjects on Reading Decoding and Reading Understanding, whereas the group performance on

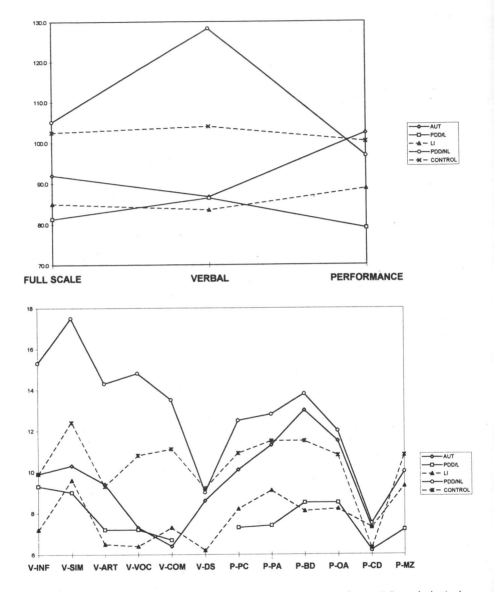

Fig. 3-2. Stony Brook PDD study: group profiles on WISC-R and Kaufman-ABC psychological measures. **Groups:** Autistic, AUT; nonautistic PDD with language impairment, PDD/L; language impaired, LI; nonautistic PDD without language impairment, PDD/NL; behavior disorder, CONT. **WISC-R:** FS, Full-Scale IQ; V, Verbal IQ; P, Performance IQ; V-INF, Information; V-SIM, Similarities; V-ART, Arithmetic; V-VOC, Vocabulary; V-COM, Comprehension; V-DS, Digit Span; P-PC, Picture Completion; P-PA, Picture Arrangement; P-BD, Block Design; P-OA, Object Assembly; P-CD, Coding; P-MZ, Mazes. **K-ABC:** K-SEQ, Sequential; K-SIM, Simultaneous; K-MPC, Mental Processing Composite; K-ACH, Achievement; K-NVB, Non-Verbal; K-AR, Arithmetic; K-RI, Riddles; K-RD, Reading Decoding; K-RU, Reading Understanding.

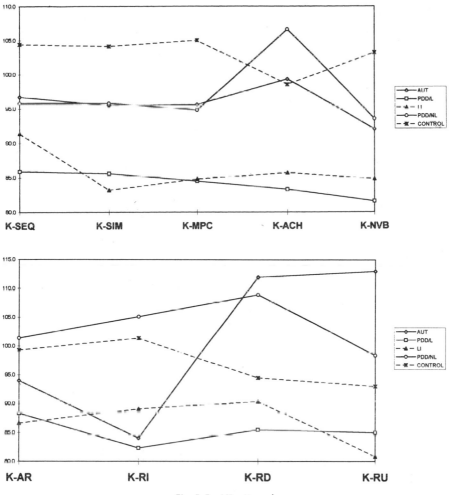

Fig. 3-2. (Continued).

the Riddles subtest was at least one standard deviation below the test mean. This discrepancy between ability on Reading Understanding and Riddles may seem paradoxical, but the former test, which might be thought to be a measure of comprehension, is also a memory task, whereas the Riddles test requires competency in abstract verbal skills. Freeman, Lucas, Forness, and Ritvo (1985) found virtually the same pattern for a high-functioning autistic group on assessment with the K-ABC and WISC-R. Given that this "autistic" cognitive profile would seem to be a consistent finding across a number of studies, it makes the comparison with the other PDD groups in this study most relevant.

Language-Impaired PDD. This group (PDD/L) differed from all other groups except the language-impaired comparison group. That is, the mean cognitive profile of this group was not only in the low average range for verbal and performance measures on the WISC-R and all scales of the K-ABC, but there were essentially no differences between PDD/L children and children with developmental receptive and expressive language disorder. The only measure that did significantly differ from the language-impaired group (see Table 3-5 for the significant differences between this and other PDD groups) was the Hand Movement task of the K-ABC (PDD/L group more deficient than language impaired). This was contradictory to initial hypotheses, as it suggested that the PDD/L group had both verbal and motor impairments constituting a truly multiply handicapped population. That is, they exhibited some of the social and behavioral problems characteristic of PDD, plus specific language and motor deficits. More significantly, this group showed none of the unique strengths that were seen in the high-functioning autistic individuals.

Non-Language-Impaired PDD. This group (PDD/NL) was an intellectually more capable group in many respects, but it should be noted that there was no significant difference between the autistic and PDD/NL groups (nor the behavioral control group) on WISC-R Full Scale and Performance IQ, nor on the Mental Processing Composite Scale (an IQ equivalent) of the K-ABC. Most striking was the significantly superior verbal IQ on the WISC-R compared with all other groups and the lack of a "high-functioning autistic profile" on the WISC-R and K-ABC. Somewhat contradictory to expectation, the PDD/NL group had a similar profile to the autistic group on the performance subtests of

Table 3-5. Stony Brook PDD Study: Comparisons of Significant Differences (p < .05) from ANOVA on all Global and Subtest Measures of Cognitive Function

	WISC-R	Kaufman
PDD/L < PDD/NL	Full Scale IQ, Verbal IQ, Performance IQ, Similarities, Vocabulary, Comprehension, Picture Completion	Achievement, Riddles, Reading Decoding
PDD/L < autistic disorder	Performance IQ, Object Assembly	Triangles, Reading Decoding, Number Recall, Reading Understanding
PDD/L < language impaired		Hand Movements
Autistic disorder < PDD/NL	Verbal IQ, Information, Similarities, Vocabulary, Comprehension	Riddles
Autistic disorder < control	Comprehension	Hand Movements, Riddles

the WISC-R, but this still constituted a marked difference between verbal and
performance abilities in the opposite direction to the high-functioning autistic
pattern. Thus, we did not observe superior abilities in tasks such as Block Design
nor deficits in measures of verbal comprehension.

To what extent this profile merely represents a more intellectually capable
high-functioning autistic group without the speech and language deficits (Tantam,
1991) is difficult to fully address with this study. However, the theories of deficits
in central coherence (proposed by Frith and typified by superiority in block
design-type tasks; see Happé, 1994) and executive function (Bishop, 1993) as core
symptoms of the autistic syndrome do not seem to be relevant to this PDD/NL
sample. This is further accentuated by an examination of the Trailmaking Tests (a
presumed measure of frontal lobe/executive function skills). In our study (see
Figure 3-3) on the Trailmaking A test there was no significant difference in time to
completion between the autistic, PDD/NL, and control groups. There was some
evidence that the skill is related to intellectual level as the two language-impaired
groups performed less well (not shown in Figure 3-3) on this task, but not
significantly different from the autistic group. However, when the Trailmaking B
test was applied, both the autistic and control groups performed less well with the
increased cognitive demand, whereas the PDD/NL subjects actually completed the
task in a shorter time than the first task, and significantly better than the autistic
subjects. Thus, at least in this measure, the PDD/NL subjects we studied did not
exhibit deficits that could be attributed to problems with executive functioning.

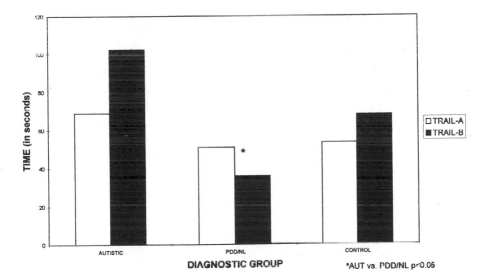

Fig. 3-3. Stony Brook PDD study: Trailmaking test comparing autistic, Asperger, and control
groups.

Discussion

The clinical/developmental and neuropsychological differences found in this study suggest that defining three subtypes of PDD in the absence of mental retardation is justifiable. The hypotheses, generated from the pilot study, that PDD subtyping would correlate with different patterns of (1) sequential and simultaneous processing, and (2) motor and language development, were not substantiated by the prospective PDD study. However, clinical concepts of atypical autism (PDD/L), classical autistic disorder, and Asperger disorder (PDD/NL) were supported by markedly different cognitive profiles among a group of children with PDD within a discrete age and IQ range. Most notably, a characteristic high-functioning autistic cognitive profile, as described by previous researchers, was replicated and was distinctly different from the profile seen in the atypical autistic groups (PDD/L) and, in most respects, from the Asperger-like (PDD/NL) group (see Table 3-5). Furthermore, there was no evidence of one continuum between the groups based on increasing intellectual ability or obvious patterns of change from the most severely impaired (autistic) to the less impaired (PDD/L/atypical autistic) to the least impaired (PDD/NL/Asperger syndrome). It is true that, in general, the Asperger-like subjects were the least intellectually impaired PDD subjects in both studies, but with respect to nonverbal functioning the Asperger and autistic groups functioned similarly. Also, the Asperger-like subjects' verbally mediated skills reflect a superiority over their nonverbal skills (at least in the Wechsler data available to us), which does not seem compatible with Tantam's (1991) theories that Asperger subjects have essentially the same disorder as autistic individuals but merely lack the structural abnormality that underlies the communication deficits apparent in autistic subjects.

The strength of this study was that we systematically and prospectively evaluated a group of young children of comparable intellectual ability at a stage of development that is not only late enough to confirm the persistence of PDD symptoms into later childhood and observe the clinical differentiation between putative PDD subtypes, but also early enough to be likely to obtain more reliable reports of the developmental characteristics of the children. Thus, differentiation of PDD subtypes based on reported functioning in preschool years, with criteria similar to those proposed in DSM-IV, does prove to predict different behavioral and cognitive outcome.

Standardized diagnostic criteria that are now available for PDD subcategories were not used in this study. An evaluation of this issue, by asking an independent child psychiatrist to blindly diagnose, from a review of the medical records, a random sample of 25 subjects, highlights the dilemma. The concordance for diagnosis by the psychiatrist with our study "diagnosis" was 60% overall and 84.6% for the autistic, language-impaired, and control groups. For the two PDD-NOS groups the concordance was only 33%. More encouragingly, the "incorrect" diagnoses still tended to differentiate the PDD-NOS groups. The discordant diagnoses given by the psychiatrist for children in the study's "atypical autistic" group were either language delayed or autistic, and for the "Asperger" group discordant diagnoses by the psychiatrist had an unusual mix of schizotypal, disintegrative, and autistic disorders. At this point it is therefore wise to consider our PDD-NOS groups as merely reflective of the different DSM-IV subtypes, but, at least, derived by consistent criteria. The psychiatrist's diagnoses would be influenced by the adequacy of the medical record and the probability that applying the diagnoses of PDD-NOS or other PDD subtypes remains a difficult clinical decision, particularly when, as in this situation, no specific training or advice regarding diagnostic decisions were given.

DSM-IV AND BEYOND

Despite accumulating evidence for the presence of PDD subtypes, many would state that the subtypes are an artifact caused by raising minor clinical variations or different developmental pathways to an undeserved nosological status, so that false conclusions are drawn regarding neurodevelopmental disorders of the same origin. The importance of differentiating between categorical and dimensional approaches to diagnosis with regard to PDD has been addressed earlier. The Stony Brook study could be said to favor a categorical approach as it shows that among children with PDD, more closely matched for age and IQ than most previous studies, there are distinct group differences when differentiation is based on early developmental history and severe impairment of language development is also set as a discriminating factor between the two types of PDD-NOS (nonautistic PDD). I have previously suggested (Pomeroy et al., 1991) that comparison studies of Asperger's disorder and autistic disorder have failed to make a distinction between Asperger's disorder and atypical autism causing potential group differences to be lost in the statistical comparisons. If these categories exist, in a meaningful manner (i.e., they are not merely subtle variants of the same neurobiological mechanisms), they must be examined for variation in course, familial pattern, outcome, associated biology, and response to treatment or intervention, as with any validation of classes of disease. Fortunately, the DSM-IV and ICD-10 diagnostic subcategorization of PDD will promote such research and there is already evidence of the emergence of interest in this topic. There have been a number of studies supporting the concept of Asperger's disorder as a distinct clinical syndrome (Klin, Volkmar, Sparrow, Cicchetti, & Rourke, 1995; Szatmari, Archer, Fisman, Streiner, & Wilson, 1995: Volkmar et al., 1996), in keeping with the observations that I have described in this chapter. Even Gillberg's group (Ehlers et al., 1997) concluded that an Asperger cognitive profile differentiating from an Autistic profile can be detected but they make slightly different interpretations of their findings invoking differences between the groups in psychological concepts known as fluid and crystallized intelligence.

The spectrum or continuum theories of classification among PDD are strongly supported in the European literature regarding Asperger syndrome and seem assumed by all of the contributors to Uta Frith's (1991) excellent text on this issue. Ironically, her translation of Asperger's original paper suggests that he also did not make such a distinction between children whom we may now identify as high-functioning autistic and those whose symptoms would place them in a category eponymously entitled after his contribution (observed also by Miller & Ozonoff, 1997). Thus, many clinicians quote examples of children who now appear to have Asperger syndrome but had early characteristics of autism or marked developmental language delay (e.g., Tantam, 1991; Gillberg, 1991). Furthermore, some family studies (e.g., Gillberg, 1991) suggest that autistic and Asperger's disorders can co-occur among siblings or first-degree relatives. The question arises as to whether the diagnostic decisions in these studies are based on valid, or idiosyncratic, opinion by the workers. It is of note that many clinical psychiatrists appear to be applying the diagnosis of Asperger's Disorder to all highly verbal, nonretarded individuals with an autistic or autistic-like disorder.

If a continuum concept is accepted, it would seem that at the extreme of least impairment these disorders blend clinically into specific developmental disorders, namely, speech and communication disorders on the atypical autism continuum and nonverbal learning disability (Rourke, 1989) on the Asperger continuum. Perhaps the most striking support for a continuum or spectrum of autistic disorder comes from two recent studies, one of family history (Bolton *et al.*, 1994) and the other of twins (Le Couteur *et al.*, 1996). In Bolton's study a comparison was made between the families of 99 autistic and 36 Down syndrome probands. This confirmed a strong familial loading for autism as well as a more broadly defined PDD. Furthermore, over 20% of first-degree relatives of the autistic probands had different patterns of subtle communication problems and/or social impairment and/or stereotypic behaviors that were below a clinical threshold to warrant a psychiatric diagnosis. Le Couteur's group studied 28 monozygotic and 20 dizygotic twin pairs in which one or both twins were autistic. Among monozygotic twins there was a 60% concordance for autism or atypical autism compared with 0% in dizygotic twins. The twins who were concordant for autism, however, showed wide discrepancy in severity of the autistic syndrome and the range of cognitive abilities. Furthermore, most of the nonautistic monozygotic twins still had evidence of a significant social and communication disorder, with one-third of these twins also having restricted, stereotyped, or repetitive behavior. Reviewing the case histories of these twins, as reported in the study, it would appear that a classic picture of Asperger's disorder was rare and only two of the "discordant" monozygotic twins would have been considered for such a diagnosis based on a relatively normal acquisition of language.

The findings from these two studies suggest that autism may eventually be viewed as a much more broadly defined entity. It is unclear whether these studies support or refute subtyping of PDD. Consideration should be given to the possibility that the definition of "true autism" still encompasses diagnostic heterogeneity. For example, at the more severe end of the spectrum, the three autistic groups with different types of social impairment described by Wing and Gould (1979) may represent a true variation, which has its counterpart in the higher-functioning end of the spectrum, as proposed by Tantam (1991), but invoked by him as evidence of varibility in the autistic syndrome, not evidence for separate diagnostic groups. These arguments have an inevitable tautological quality and can only be addressed by continued study. We need to learn more about variation in course and outcome for children who have a disorder within this broader spectrum of PDD which has been identified and categorized early, thereby allowing a systematic long-term follow-up. We may then be able to judge to what degree these PDD subtypes prove to have any distinctive characteristics.

CONCLUSION

Clinicians who provide service to children and adults with PDD report an increase in the rate of referral for these disorders. Is this a consequence of a true increase in incidence, a broader diagnostic inclusiveness, improved identification, or a mix of all of these factors? There has certainly been a rise in the generally accepted incidence of autism, as well as preliminary evidence that the rate of higher-functioning (nonretarded) autism may have been underestimated in older studies (Honda, Shimizu, Misumi, Niimi, & Ohashi, 1996). Opinion regarding an autistic spectrum and/or PDD subtyping remains inconclusive, but some useful knowledge has been gained. My clinical and research observations support subcategories of PDD when the extreme (or most typical) clinical histories are considered.

I believe that children and adolescents with classical autistic development and profiles, in association with good intelligence, usually continue to exhibit as young adults the core cognitive deficits described in our studies and others. They also appear more socially impaired, perseverative, and ritualistic than the other PDD groups, and their language is often still characterized by its unusual voice production and quality, with less severe but still apparent problems with comprehension and expression (e.g., echolalia may still be evident to some degree). Siegel, Minshew, and Goldstein (1996) advocated caution in using any specific IQ profile (e.g., verbal–performance discrepancy) for diagnostic purposes, as they found marked variability in such measures among a well-diagnosed group of high-functioning autistic children and adults. I would strongly support the statement that IQ profiles should not be used for diagnostic purposes but this group's data offer other interpretation. Despite the observation that a verbal–performance discrepancy was not a consistent finding, there was a significant difference on Wechsler IQ measures between low comprehension (abstract verbal skills) and high Block Design/Object Assembly (visuospatial skills) for the children, as described in other studies. This was less evident in the adult group, which raises the possibility of developmental changes in IQ profiles in higher-functioning autistic individuals. Thus, maturational effects could coincide with measureable cognitive changes that are associated also with improved language and social skills. Such changes might account for case histories that purport to show that autistic individuals can develop Asperger syndrome in adult years.

In 1987, Friedman and I (Pomeroy & Friedman, 1987) listed the characteristics we saw as defining Asperger syndrome. These included unusual, rigid, omnipotent personality characteristics; normal intelligence, but significant social and academic problems; relatively normal language development; evidence of developmental motor problems; preoccupation with self-interests; abnormalities in expressive speech; and neuropsychological profiles that are compatible with poor abstract thinking and probably non-dominant-hemisphere dysfunction. Some reanalysis of the neuropsychological observations is necessary based on the PDD study findings, but, whereas I concur with Siegel *et al.* (1996) that a low verbal–high performance IQ split has no clinical specificity, I cannot recall seeing a referred child with the opposite discrepancy (high verbal–low performance) who did not exhibit some evidence of social–emotional deficits. Commonly their physical clumsiness is matched by an awkward, gauche social manner, even if they may not be considered to have PDD.

Some of the features of Asperger syndrome that I have observed more consistently in my recent clinical evaluations are the tendency to present clinically in late childhood or adolescence; severe lack of insight into their evident social and emotional problems which often leads to an early breakdown in efforts to treat or help these young (mostly) boys; a tendency to grandiosity, sensitivity to personal slights, but a lack of empathy for others' feelings; and emergence of other psychiatric symptoms including affective and paranoid illnesses. I have also been struck by the marked variability in degree of associated handicaps. Some children seem relatively calm and handicapped only by their cognitive and social deficits, whereas other children with the same developmental and cognitive profile have a range of severe behavioral deficits such as hyperactivity, impulsivity, aggression, vocal and motor tics, need to control others, and idiosyncratic thought and behavior that requires intensive and prolonged behavioral, psychiatric, and educational interventions. These young patients are much more likely to be identified in psychiatric settings than programs for developmentally disabled individuals, and may ultimately be presenting more commonly to adult psychiatric services than is presently realized.

Although differential diagnosis between Asperger syndrome and HFA seems to emerge as an issue at a later stage of development, I have had a small number of recent referrals for assessment of preschoolers who pass diagnostic criteria for Asperger's disorder, and our own study made diagnostic differentiation based on development in the first 5 years of life. Therefore, there is support for the fact that children with Asperger's disorder can be differentiated in the preschool years, and Szatmari's most recent study (Szatmari *et al.*, 1995) identified a relatively large cohort of 4- to 6-year-olds whom he diagnosed as Asperger subjects.

With regard to atypical autism the issues of differential diagnosis are more relevant to the first 3 years of life. The PDD study would support the idea that an autistic variant exists in which severe speech and language impairment is associated with a range of autistic-like behaviors (particularly in the social domain). These disorders have been previously described (Paul, Cohen, & Caparulo, 1983; Rutter & Schopler, 1987; Brook & Bowler, 1992) with varying opinion about their diagnostic placement. The PDD study seems to confirm their status as a clinical bridge between autistic disorder and severe developmental receptive and expressive language disorder. There does appear to be some shared features in the type of language deficits seen in HFA and severe developmental language disorders (Rapin, 1996), but Minshew, Goldstein, and Siegel (1995) argued that the language deficits in HFA can be differentiated from those seen in developmental language disorders. Cognitively, the atypical autistic profile in the PDD study was similar to the language impaired group, but it is my impression that, prior to age 3, children in this clinical group are difficult to distinguish from children who will develop more classical autistic disorder. To some degree a subjective impression of less severe social deficits, better joint attention and less ritualistic qualities seems to define the atypical autistic group but they may still pass the descriptive diagnostic criteria for an autistic disorder in the early years of development. These clinical observations are beginning to be assessed in research studies (e.g., Mayes, Volkmar, Hooks, & Cicchetti, 1993; McArthur & Adamson, 1996), and have important implications for the measurement of effects of early intervention and outcome research. This group of children probably outnumbers the children who will ultimately develop autism and we need improved diagnostic approaches to adequately differentiate these diagnostic groups. Fortunately, work is also progressing on this issue (Lord, 1995; DiLavore, Lord, & Rutter, 1995).

Atypical autism and Asperger's disorder appear to have significant enough defining features throughout the age range to warrant subcategorization of PDD. This does not yet prove that they are neurobiologically or etiologically distinct categories and many clinicians can present case histories of children who have contradictory symptomatology or history (e.g., "Asperger cases" where there is exceptional arithmetic ability, or history of language delay, or a sibling with an autistic disorder). In the preschool years these diagnostic groups may be difficult to differentiate in individual cases but their ongoing development does seem to lead to different patterns that suggest inborn differences that may be influenced by the treatments and intervention we apply. The issue of accurate diagnosis in deciding if new, dramatic, treatments are able to change the autistic process is already leading to heated debate (e.g., Shapiro & Hertzig, 1995). Theories of continuum and spectrum cannot be excluded and the fascinating similarities between some children with more subtle learning disorders (verbal and nonverbal) and those with high-functioning PDD have to be explained. A more radical issue is consideration of the degree to which symptoms of PDD are distinct. Those of us who work in child and adolescent psychiatry services are aware that social and behavioral characteristics typically seen in PDD are detectable in a wider range of disorders than would normally be considered the autistic spectrum. This includes childhood psychosis and what are called borderline disorders by some researchers (Towbin, Dykens, Pearson, & Cohen, 1993; Alaghbad-Rad et al., 1995). Thus, a less rigid view of the specificity of PDD symptoms might have to be considered by clinicians and clinical researchers in the future. Ultimately, we may be able to consider specific aspects of the PDD profile from a more neurodevelopmental or neuroanatomical perspective. Such an approach may also assist in helping us understand why individual children present with contradictory symptoms that confound the efforts to neatly define diagnostic subcategories.

ACKNOWLEDGMENTS

The PDD study was aided by Social and Behavioral Sciences Research Grant No. 12-216 from the March of Dimes Birth Defects Foundation. I would like to thank and acknowledge my colleagues who worked with me on these studies. The pilot study was assisted by Dr. James Falk, and the PDD study group included Drs. Laurie Stephens, Carol Friedman, Pat Quinn, and John Amato. My appreciation is also extended to Drs. Gabrielle Carlson and Ken Gadow for their review and comments on the chapter, and Kathy Grzymala for secretarial support.

REFERENCES

Adams, P. L. (1973). *Obsessive children: A sociopsychiatric study*. London: Butterworths.
Alaghbad-Rad, J., McKenna, K., Gordon, C. T., Albus, K. E., Hamburger, S. D., Rumsey, J. M., Frazier, J. A., Lenane, M. C., & Rapoport, J. L. (1995). Childhood-onset schizophrenia: The severity of premorbid course. *Journal of the American Academy of Child and Adolescent Psychiatry, 34,* 1273–1283.
American Psychiatric Association. (1980). *Diagnostic and statistical manual of mental disorders* (3rd ed.). Washington, DC: Author.
American Psychiatric Association. (1987). *Diagnostic and statistical manual of mental disorders* (rev. 3rd ed.). Washington, DC: Author.
American Psychiatric Association. (1994). *Diagnostic and statistical manual of mental disorders* (4th ed.). Washington, DC: Author.
Bishop, D. V. M. (1993). Autism, executive functions and theory of mind: A neuropsychologic perspective. *Journal of Child Psychology and Psychiatry, 34,* 279–293.
Bolton, P., MacDonald, H., Pickles A., Rios, P., Goode, S., Crowson, M., Bailey, A., & Rutter, M. (1994). A case–control family history study of autism. *Journal of Child Psychology and Psychiatry, 35,* 877–900.

Brook, S. L., & Bowler, D. M. (1992). Autism by another name? Semantic and pragmatic impairments in children. *Journal of Autism and Developmental Disorders*, *22*, 61–81.

Childers, A. T. (1931). A study of some schizoid children. *Mental Hygiene*, *15*, 106–134.

Cull, A., Chick, J., & Wolff, S. (1984). A consensual validation of schizoid personality in childhood and adult life. *British Journal of Psychiatry*, *144*, 646–648.

DiLavore, P. C., Lord, C., & Rutter, M. (1995). The pre-linguistic autism diagnostic observation schedule. *Journal of Autism and Developmental Disorders*, *25*, 355–379.

Eaves, L. C., Ho, H. H., & Eaves, D. M. (1994). Subtypes of autism by cluster analysis. *Journal of Autism and Developmental Disorders*, *24*, 3–22.

Ehlers, S., Nyden, A., Gillberg, C., Dahlgren, S.-O., Sandberg, A., Hjelmquist, E., & Oden, A. (1997). Asperger syndrome, autism and attention disorders: A comparative study of the cognitive profiles of 120 children. *Journal of Child Psychology and Psychiatry*, *37*, 207–217.

Fein, D., Waterhouse, L., Lucci, D., & Snyder, D. (1985). Cognitive subtypes in developmentally disabled children: A pilot study. *Journal of Autism and Developmental Disorders*, *15*, 77–95.

Fennig, S., Pomeroy, J. C., Stephens, L., Fennig, S., & Friedman, C. (1994). *Stony Brook PDD study: Validation of sub-categories of PDD-Asperger's disorder*. Poster presented at the annual meeting of the American Academy of Child and Adolescent Psychiatry, New York.

Freeman, B. J., Lucas, J. C., Forness, S. R., & Ritvo, E. R. (1985). Cognitive processing of high functioning autistic children: Comparing the K-ABC and the WISC-R. *Journal of Psychoeducational Assessment*, *4*, 357–362.

Frith, U. (Ed.). (1991). *Autism and Asperger syndrome*. Cambridge: Cambridge University Press.

Gillberg, C. (1989). Asperger syndrome in 23 Swedish children. *Developmental Medicine and Child Neurology*, *31*, 520–531.

Gillberg, C. (1991). Clinical and neurobiological aspects of Asperger syndrome in six family studies. In U. Frith (Ed.), *Autism and Asperger syndrome* (pp. 122–146). Cambridge: Cambridge University Press.

Gillberg, I. C., & Gillberg, C. (1989). Asperger syndrome — some epidemiological considerations: A research note. *Journal of Child Psychology and Psychiatry*, *30*, 631–638.

Happé, F. G. E. (1994). Current psychological theories of autism: The "theory of mind" account and rival theories. *Journal of Child Psychology and Psychiatry*, *35*, 215–239.

Heston, L. L. (1970). The genetics of schizophrenia and schizoid disease. *Science*, *167*, 249–255.

Honda, H., Shimizu, Y., Misumi, K., Niimi, M., & Ohashi, Y. (1996). Cumulative incidence and prevalence of childhood autism in children in Japan. British Journal of Psychiatry, *169*, 228–235.

Jenkins, R. L., & Glickman, S. (1946). Common syndromes in child psychiatry. *American Journal of Orthopsychiatry*, *16*, 244–256.

Kanner, L. (1943). Autistic disturbances of affective contact. *Nervous Child*, *2*, 217–250.

Kaufman, A. S., O'Neil, M. R., Avant, A. H., & Long, S. W. (1987). Introduction to the Kaufman Assessment Battery for Children (K-ABC) for pediatric neuroclinicians. *Journal of Child Neurology*, *2*, 3–16.

Kerbeshian, J., Burd, L., & Fisher, W. (1990). Asperger's syndrome: To be or not to be? *British Journal of Psychiatry*, *156*, 721–725.

Kety, S. S., Rosenthal, D., Wender, P. H., & Schulsinger, F. (1968). The types and prevalence of mental illness in the biologic and adoptive families of adopted schizophrenics. In D. Rosenthal & S. S. Kety (Eds.), *The transmission of schizophrenia* (p. 345). London: Pergamon Press.

Klin, A., Volkmar, F. R., Sparrow, S. S., Cicchetti, D. V., & Rourke, B. P. (1995). Validity and neuropsychological characterization of Asperger syndrome: Convergence with nonverbal learning disabilities syndrome. *Journal of Child Psychology and Psychiatry*, *36*, 1127–1140.

Kolvin, I., Ounsted, C., Humphrey, M., & McNay, A. (1971). II. The phenomenology of childhood psychoses. *British Journal of Psychiatry*, *118*, 385–395.

Le Couteur, A., Bailey, A., Goode, S., Pickles, A., Robertson, S., Gottesman, I., & Rutter, M. (1996). A broader phenotype of autism: The clinical spectrum in twins. *Journal of Child Psychology and Psychiatry*, *37*, 785–801.

Lord, C. (1995). Follow-up of two-year-olds referred for possible autism. *Journal of Child Psychology and Psychiatry*, *36*, 1365–1382.

Mayes, L., Volkmar, F., Hooks, M., & Cicchetti, D. (1993). Differentiating Pervasive Developmental Disorder Not Otherwise Specified from autism and language disorder. *Journal of Autism and Developmental Disorders*, *23*, 79–90.

McArthur, D., & Adamson, L. B. (1996). Joint attention in preverbal children: Autism and developmental language disorder. *Journal of Autism and Developmental Disorders*, *26*, 481–496.

Mednick, S. A. (1970). Breakdown in individuals at high risk for schizophrenia: Possible predispositional perinatal factors. *Mental Hygiene*, *54*, 50–63.

Mednick, S. A., & Schulsinger, F. (1970). Factors related to breakdown in children at high risk for schizophrenia. In M. Roft & D. F. Ricks (Eds.), *Life history research in psychopathology*. Minneapolis: University of Minnesota Press.

Miller, J. N., & Ozonoff, S. (1997). Did Asperger's cases have Asperger disorder? A research note. *Journal of Clinical Psychology and Psychiatry*, *38*, 247–251.

Minshew, N. J., Goldstein, G., & Siegel, D. J. (1995). Speech and language in high-functioning autistic individuals. *Neuropsychology*, *9*, 255–261.

Nagy, J., & Szatmari, P. (1986). A chart review of schizotypal personality disorders in children. *Journal of Autism and Developmental Disorders*, *16*, 351–367.

Paul, R., Cohen, D. J., & Caparulo, B. K. (1983). A longitudinal study of patients with severe developmental disorder of language learning. *Journal of American Academy of Child Psychiatry*, *22*, 525–534.

Paykel, E. S. (1981). Have multivariate statistics contributed to classification? *British Journal of Psychiatry*, *139*, 357–362

Petti, T. A., & Vela, R. M. (1990). Borderline disorder of childhood: An overview. *Journal of the American Academy of Child and Adolescent Psychiatry*, *29*, 327–337.

Pomeroy, J. C. (1984). Non-autistic psychosis and severe developmental disorders in children. Unpublished manuscript, J. Franklin Robinson Award.

Pomeroy, J. C., & Friedman, C. (1987). *Asperger syndrome — a clinical subtype of PDD: The neuropsychologic evidence*. Poster presented at the annual meeting of the American Academy of Child and Adolescent Psychiatry, Washington, DC.

Pomeroy, J. C., Friedman, C., & Stephens, L. (1990). Further thoughts on autistic tendencies [Letter to the editor]. *Developmental Medicine and Child Neurology*, *32*, 832–833.

Pomeroy, J. C., Friedman, C., & Stephens, L. (1991). Autism and Asperger's: Same or different? [Letter to the editor]. *Journal of the American Academy of Child and Adolescent Psychiatry*, *30*, 152–153.

Pomeroy, J. C., Stephens, L., Fennig, S., & Friedman, C. (1994). *Stony Brook PDD study: Validation of PDD sub-categories — atypical autism*. Poster presented at the annual meeting of the American Academy of Child and Adolescent Psychiatry, New York, NY.

Quitkin, F., & Klein, D. F. (1969). Two behavioral syndromes in young adults related to possible minimal brain dysfunction. *Journal of Psychiatric Research*, *7*, 131–142.

Rapin, I. (1996). Practitioner review: Developmental language disorders: A clinical update. *Journal of Child Psychology and Psychiatry*, *37*, 643–655.

Rescorla, L. (1988). Cluster analytic identification of autistic preschoolers. *Journal of Autism and Developmental Disorders*, *18*, 475–492.

Robinson, J. F., & Vitale, L. J. (1954). Children with circumscribed interest patterns. *American Journal of Psychiatry*, *24*, 755–767.

Rourke, B. P. (1989). *Nonverbal learning disabilities*. New York: Guilford Press.

Rumsey, J. M. (1992). Neuropsychological studies of high-level autism. In E. Schopler & G. B. Mesibov (Eds.), *High-functioning individuals with autism* (pp. 41–64). New York: Plenum Press.

Rutter, M. (1971). The description and classification of infantile autism. In D. W. Churchill, G. D. Alpern, & M. K. DeMyer (Eds.), *Infantile autism.* Springfield, IL: Thomas.

Rutter, M., & Schopler, F. (1987). Autism and pervasive developmental disorders: Concepts and diagnostic issues. *Journal of Autism and Developmental Disorders, 17,* 159–186.

Sevin, J. A., Matson, J. L., Coe, D., Love, S. R., Matese, M. J., & Benavidez, D. A. (1995). Empirically derived subtypes of pervasive developmental disorders: A cluster analytic study. *Journal of Autism and Developmental Disorders, 25,* 561–578.

Shapiro, T., & Hertzig, M. (1995). Applied behavioral analysis: Astonishing results? [Letter to the editor]. *Journal of the American Academy of Child and Adolescent Psychiatry, 34,* 1255.

Shea, V., & Mesibov, G. B. (1985). Brief report: The relationship of learning disabilities and higher-level autism. *Journal of Autism and Developmental Disorders, 15,* 425–435.

Sherman, M., Shapiro, T., & Glassman, M. (1983). Play and language in developmentally disordered preschoolers: A new approach to classification. *Journal of the American Academy of Child and Adolescent Psychiatry, 22,* 511–524.

Siegel, B., Anders, T. F., Ciaranello, R. D., Bienenstock, B., & Kraemer, H. C. (1986). Empirically derived subclassification of the autistic syndrome. *Journal of Autism and Developmental Disorders, 16,* 275–293.

Siegel, D. J., Minshew, N. J., & Goldstein, S. (1996). Wechsler IQ profiles in diagnosis of high functioning autism. *Journal of Autism and Developmental Disorders, 26,* 389–406.

Szatmari, P., Archer, L., Fisman, S., Streiner, D. L., & Wilson, F. (1995). Asperger's syndrome and autism: Differences in behavior, cognition and adaptive functioning. *Journal of the American Academy of Child and Adolescent Psychiatry, 34,* 1662–1671.

Szatmari, P., Tuff, L., Finlayson, M. A. J., & Bartolucci, G. (1990). Asperger's syndrome and autism: Neurocognitive aspects. *Journal of the American Academy of Child and Adolescent Psychiatry, 29,* 130–136.

Tanguay, P. E, (1984). Toward a new classification of serious psychopathology in children. *Journal of the American Academy of Child Psychiatry, 23,* 373–384.

Tantam, D. (1991). Asperger syndrome in adulthood. In U. Frith (Ed.), *Autism and Asperger syndrome* (pp. 147–183). Cambridge: Cambridge University Press.

Towbin, K. E., Dykens, E. M., Pearson, G. S., & Cohen, D. J. (1993). Conceptualizing "Borderline Syndrome of Childhood" and "Childhood Schizophrenia" as a developmental disorder. *Journal of the American Academy of Child and Adolescent Psychiatry, 32,* 775–782.

Van Krevelen, D. A. (1971). Early infantile autism and autistic psychopathy. *Journal of Autism and Childhood Schizophrenia, 1,* 82–86.

Voeller, K. K. S. (1986). Right hemisphere deficit syndrome in children. *American Journal of Psychiatry, 143,* 1004–1009.

Volkmar, F. R., Klin, A., Schultz, R., Bronen, R., Marans, W. D., Sparrow, S., & Cohen, D. J. (1996). Asperger's syndrome. *Journal of the American Academy of Child and Adolescent Psychiatry, 35,* 118–123.

Watkins, J. M., Asarnow, R. F., & Tanguay, P. E. (1988). Symptom development in childhood onset schizophrenia. *Journal of Child Psychology and Psychiatry, 29,* 865–878.

Weintraub, S., & Mesulam, M.-M. (1983). Developmental learning disabilities of the right hemisphere. *Archives of Neurology, 40,* 463–468.

Wing, L. (1981a). Asperger's syndrome: A clinical account. *Psychological Medicine, 11,* 115–129.

Wing, L. (1981b). *The severe social and communication disorders of early childhood: Diagnosis and classification.* Paper read at the League School International Symposium, New York.

Wing, L. (1984). Schizoid personality in childhood [Letter to the editor]. *British Journal of Psychiatry, 145,* 444.

Wing, L. (1991). The relationship between Asperger's syndrome and Kanner's autism. In U. Frith (Ed.), *Autism and Asperger syndrome* (pp. 93–121). Cambridge: Cambridge University Press.

Wing, L., & Gould, J. (1979). Severe impairments of social interaction and associated abnormalities in children: Epidemiology and classification. *Journal of Autism and Developmental Disorders, 9,* 11–29.

Wolff, S. (1964). *Schizoid personality in childhood.* Paper read at the Sixth International Psychotherapy Congress, London.

Wolff, S., & Chick, J. (1980). Schizoid personality in childhood: A controlled follow-up study. *Psychological Medicine, 10,* 85–100.

World Health Organization (1992). *International classification of diseases* (10th ed.). Geneva: Author.

APPENDIX

Question items (from the McMaster University Structured Interview for Social and Communication Disorders) used to subcategorize PDD groups in the Stony Brook PDD study.

A. Within the first 3 years of life:
  1. Did he/she like having other people around?
  2. Did he/she enjoy the attention of other people?
  3. Did he/she ignore or resist other people? (Abnormal or different from other children?)
  4. During infancy, did he/she show little urge to communicate (e.g., babble or smile)?
  5. Did he/she tend to avoid looking at people?
  6. Was there ever anything unusual about his/her language like:
      a. Often repeating words or phrases he/she had just heard, in place of responding to what was said?
      b. Often using the wrong pronoun such as saying he/she wants a cracker rather than I want a cracker.
  7. Did he/she have any repetitive and unproductive patterns of behavior, such as hand movements, clapping, twirling?
  8. Did he/she have rituals that must be adhered to or else he/she became upset?
B. Within the first 5 years of life and present behavior:
  1. Does (or did) he/she insist on doing things in the same way (e.g., dressing in the same order)?
  2. Does he/she take only a passive role in social interaction?
  3. When he/she speaks to people, does he/she look at them?
  4. Does he/she have a monotonous way of talking, that is does he/she not often change the tone of his/her voice as he/she is speaking?
  5. Does he/she have repetitive patterns of speech, such as:
      a. reverts to the same topic of conversation again and again?
      b. makes irrelevant remarks in conversations which recur?
  6. Does he/she employ an odd pitch or tone to his/her conversation?
  7. Would you say that he/she is non-communicative?
  8. Does he/she keep returning to a subject time and again, even if it is inappropriate?
  9. Did he/she play various roles such as Batman by inventing pretend play?

Using these items, a reviewer, blind to the identification of subjects, selected those who would pass criteria for Autistic Disorder based on DSM-III-R. Thirteen other items addressing schizotypal and psychotic symptomatology were reviewed to ensure that no child who could be considered psychotic (schizophrenic) was included in the study.

4

Differential Diagnosis of Asperger Disorder

PETER SZATMARI

INTRODUCTION

Asperger syndrome (AS) refers to a constellation of behaviors characterized by unusual social interactions, difficulties in both verbal and nonverbal communication, and an intense interest in very circumscribed topics. The condition is currently classified as a type of pervasive developmental disorder (PDD) and shares with other PDDs the impairments in reciprocal social interaction, the qualitative impairments in communication, and a pattern of repetitive stereotypic activities. The disorder is "pervasive" insofar as the difficulties pervade all aspects of the child's life and it is also a developmental disability with an early onset and a pattern that changes with maturation. Asperger disorder has now been included in both DSM-IV (APA, 1994) and ICD 10 (WHO, 1992) even though its nosologic validity is uncertain and controversial. Nevertheless, with such "official" recognition, it is expected that many more children and adolescents will be receiving this diagnosis so it is important that practical guidelines for differential diagnosis be outlined.

The differentiation of AS from other conditions is helpful, however, only if it provides clinically relevant information on etiology, outcome, or response to treatment. Insofar as AS is a type of PDD, it is certainly important to

PETER SZATMARI • Department of Psychiatry, McMaster University, Hamilton, Ontario, L8N 3Z5, Canada.

Asperger Syndrome or High-Functioning Autism?, edited by Schopler et al. Plenum Press, New York, 1998.

distinguish it from other conditions *outside* the PDD spectrum. AS can be confused with social phobia, semantic–pragmatic language disorders, obsessive-compulsive disorder(OCD), schizotypal personality disorders, and others. Because the etiology, outcome, and response to treatment for at least some of these latter disorders may be different than those for PDD, it is important to have an accurate diagnosis. It is less clear that the differentiation of AS from other PDDs is as clinically useful because there is no consensus that AS has a specific etiology, outcome, or treatment different from higher-functioning autism.

Moreover, there is very little information on empirical distinctions that can be made between AS, autism, and other disorders within the PDD spectrum. A systematic review of the literature conducted using MEDLINE and consulting key references identified only a small number of studies on this issue. The objective of this chapter is to review these studies and to supplement this information with more anecdotal evidence from clinical experience.

THE DIAGNOSIS OF ASPERGER SYNDROME

Diagnostic Criteria

A review of the literature prepared for the DSM-IV committee of the American Psychiatric Association (Szatmari, 1992) provided information that supported the inclusion of AS within the PDDs. However, little empirical data were available to specify the most reliable and valid diagnostic criteria. As pointed out by Ghaziuddin, Tsai, and Ghaziuddin (1992), the criteria previously used by other authors to diagnose children with AS were quite variable and identified different groups of children. The criteria in DSM-IV (APA, 1994) and ICD-10 (WHO, 1992), although virtually identical, are different again from those in the literature and specify that children with AS have to meet the same threshold criterion as autism for impairments in reciprocal social interaction and restricted, repetitive, stereotyped patterns of behaviors. However, there must not be any clinically significant general delay in language or in cognitive development. Furthermore, the child cannot meet criteria for another PDD, including autism, or schizophrenia.

Unfortunately, this may be an overly restrictive definition. In a study investigating the outcome of higher-functioning preschool children with PDD (Szatmari, Archer, Fisman, Streiner, & Wilson, 1995), only 1 of 68 subjects met these DSM-IV criteria for Asperger disorder. Of the 21 children given a "clinical" diagnosis of AS, 14 met the reciprocal social impairment threshold for autism, 18 met the communication threshold, 17 met the repetitive activity domain, and all 21 met the age of onset criterion. In sum, 12 met the overall criteria for autism. Twelve of the fourteen children who scored above the threshold on social impairment also met the communication and repetitive activity thresholds and thus qualified for a diagnosis of autism. In other words, it is virtually impossible for a child to meet the same social and repetitive behavior criteria as autism and not meet the other two criteria as well. It may be that either the social impairment threshold should be lowered or else the decision that autism takes precedence over AS might need to be reconsidered.

Can AS Be Differentiated from Other PDDs?

The first question is whether AS can be reliably differentiated from other conditions both within and outside the PDD spectrum. As part of a family-genetic study of the PPD, Mahoney *et al.* (in press) conducted an analysis of clinician agreement of PDD subtypes. Extensive clinical information including a semis-tructured interview (the Autism Diagnostic Interview), a child observation (the Autism Diagnostic Observation Schedule), previous medical records, and infor-mation on adaptive functioning and intelligence was given to three raters with an average of 20 years' experience in the assessment and diagnosis of autism. They independently reviewed all of the clinical data (with previous diagnostic information excluded) and arrived at a diagnosis of either PDD or not PDD. If a diagnosis of PDD was given, then an attempt was made to subtype the form of PDD into one of the DSM-IV categories. If a PDD child used spontaneous verbal phrases in a useful way before 3 years of age and had an IQ above 70, he or she was given a diagnosis of AS instead of autism (even if the criteria for autism were met).

The clinicians had no difficulty in distinguishing PDD children from those with other developmental disabilities (κ = .67). The rates of a diagnosis of AS for the three clinicians were 9, 10, and 12%, respectively. For 6 of 93 PDD cases, all three clinicians agreed that the child had AS, whereas for 79 cases they unanimously agreed that the child did *not* have AS. The observed level of agreement was 94% and κ (which corrects for chance agreement) was .68. These data indicate that using a modified version of the DSM-IV criteria for AS, it is possible to get excellent levels of agreement. These modified DSM-IV criteria for AS appear to have adequate measurement potential (at least when used by three experts) and can differentiate AS from other PDDs.

The Approach to Differential Diagnosis

The assessment of children with PDD must be comprehensive and should include a careful developmental history focusing specifically on delayed social and communication milestones as well as examples of possible deficits in reciprocal social interaction and communication. A careful assessment of play is also necessary paying particular attention to preoccupation with parts of objects, circumscribed interests, and unusual preoccupation or obsessions. Information from the child's teacher is very helpful as there is evidence that a child with PDD may behave differently at school than at home (Szatmari, Archer, Fisman, & Streiner, 1994).

It is also important to conduct an assessment of the child him- or herself. Particular attention must be paid to the degree of expressive language, curiosity about the environment, cognitive and self-help abilities, the presence of tics, and so forth. Assessments of motor imitation, turn taking, sharing, and asking for help are all useful indicators of possible impairments in reciprocal social interaction. Many of these characteristics are captured in structured observation schedules such as the Autism Diagnostic Observation Schedule (Lord et al., 1989) and its various formats.

In order to differentiate AS from those psychiatric disorders that are outside the PDD spectrum, a more standard psychiatric interview should be conducted with both the child and his or her parents. Symptoms of anxiety can be detected by asking how the child responds in various situations. The differentiation of AS from social phobia can be accomplished by paying particular attention to the child's performance in public situations, a previous history of selective mutism, and experiences of embarrassment. PDD children, even those with AS, rarely, if ever, experience embarrassment or humiliation unless they are older or very high functioning. The psychiatric interview should also focus on obsessions and compulsions and the possibility of accompanying distress. A history of Tourette's syndrome, experiences of hallucinations or delusions, and symptoms of schizotypal personality disorder can also be ascertained during the parent and child interview. It is, however, worth noting that the test–retest reliability of interviewing a child under 12 years of age is extremely low (Fallon & Schwab-Stone, 1994). It is likely to be even lower when interviewing children with significant language and cognitive impairments such as in PDD.

Accessory Diagnostic Tests

Accessory diagnostic tests refer to assessments that can be used in differential diagnosis. They provide information about *correlates* of the diagnostic distinction but are not themselves part of the diagnostic criteria. Examples include certain genetic markers, brain imaging, blood tests, family history, and neuropsychological testing.

Motor clumsiness has been frequently referred to in the literature as a marker that differentiates children with AS from those with autism. Asperger (1944) himself considered that the children were extremely clumsy, and indeed, this feature is part of the diagnostic criteria for AS proposed by Gillberg and Gillberg (1989). However, there are no empirical data to suggest that children with AS are clumsier than those with higher-functioning autism. In fact, two separate studies (Ghaziuddin, Butler, Tsai, & Ghaziuddin, 1994; Marjiviona & Prior 1995) found that motor clumsiness was not more frequent among children with AS versus those with autism.

There are some data, however, on neuropsychological measures that could be used to differentiate the groups. An early report by Ozonoff, Rogers, and Pennington (1991) found that children with AS were able to pass simple theory of mind tasks whereas those with higher-functioning autism could not. However, ability on theory of mind tests is very highly correlated with verbal ability (Ozonoff, Rogers, and Pennington, 1991) and insofar as those with AS have better verbal ability than those with autism, these results may be a function of how the groups were differentiated in the first place.

Perhaps the most robust cognitive difference between children with AS and autism is found in language. Szatmari *et al.* (1989, 1995) showed, using two different samples of PDD children (one group of preschoolers and an older group), that children with autism score more poorly on language tests than children with AS. In general, on measures of both expressive and receptive language, the autistic group tended to score two standard deviations below the mean whereas the AS group tended to score within the average range or within a standard deviation of the population mean (Szatmari *et al.*, 1995).

There are also data on patterns of verbal–performance abilities. Papers by Pomeroy and Friedman (1987) and Klin, Volkmar, Sparrow, Cicchetti, and Rourke (1995) reported that children with AS are more impaired on visual-spatial, visual-perceptual, and visual-motor indices than children with autism. The usual verbal–performance splits seen in autism are not apparent in those with AS. Rather, performance IQ measures tend to be lower than verbal IQ measures. Klin *et al.* (1995) suggested that this pattern of deficits is similar to that seen in nonverbal forms of learning disability and may reflect dysfunction in the right hemisphere.

There are, however, contradictory data. In an early report, Szatmari, Tuff, Finlayson, and Bartolucci (1990) found no significant differences between high-functioning children with autism and AS on a battery of nonverbal neuropsychological tests, although there was a large discrepancy between the groups in chronological age. Thus, the lack of differences may have been confounded by changes in neuropsychological functioning with age. In a study of 4- to 6-year-olds with autism and AS, both groups performed at similar levels on tests of visual-motor functioning (Szatmari *et al.*, 1995).

It is a little difficult to reconcile these conflicting findings. The Klin *et al.* (1995) study used motor clumsiness as an inclusion criterion for AS and this may have influenced the extent to which differences on visual-motor functioning emerged in the analyses. The Szatmari *et al.* (1990, 1995) studies did not include this criterion. In addition, both the Pomeroy and Friedman and Klin *et al.* studies looked at older children, so it may be that the differences observed are a function of chronological age. Longitudinal assessments of neuropsychological functioning in children with PDD would be important to resolve these contradictory findings.

Another accessory diagnostic tool that might be helpful in differentiating AS from autism is the Vineland Adaptive Behavior Scales (Sparrow, Balla, and Cicchetti, 1984). This instrument has been employed in a number of studies of autistic children and was found to be a reliable and valid index of competence in social-communication functioning (Volkmar *et al.,* 1987). Autistic children tend to score very low on the socialization and communication domains compared with the motor and activities of daily living domains and standardized measures of intelligence. Children with AS, on the other hand, tend to perform better in communication than in socialization. For example, Szatmari *et al.* (1995) reported that there is an average 12-point difference between the communication and socialization domains for children with AS. Among children with autism, there was little or no discrepancy between these domains. Thus, theory of mind tests, measures of receptive and expressive language, and the pattern of performance on IQ and the Vineland Adaptive Behavior Scales might be useful diagnostic tools in differential diagnosis.

DIFFERENTIAL DIAGNOSIS

In this section, guidelines are presented for the differentiation of AS from other types of PDD, and then from developmental and psychiatric disorders that can be confused with AS.

Differentiation of AS from Other PDDs

Autism

Given that both autism and AS are types of PDD, it follows that they would share many clinical features. These behaviors fall under the category of impairments in reciprocal social interaction, of verbal and nonverbal communication, and of repetitive stereotypic activities. There is evidence, however, that even within these commonalities, there are several features on which children with AS and autism differ.

It has long been recognized that high- and low-functioning children with autism differ on their clinical features. Because children with AS by definition have "normal" cognitive development, the key issue is to distinguish higher-functioning children with autism from those with AS. A previous review of the literature up to 1992 indicated that children with AS are more often verbal, less often have delayed echolalia and pronoun reversal, less evidence of impairments in reciprocal social interaction, but have a higher rate of bizarre and unusual obsessions (Szatmari, 1992).

Since that review was published, two further studies have appeared comparing children with AS and higher-functioning autism. In the DSM-IV field trial, 42 children were identified as having AS (Volkmar *et al.,* 1994). They differed from autistic children in terms of more often having higher verbal than performance IQ, fewer examples of repetitive stereotypic behaviors such as rituals or resistance to change, and less social impairment.

Szatmari *et al.* (1995) also compared 21 children with AS and 47 with higher-functioning autism. The children were between 4 and 6 years of age and all were functioning in the nondevelopmentally handicapped range of IQ. Of 30 items from the Autism Diagnostic Interview (excluding those language items that were used to differentiate the groups in the first place), there were differences on 9 individual items. Of these, a regression analysis indicated that three variables independently predicted group membership: abnormal social development at 36 months, lack of social reciprocity, and lack of social intentionality. These three variables correctly classified 93.6% of the autistic group and 57.1% of the AS group and provided a good fit to the model.

Only one study has compared the outcome of children with AS and higher-functioning autism (Szatmari *et al.,* 1997). This is an important design because if the clinical differentiation is largely related to measurement error or is of uncertain clinical significance, one would expect that over time, the clinical differences would attenuate and the groups would become more similar. In fact, the outcome results were consistent in demonstrating that the differences in autistic symptoms, language, and adaptive behavior seen previously between the children with AS and autism were also apparent 2 years later.

A closer inspection of individual findings, however, indicated that there was greater variation in the outcome measures for the children with autism than for those with AS. This variation in outcome appeared to be associated with variation in expressive language as measured by a test of oral vocabulary. Virtually all of the children with AS improved in their expressive language over 2 years whereas only half of those with autism did. If the autism group was stratified according to whether or not there was improvement on the measure of oral vocabulary, important differences in outcome were observed. The autistic children who improved in their expressive abilities appeared to resemble more and more the children with AS in terms of the number of autistic symptoms and level of functioning in socialization and communication. The autistic children who failed to improve in their expressive language appeared to fall behind the rest of the cohort on these measures.

In other words, although there appear to be robust and stable differences between AS and autistic children, the key difference may be in the *attainment* of certain developmental milestones. By definition, the children with AS have some expressive language by 3 years of age. This places them on a certain developmental trajectory associated with milder impairments in reciprocal social interaction and repetitive stereotypic activities. Some children with autism reach this developmental milestone of expressive language but at a later age. Presumably they then begin a new developmental pathway and also appear to have fewer impairments in reciprocal social interaction and repetitive activities than they did previously. They may now be on the same developmental pathway as the children with AS. Children with autism who do not develop a certain level of expressive language abilities remain on the original developmental pathway and fall further and further behind the cohort of PDD children with expressive language. This model needs to be corroborated by further follow-up assessments and a clearer understanding of what basal level of expressive language abilities is needed in order to jump to another developmental trajectory. Nevertheless, the model does provide a hypothesis about the differences between AS and autism in terms of development over time rather than in terms of static cross-sectional comparisons.

Atypical Autism

Atypical autism refers to another condition within the spectrum of PDD. The children may be "atypical" in several ways; they may have fewer symptoms overall, they may be "subthreshold" for one of the three domains of socialization, communication, or repetitive behaviors, or else their age of onset may be after 36 months of age (but they do not qualify for a diagnosis of disintegrative disorder or Rett's disorder). Atypical autism has usually been applied to a heterogeneous group of both high- and low-functioning individuals with PDD (Szatmari, 1992). It is not at all clear that high-functioning atypical children are different from those with AS. DSM-IV states that the term *atypical autism* is most often applied to individuals who are very *low* functioning. Such individuals may manifest fewer symptoms of autism because of limited capacity to communicate or to notice changes and so be resistant to them.

In fact, it is extremely difficult to reliably differentiate children with atypical autism from those with other PDDs. In the study referred to previously (Mahoney et al., in press), the three clinicians also made diagnoses of atypical autism. It was clear that the differentiation of atypical autism from the other types of PPDs was no better than chance. Of 93 PDD cases, for example, the three clinicians only agreed unanimously that 1 child had atypical autism. The pattern of disagreement for the others seemed quite random. It appears that if a child has enough PDD symptoms to be around the diagnostic threshold but is not obviously autistic, it is extremely difficult to decide whether or not the criteria for a domain have been met.

Given these considerations, it is perhaps best to be very conservative in using the term *atypical autism*, and to apply it largely to lower-functioning individuals. This would of course make the differential diagnosis of atypical autism from AS very simple as the latter condition cannot be diagnosed in the presence of significant cognitive delay.

Differentiation of AS from Disorders outside the PDD Spectrum

Schizoid and Schizotypal Disorders of Childhood

DSM-IV describes schizoid personality disorder as a constellation of enduring traits characterized by little desire for close relationships, a preference for solitary activities, little interest in heterosexual experiences, few close friends, indifference to praise or criticism, emotional coldness, and detached or flattened affect. Schizotypal personality disorder differs from schizoid disorder by including other symptoms such as odd beliefs, magical thinking, ideas of reference, perceptual illusions, depersonalization and realization, as well as odd thinking and unusual speech patterns. Phenomenologically, the latter symptoms resemble subthreshold psychotic symptoms such as thought disorder, hallucinations, delusions, and paranoid beliefs. Indeed, several studies have indicated that schizoid–schizotypal disorders in adults are genetically related to schizophrenia although there is no evidence that this is also true for *children* with schizoid–schizotypal disorders.

It is apparent that many schizoid and schizotypal characteristics are also found in children with AS. An important issue then is the extent to which these disorders (at least in childhood) are distinct from AS. Nagy and Szatmari (1986) reported on 28 children with "schizotypal personality disorders that met the DSM-III criteria for this condition." It was clear that virtually all of the children had many features of PDD and would have met the current DSM-IV criteria for either autism or AS. Indeed, Sula Wolff (who has done the most work on these disorders in childhood) regards AS and schizoid–schizotypal disorders as interchangeable terms that identify roughly the same group of children (Wolff, 1995).

There is a very strong implication in DSM-IV and elsewhere in the literature that schizoid–schizotypal disorders have a genetic relationship with schizophrenia. If the term is applied to childhood disorders, it would seem important to maintain this conceptual link. There are some children who meet criteria for schizoid–schizotypal disorders who also have developmental histories that are relatively free of delayed milestones and impairments in reciprocal social interaction and communication (but not repetitive activities). Therefore, although the official ICD-10 and DSM-IV criteria do not include this criterion, it may be most appropriate to apply these labels to children who develop schizoid–schizotypal symptoms after the preschool years, i.e., after 5 or 6 years of age. Alternatively, one could use AS or another PDD as an exclusionary diagnosis. This would clearly separate out the PDDs from schizoid–schizotypal disorders. Further follow-up studies of this latter group of children would be needed to see whether they are, in fact, at greater risk for schizophrenia.

Schizophrenia with Childhood Onset

Schizophrenia with childhood onset refers to the clinical presentation of psychotic features in children under 15 years of age or before puberty. DSM-IV does not have separate diagnostic criteria for schizophrenia of childhood onset. Several clinical studies, however, have indicated that the phenomenology is affected by developmental factors (Russell,1989; McKenna, Bott, & Sammons, 1994) although the etiology and response to treatment of childhood-onset schizophrenia are similar to those of the adult-onset variety. The course appears to be more variable in childhood onset and a substantial proportion of those given a diagnosis of childhood schizophrenia often have a more clearly bipolar affective presentation later on (Werry, McClellan, & Chand, 1991).

To meet the DSM-IV criteria for schizophrenia, a child must experience at least two of the following: delusions, mood-incongruent hallucinations, disorganized speech, disorganized or catatonic behavior, and negative symptoms such as flat affect, poverty of speech, and an inability to initiate and sustain goal-directed activities. With childhood onset, there may be a failure to achieve expected levels of social and educational functioning. Finally, the symptoms must have been present for at least 6 months. It is apparent that children with AS share many clinical features with schizophrenia. The conversation of children with AS may sound "disorganized," difficulties in behavior may be judged "catatonic," and the impairments in non-verbal communication could include flat affect and avolition. Furthermore, it can often be difficult to distinguish "true" hallucinations from pseudohallucinations, particularly if the child with AS has cognitive problems or difficulties expressing him- or herself. Furthermore, under periods of intense stress, a child with AS may experience intense anxiety and express ideas of reference that could be misinterpreted as "delusional." Another complicating feature is that children with schizophrenia have developmental histories often characterized by social withdrawal, poor peer relations, and a restricted range of interests. IQ is often below normal and there can be a history of language delay and motor abnormalities. In fact, Watkins, Asarnow, and Tanguay (1987) reported that 39% of children with schizophrenia had symptoms of autism.

There are three key features that can be used in differential diagnosis. First, the presence of true hallucinations and delusions (as opposed to pseudohallucinations and ideas of reference) strongly suggests a diagnosis of schizophrenia. These symptoms should not be confused with talking to oneself or reenacting scenes from favorite videos, behaviors often seen in PDD children. Thought disorder should also be evaluated extremely carefully in view of a developmental history of communication abnormalities (see Caplan, Guthrie, Fish, Tanguay, & David-Lando, 1989). The second key feature is duration. Children with PDD can act in a bizarre manner under conditions of extreme stress. However, the psychotic symptoms of schizophrenia need to last for a full month (unless partially treated with medication). The "psychotic" symptoms of children with AS are usually much more transient and last hours, or, at most, days. Removal of the stress should result in complete resolution of these bizarre behaviors and should clarify the diagnosis quickly. The third differentiating feature is age of onset and course. Although it is true that many individuals with schizophrenia have delayed milestones and a restricted range of interests in early childhood, the presence of true psychotic phenomena usually only occurs after 9 years of age (Russell *et al.*, 1989). In contrast, the developmental histories of children with PDD demonstrate significant developmental abnormalities prior to 5 years of age, and if the child is higher functioning, there is also significant improvement over time. In childhood schizophrenia, on the other hand, there appears to be a deterioration of functioning and an exacerbation of symptoms over time.

Semantic–Pragmatic Language Disorder

Semantic–pragmatic disorder is a subtype of developmental language disorders. It is characterized by near-normal vocabulary, grammar, and phonology, but language *use* is abnormal in content and function and comprehension is also impaired. There are considerable difficulties in initiating and sustaining a conversation, maintaining cohesive links in conversation from topic to topic, and words are used out of context. The speech of children with semantic–pragmatic disorders often resembles the tangential speech of jargon aphasia.

Bishop and Rosenblum (1987) reported that children diagnosed with semantic–pragmatic disorder also tend to have the types of social-communication impairments seen in PDD. However, Bishop (1989) concluded that children with this language disorder would not meet criteria for autism. It may be that semantic–pragmatic disorder should be considered a type of PPD rather than a pure language disorder.

Children with semantic–pragmatic disorders usually have delayed milestones in language, that is, they develop single words well after 12 months and phrases after 36 months. Thus, the differentiation of children with semantic–pragmatic disorder from those with AS is clear-cut, although it depends on the parents' ability to accurately report these developmental milestones. There are, of course, children who develop phrase speech either just before or after 36 months and their classification as AS or semantic–pragmatic disorder is unclear. Unfortunately, there is a paucity of empirical data on children with semantic–pragmatic disorder and research with this group of children is urgently needed. If the nosologic status of AS is unclear, the same must be said for semantic–pragmatic disorder. The differentiation of this condition from atypical autism in the presence of normal IQ would seem to be particularly problematic.

Obsessive-Compulsive Disorder

Children with AS often display ritualistic behavior and resistance to change. These repetitive behaviors refer to a fixed sequence of behaviors that are nonfunctional and have been developed by the child without prompting from an adult or caregiver. Thus, it is not appropriate to refer to a bedtime routine as a "ritual" because it serves a functional purpose. Compulsions are repetitive behaviors in which the individual feels driven to perform the behavior so as to reduce the anxiety associated with an obsessive thought or to prevent some unpleasant situation. Thus, individuals who have persistent thoughts of bacterial infection will often wash their hands and engage in other repetitive cleaning behaviors in an effort to reduce the distress associated with the obsession. By definition, individuals with OCD (at least adults) recognize that the behavior is excessive, unreasonable, and unnecessary. However, they are driven by anxiety to perform the repetitive behaviors. Such insight into the unrealistic nature of obsessions or compulsions is often lacking in children with OCD.

These behaviors can be very difficult to distinguish from the types of obsessive interests and ritualistic behavior that are commonly seen in children with AS. It is important to distinguish the obsessive *interests* seen in children with AS from the obsessive *thoughts* in OCD. AS children have a very circum-scribed range of interests and usually show intense interest in one or two hobbies or activities. Although these are referred to as "obsessive," they are not experienced by the child as ego dystonic, excessive, or unreasonable. In fact, engaging in these activities tends to reduce anxiety and give the children pleasure rather than dysphoria. Some AS children will also engage in ritualistic behavior. If they are interrupted, this will cause extreme behavioral disturbances and excess anxiety. Such ritualistic behavior can be very difficult if not impossible to distinguish from that seen in OCD. McDougle *et al.* (1995) conducted an interesting case–control study trying to differentiate the obsessions and compulsions in OCD from those seen in autism. They reported that in autism, the obsessions and compulsions have a much less elaborated content and tend to be more concrete and stereotypic. Most PDD individuals lack insight into the unreasonable nature of their behavior.

The developmental history can also be extremely important. Usually children with OCD do not have a very early onset of their preoccupations or obsessions, and have a relatively preserved developmental history. Children with OCD who also have Tourette's syndrome or some other organic condition such as cerebral palsy or epilepsy are the exception to this rule. The key issue in differential diagnosis is to pay very close attention to the presence or absence of impairments in reciprocal social interaction. Evidence of poor social-emotional reciprocity, empathy, sharing and turn taking, lack of social skills, and the like would all support a diagnosis of AS because they are not part of the diagnostic picture of OCD.

Social Phobia

Social phobia is defined as a "persistent fear of one or more situations (the social phobic situation) in which the person is exposed to possible scrutiny by others and fears that he or she may do something or act in a way that would be humiliating or embarrassing" (APA, 1994). Social phobia is a common psychiatric disorder in adults, but unfortunately, there is little relevant information in children. Biedel (1991) reported that children with social phobia exhibited clinical features that were very similar to the symptoms of adults, indicating that the disorder can be seen in young children.

At first, it may seem unnecessary to consider social phobia in the differential diagnosis of AS. Nevertheless, it is true that many high-functioning children with PDD show symptoms of anxiety in social situations as manifested by poor eye gaze and lack of social initiative. Furthermore, if the child with social phobia has a history of developmental delays such as a learning disability or clumsiness, the presence of the comorbidity may suggest a diagnosis of AS. This confusion may be even more apparent in girls with AS, as there is some evidence that higher-functioning PDD girls show less in the way of social impairments than higher functioning PDD boys (McLennan, Lord, & Schopler, 1993).

The key to differential diagnosis is the early onset of significant impairments in reciprocal social interaction and communication prior to 5 years of age in PDD. In children with social phobia, the anxiety about social situations usually does *not* occur until after the preschool years. Furthermore, children with AS develop unusual obsessions, a restricted range of interests, and preoccupations. This is *not* apparent in children with social phobia. It is also important to inquire about various situations in which the social anxiety may arise. Social phobia is most acutely experienced outside the home, whereas inside the home, with parents and familiar adults, relationships are usually warm and satisfying. Although children with AS may be more comfortable at home than outside the home, there are still very subtle impairments in social-emotional reciprocity, social intentionality, sharing and turn taking that are present even with parents and caregivers. Thus, a careful delineation of the symptoms, their context and developmental course is very useful in differentiating social phobia from AS.

CONCLUSION

In some ways, a chapter on the differential diagnosis of AS may be premature given that the current diagnostic criteria for AS may not be the "right" ones. For example, there are no studies that have compared various diagnostic criteria for AS in terms of their agreement, their measurement properties (i.e., sensitivity, specificity, and reliability), or the extent to which they identify homogeneous subgroups with specific etiologies, outcome, or response to treatment. Further, with the exception of autism, there are no case–control studies that have compared the clinical features of AS with other disorders that might be confused with it. Presumably, the "best" criteria for AS would be those that could be reliably assessed, provide adequate coverage to diagnose sufficient numbers of children, and provide the greatest differentiation from other disorders in terms of clinical features, etiology, outcome, and/or response to treatment.

This chapter has reviewed data suggesting that the current DSM-IV criteria for AS may be overly restrictive. On the other hand, using a modified version of these criteria, clinicians can generally agree on whether or not a child with PDD has AS. It is also clear that differentiating AS from conditions outside the PDD spectrum is useful as this provides important information about treatment approaches that are consistent with those used for PDD children in general. It is less clear that the differentiation of AS from autism is as clinically useful. There are some data suggesting that PDD children with normal cognitive and language development (i.e., children with AS) have a different outcome than autistic children without these characteristics. There are also data suggesting that better outcome is associated with less impairment in reciprocal social interaction. Insofar as these data are valid, it would suggest that the clinical characteristics differentiating autism from AS are providing a useful distinction. However, it may be misleading to think of AS as a disorder dinstinct from autism if by that we mean the two conditions have a different etiology. This may be true but the necessary family-genetic studies have not yet been carried out to substantiate this hypothesis. The current evidence suggests that the diagnosis of AS may serve rather as a prognostic indicator within the spectrum of conditions known as PDD. In other words, the clinical label may serve to mark off a group of PDD children who mature along a particular developmental pathway different from that for most children with autism. If children with autism develop fluent and useful language, they too may join this pathway but will do so at a later age maintaining the differences seen earlier on a cross-sectional basis. Whether a prognostic indicator, such as AS, deserves status as a "disorder" is more a matter of policy and clinical judgment than it is a matter of scientific evidence. The real problem lies in what our conception of a "disorder" is in child psychiatry, not in what signs and symptoms a child presents with. The clinician should not lose sight of both the advantages and disadvantages of making a specific diagnosis in a child who presents with impairments in socialization and communication. A diagnosis of AS may provide a powerful interpretation of a child's unusual behavior, but a label should not be considered an explanation and given more status than it deserves.

REFERENCES

American Psychiatric Association. (1994). *Diagnostic and statistical manual of mental disorders* (4th ed.). Washington, DC. Author.

Asperger, H. (1944). Die "autistischen Psychopathen" in Kindesalter. *Archiv für Psychiatrie und Nervenkrankheiten, 117*, 76–136.

Biedel, D. C. (1991). Social phobia and overanxious disorder in school-age children. *Journal of the American Academy of Child and Adolescent Psychiatry, 30*, 545–552.

Bishop, D. V. M. (1989). Autism, Asperger's syndrome and semantic–pragmatic disorder: Where are the boundaries? *British Journal of Disorders of Communication, 24*, 107–121.

Bishop, D. V. M., & Rosenbloom, L. (1987). Classification of childhood language disorders. In W, Yule and M. Rutter (Eds.), *Language development and disorders* (pp. 16–41). London: Mac Keith Press.

Caplan, R., Guthrie, D., Fish, B., Tanguay, P. E., & David-Lando, G. (1989). The Kiddie Formal Thought Disorder Rating Scale (K-FTDS): Clinical assessment, reliability and validity. *Journal of the American Academy of Child and Adolescent Psychiatry, 28*, 408.

Ehlers, S., & Gillberg, C. (1993). The epidemiology of Asperger syndrome: A total population study. *Journal of Child Psychology and Psychiatry, 34*, 1327–1350.

Fallon, T., & Schwab-Stone, M. (1994). Determinants of reliability in psychiatric surveys of children aged 6–12. *Journal of Child Psychology and Psychiatry, 35*, 1391–1408.

Ghaziuddin, M., Butler, E., Tsai, L., & Ghaziuddin, N. (1994). Is clumsiness a marker for Asperger syndrome? *Journal of Intellectual Disabilities Research, 38*, 519–527.

Ghaziuddin, M., Tsai, L. Y., & Ghaziuddin, N. (1992). Brief report: A comparison of the diagnostic criteria for Asperger syndrome. *Journal of Autism and Developmental Disorders, 22*, 643–649.

Gillberg, C. (1989). Asperger's syndrome in 23 Swedish children. *Developmental Medicine and Child Neurology 31*, 520–531.

Gillberg, I. C., & Gillberg, C. (1989). Asperger syndrome—some epidemiological considerations: A research note. *Journal of Child Psychology and Psychiatry, 30*, 631–638.

Klin, A., Volkmar, J. F. R., Sparrow, S. S., Cicchetti, D. V., & Rourke, B. P. (1995). Validity and neuropsychological characterization of Asperger syndrome: Convergence with nonverbal learning disabilities syndrome. *Journal of Child Psychology and Psychiatry, 36*, 1127–1140.

Le Couteur, A., Rutter, M., Lord, C., Rios, P., Robertson, S., Holdgrater, M., & McLennan, J. D. (1989). Autism Diagnostic Interview. *Journal of Autism and Developmental Disorders, 19*, 363–388.

Lord, C., Rutter, M., Gode, S., Heemsbergen, J., Jordan, H., Mawhood, L., & Schopler, E. (1989). Autism diagnostic observation schedule. A standardized observation of communicative and social behavior. *Journal of Autism and Developmental Disorders, 19*, 185–212.

Mahoney, W., Szatmari, P., Bryson, S., Bartolucci, G., Walter, S. D., MacLean, J., Hoult, L., & Jones, M. B. (in press). Reliability and accuracy of differentiating pervasive developmental disorder subtypes. *Journal of the American Academy of Child and Adolescent Psychiatry.*

Marjiviona, J., & Prior, M. (1995). Comparison of Asperger syndrome and high-functioning autistic children on a test of motor impairment. *Journal of Autism and Developmental Disorders, 25*, 23–39.

McDougle, C. J., Kresch, L. E., Goodman, W. K., Naylor, S. T., Volkmar, F. R., Cohen, D. J., & Price, L. H. (1995). A case-controlled study of repetitive thoughts and behavior in adults with autistic disorder and obsessive–compulsive disorder. *American Journal of Psychiatry, 152*, 772–776.

McKenna, K., Gordon, C. T., Lenane, M., Kaysen, D., Fahey, K., & Rapoport J. L. (1994). Looking for childhood-onset schizophrenia: The first 71 cases screened. *Journal of the American Academy of Child and Adolescent Psychiatry, 33*, 636–644.

McLennan, J. D., Lord, C., & Schopler, E. (1993). Sex differences in higher-functioning people with autism. *Journal of Autism and Developmental Disorders, 23*, 217–227.

Nagy, J., & Szatmari, P. (1986). A chart review of schizotypal personality disorders in children. *Journal of Autism and Developmental Disorders, 16*, 351–367.

Ozonoff, S., Pennington, B. F., & Rogers, S. J. (1991). Executive function deficits in high-functioning autistic individuals: Relationship to theory of mind. *Journal of Child Psychology and Psychiatry, 32*, 1081–1105.

Ozonoff, S., Rogers, S. J., & Pennington, B. F. (1991). Asperger's syndrome: Evidence of an empirical distinction from high-functioning autism. *Journal of Child Psychology and Psychiatry, 21,* 1107–1122.

Pomeroy, J., & Friedman, C. A. (1987). A*sperger's syndrome: A clinical subtype of pervasive developmental disorder.* Paper presented at the 30th annual meeting of the American Academy of Child and Adolescent Psychiatry, Los Angeles.

Russell, A., Bott, L., & Sammons, C. (1989). The phenomenology of schizophrenia occurring in childhood. *Journal of the American Academy of Child and Adolescent Psychiatry, 29,* 399–407.

Sparrow, S. S., Balla, D., & Cicchetti, D. (1984). *Vineland Adaptive Behavior Scales* (Survey Form). Circle Pines, MN: American Guidance Service.

Szatmari, P. (1992). The validity of autistic spectrum disorders: A literature review. *Journal of Autism and Developmental Disorders, 22,* 583–600.

Szatmari, P., Archer, L., Fisman, S., & Streiner, D. L. (1994). Parent and teacher agreement in the assessment of pervasive developmental disorders. *Journal of Autism and Developmental Disorders, 24,* 703–717.

Szatmari, P., Archer, L., Fisman, S., Streiner, D. L., & Wilson, F. (1995). Asperger's syndrome and autism: Differences in behavior, cognition and adaptive functioning. *Journal of the American Academy of Child and Adolescent Psychiatry 34,* 1662–1671.

Szatmari, P., Bartolucci, G., & Bremner, R. (1989). Asperger's syndrome and autism: Comparisons on early history and outcome. *Developmental Medicine and Child Neurology, 31,* 709–720.

Szatmari, P., Streiner, D. L., Bryson, S. B., Ryerse, C., Wilson, F., & Archer, L. (1997). The two-year outcome of preschool children with autism and Asperger syndrome. Paper presented at the annual meeting of The American Academy of Child and Adolescent Psychiatry, Toronto, Ontario, October 1997.

Szatmari, P., Tuff, L., Finlayson, A. J., & Bartolucci, G. (1990). Asperger's syndrome and autism: Neurocognitive aspects. *Journal of the American Academy of Child and Adolescent Psychiatry, 29,* 1:130–136.

Volkmar, F. R., Klin, A., Siegel, B., Szatmari, P., Lord, C., Campbell, M., Freeman, B. J., Cicchetti, D. V., Rutter, M., Kline, W., Buitelaar, J., Hattab, Y., Fombonne, E., Fuentes, J., Werry, J., Stone, W., Kerbeshian, J., Hoshino, Y., Bregman, J., Loveland, K., Szymanski, L., & Towbin, K. (1994). Field trial for Autistic Disorder in DSM-IV. *American Journal of Psychiatry, 151,* 1361–1367.

Volkmar, F. R., Sparrow, S. S., Goudreau, D., Cicchetti, D., Paul, R., & Cohen, D. J. (1987). Social deficits in autism: An operational approach using the Vineland Adaptive Behavior Scales. *Journal of the American Academy of Child Psychiatry, 26,* 156–161.

Watkins, J., Asarnow, R. F., & Tanguay, P. (1988). Symptom development in childhood onset schizophrenia. *Journal of Child Psychology and Psychiatry, 29,* 865–878.

Werry, J. S., McClellan, J. M., & Chand, L. (1991). Childhood and adolescent schizophrenic, bipolar and schizoaffective disorders: A clinical and outcome study. *Journal of the American Academy of Child and Adolescent Psychiatry, 30,* 457–465.

Wolff, S. (1995). How can we best understand the condition? *Loners; The life path of unusual children.* London: Routledge.

World Health Organization. (1992). *The ICD-10 classification of mental and behavioural disorders. Clinical descriptions and diagnostic guidelines.* Geneva: Author.

Diagnostic and Assessment Issues

High-Functioning People with Autism and Asperger Syndrome

A Literature Review

CHRISTOPHER GILLBERG and STEPHAN EHLERS

INTRODUCTION

The number of papers on Asperger syndrome (AS) and high-functioning autism (HFA) is growing at a fast pace. At least 140 articles have appeared in the English language over the last 14 years. More than two-thirds of these were published in the last 5 years. This chapter aims to review (1) the history of AS and HFA, (2) current diagnostic concepts and criteria, (3) some of the controversial issues pertaining to diagnosis, and then to (4) selectively review the studies in the field with a view to identifying possible unifying/differentiating features of these two disorders. Finally, there is also a brief section on intervention guidelines based mostly on the authors' many years of clinical experience with individuals with HFA/AS.

In the literature published before the 1980s, apart from the writings by Asperger himself (e.g., Asperger, 1944, 1952), we have only been able to find four (non-book chapter) papers specifically referring to "autistic psychopathy" as originally coined by Asperger (van Krevelen & Kuipers, 1962; van Krevelen, 1971; Wurst, 1974; Dauner & Martin, 1978). However, Robinson and Vitale (1954) working in the United States (Pennsylvania) described three children with circum-

CHRISTOPHER GILLBERG and STEPHAN EHLERS • Department of Child and Adolescent Psychiatry, Annedals Clinics, S-413 45 Göteborg, Sweden.

Asperger Syndrome or High-Functioning Autism?, edited by Schopler *et al.* Plenum Press, New York, 1998.

scribed interest patterns, and at least one, possibly all three, of these met current diagnostic criteria for AS. This paper was discussed by Kanner (1954), who referred to work—published in the German language—by Schneerson in Tel Aviv on 64 children (48 boys and 16 girls) ranging in age between 8 and 13 years showing similar traits. Kanner did not mention Asperger's work, but Asperger was struck by the similarity of his own and Kanner's cases (Asperger, 1950), even though he later stated that he was referring to a "completely different condition." Interestingly, Kretschmer's concept of "schizothymia," particularly the variant referred to as "detached idealism," shares many features with AS (Kretschmer, 1924).

After completion of work on this chapter, a translation of a paper on schizoid personality disorder in children by Ssucharewa (1926) was published by Wolff (1996). It seems that this disorder might be equivalent to AS (Wolff, 1996).

No papers published before 1980 referred expressly to HFA (although indirectly, a considerable number of cases with HFA have been implicated in the large body of general autism research). According to our review (aided by S. M. Levy), DeMyer, Hingtgen, and Jackson (1981) were first to use the HFA label. In England, Elisabeth Newson has long been referring to "more able" autistic people (e.g., Newson & Newson, 1979).

Beginning with Wing's seminal paper (Wing, 1981a)—in which she coined the term Asperger's syndrome—interest has grown, and there are now (December 1995) at least 90 papers published in the English language explicitly dealing with AS. One book has been entirely devoted to the subject (Frith, 1991). In addition, we have found 55 papers referring to HFA or a similar diagnostic label published from 1980 to the present. The bulk of the papers referring to AS originated in the United Kingdom, Canada, and Scandinavia, but recently the concept has become endorsed in Australia and the United States as well. HFA and Pervasive Developmental Disorder Not Otherwise Specified (PDD-NOS) (APA, 1987, 1994) appear to have been more generally adopted in the United States. It is only in the last few years that AS has become part of the generally accepted diagnostic international nomenclature (WHO, 1992, 1993; APA, 1994), and it is expected that as operationalized diagnostic criteria (Gillberg & Gillberg, 1989; Szatmari, 1989; Gillberg, 1991; WHO, 1993; APA, 1994) become available, the literature will expand at an even higher rate.

However, the fact that PDD-NOS, Rett's syndrome, and AS (or "Asperger disorder") are all classified as "299.80" in the DSM-IV may contribute to further diagnostic confusion.

It is of some interest that most papers on AS have referred to children and adolescents [with the exception of Tantam's papers on adults, e.g., Tantam (1988), and Wolff's on schizoid children grown up, e.g., Wolff, Townsend, McGuire, & Weeks (1991)], whereas most papers on HFA have included samples of adults (mostly men). This could be a function of AS being a "newer" diagnostic concept (and, hence, being applied more often in "new," younger cases) and HFA being used mostly in the follow-up studies (often in young adulthood) of individuals diagnosed, many years ago, according to criteria set out for autism.

DIAGNOSTIC DEFINITIONS AND ISSUES

At the present time, it is not at all clear that AS and HFA represent distinct conditions (Klin, 1993). Yet, most of the published work employs diagnostic criteria that would tend to make dual diagnosis impossible (WHO, 1993; APA, 1994). Gillberg's position is different and accepting the possibility that in some individuals it might be appropriate to diagnose autism at one point in time and AS at another in the same individual.

Even though we hold that the evidence is not there to suggest that HFA and AS are either completely overlapping, partly overlapping, or distinct conditions, in this chapter we will do our best to keep them separate so as to better identify possible commonalities and differentiating features.

The various sets of published diagnostic criteria for AS are outlined in Table 5-1.

There are currently no explicit diagnostic guidelines for HFA, although, in our view, it would seem appropriate to diagnose this condition in cases for which autistic disorder (APA, 1987, 1994)/childhood autism (WHO, 1993) criteria apply and the total IQ is above 65–70. In the literature this has been the most commonly used "definition." Alternatively, a case could be made for a diagnosis of HFA in those individuals who are perceived to have "mild" autism [e.g., according to Childhood Autism Rating Scale (CARS) interview (Schopler, Reichler, & Renner, 1988)]. Whether or not such cases are identical to or essentially different from those diagnosed with AS is open to speculation. However, the few comparative studies that have been performed (Szatmari, Bartolucci, & Brenner, 1989; Gillberg, 1989; Ramberg, Ehlers, Nydén, Gillberg, & Johansson, 1996; Ehlers et al., 1997) suggest that it is IQ per se that distinguishes AS (with higher verbal and full-scale IQ) from HFA (with lower full-scale IQ). However, it could also be a matter of verbal (particularly vocabulary) abilities per se being better in AS than in HFA. It is possible that a family history of AS or AS-like symptoms is more typical of AS, and that a family history is less obvious in HFA (Gillberg, 1989). It is also likely that, at least with overall IQ uncontrolled, motor clumsiness may be a typical feature of AS, but not of HFA (Gillberg, 1989). Nevertheless, it is not generally agreed that motor clumsiness is specific to AS and not HFA (Ghaziuddin, Tsai, & Ghaziuddin, 1992). In a recent study by Ghaziuddin and co-workers, there were no overall differences on the Bruininks–Oseretsky test for motor functioning between a small group of children with HFA and another small group of children with AS (Ghaziuddin, Butler, Tsai, & Ghaziuddin, 1994). However, in that study the children with AS were older and had higher IQ and the difference between IQ and motor skills was considerably greater in the AS group. Motor functions were strongly correlated with IQ in the HFA group, but the correlation was very low in the AS group. It is conceivable that AS individuals may be so much more "high functioning" than those with HFA that abnormal *social* motor control and apraxia may be more

Table 5-1. Asperger Syndrome Diagnostic Criteria

Gillberg and Gillberg's (1989) diagnostic criteria (elaborated by Gillberg, 1991)
1. Social impairment (extreme egocentricity) (at least two of the following):
   (a) Inability to interact with peers
   (b) Lack of desire to interact with peers
   (c) Lack of appreciation of social cues
   (d) Socially and emotionally inappropriate behavior

2. Narrow interest (at least one of the following):
   (a) Exclusion of other activities
   (b) Repetitive adherence
   (c) More rote than meaning

3. Repetitive routines (at least one of the following):
   (a) On self, in aspects of life
   (b) On others

4. Speech and language peculiarities (at least three of the following):
   (a) Delayed development
   (b) Superficially perfect expressive language
   (c) Formal pedantic language
   (d) Odd prosody, peculiar voice characteristics
   (e) Impairment of comprehension including misinterpretations of literal/implied meanings

5. Nonverbal communication problems (at least one of the following):
   (a) Limited use of gestures
   (b) Clumsy/gauche body language
   (c) Limited facial expression
   (d) Inappropriate expression
   (e) Peculiar, stiff gaze

6. Motor clumsiness:
   Poor performance on neurodevelopmental examination

Diagnostic criteria of Szatmari et al. (1989)

1. Solitary (two of):
   No close friends
   Avoids others
   No interest in making friends
   A loner

2. Impaired social interaction (one of):
   Approaches others only to have own needs met
   A clumsy social approach
   One-sided responses to peers
   Difficulty sensing feelings of others
   Detached from feelings of others

3. Impaired nonverbal communication (one of):
   Limited facial expression
   Unable to read emotion from facial expressions of child
   Unable to give message with eyes
   Does not look at others
   Does not use hands to express oneself

Table 5-1. *(Continued)*

Gestures are large and clumsy
Comes too close to others

4. Odd speech (two of):
Abnormalities in inflection
Talks too much
Talks too little
Lack of cohesion to conversation
Idiosyncratic use of words
Repetitive patterns of speech

5. Does not meet DSM-III-R criteria for:
Autistic disorder

ICD-10 (1993) research criteria

A. There is no clinically significant general delay in spoken or receptive language or cognitive development. Diagnosis requires that single words should have developed by 2 years of age or earlier and that communicative phrases be used by 3 years of age or earlier. Self-help skills, adaptive behavior, and curiosity about the environment during the first 3 years should be at a level consistent with normal intellectual development. However, motor milestones may be somewhat delayed and motor clumsiness is usual (although not a necessary diagnostic feature). Isolated special skills, often related to abnormal preoccupations, are common, but are not required for diagnosis.

B. There are qualitative abnormalities in reciprocal social interaction in at least two of the following areas (criteria as for autism):
   (a) Failure adequately to use eye-to-eye gaze, facial expression, body posture, and gesture to regulate social interaction
   (b) Failure to develop (in a manner appropriate to mental age, and despite ample opportunities) peer relationships that involve a mutual sharing of interest, activities, and emotions
   (c) Lack of social-emotional reciprocity as shown by an impaired or deviant response to other people's emotions, or lack of modulation of behavior according to social context; or a weak integration of social, emotional, and communicative behaviors
   (d) Lack of spontaneous seeking to share enjoyment, interests, or achievements with other people (e.g., a lack of showing, bringing, or pointing out to other people objects of interests to the individual)

C. The individual exhibits an unusually intense, circumscribed interest or restricted, repetitive, and stereotyped patterns of behavior, interests, and activities in at least one of the following areas (criteria as for autism; however, it would be less usual for these to include either motor mannerisms or preoccupations with part-objects or nonfunctional elements of play materials):
   (a) An encompassing preoccupation with one or more stereotyped and restricted patterns of interest that are abnormal in their intensity and circumscribed nature though not in their content of focus
   (b) Apparently compulsive adherence to specific, nonfunctional routines or rituals
   (c) Stereotyped and repetitive motor mannerisms that involve either hand or finger flapping or twisting or complex whole-body movements
   (d) Preoccupations with part-objects or nonfunctional elements of play materials (such as their odor, the feel of their surface, or the noise or vibration that they generate)

(continued)

Table 5-1. *(Continued)*

D. The disorder is not attributable to the other varieties of pervasive developmental disorder; simple schizophrenia (F20.6); schizotypal disorder (F 21); obsessive-compulsive disorder (F42); anankastic personality disorder (F60.5); reactive and disinhibited attachment disorders of childhood (94.1 and F94.2, respectively).

DSM-IV (1994) criteria

A. Qualitative impairment in social interaction, as manifested by at least two of the following:
1. Marked impairment in the use of multiple nonverbal behaviors such as eye-to-eye gaze, facial expression, body postures, and gesture to regulate social interaction
2. Failure to develop peer relationships appropriate to developmental level
3. A lack of spontaneous seeking to share enjoyment, interests, or achievements with other people (e.g., by a lack of showing, bringing, or pointing out objects of interest to other people)
4. Lack of social or emotional reciprocity

B. Restricted repetitive and stereotyped patterns of behavior, interests, and activities, as manifested by at least one of the following:
1. Encompassing preoccupation with one or more stereotyped and restricted patterns of interest that is abnormal either in intensity or in focus
2. Apparently inflexible adherence to specific, nonfunctional routines or rituals
3. Stereotyped and repetitive motor mannerisms (e.g., hand or finger flapping or twisting, or complex whole-body movements)
4. Persistent preoccupation with part-objects

C. The disturbance causes clinically significant impairment in social, occupational, or other important areas of functioning

D. There is no clinically significant general delay in language (e.g., single words used by age 2 years, communicative phrases used by age 3 years)

E. There is no clinically significant delay in cognitive development or in the development of age-appropriate self-help skills, adaptive behavior (other than in social interaction), and curiosity about the environment in childhood.

F. Criteria are not met for another specific Pervasive Developmental Disorder or Schizophrenia.

evident, because of the wider range of abilities shown (and demanded to be shown) by people with AS than by those with HFA.

Currently, the most controversial issues in the diagnosis of AS versus HFA appear to be whether or not:

1. Motor skills should be regarded as a differentiating feature
2. AS or HFA could be associated with cognitive disability (including overall mental retardation)
3. Language development is impaired in HFA but spared, or even hyper-functioning, in AS
4. A diagnosis of HFA and one of AS can be made in the same individual at different stages of development (e.g., HFA in early childhood "turning into" AS in later school years, or vice versa)
5. HFA and AS refer to the same or distinct groups of individuals

The exploration of issue 1 is rendered difficult by the circularity of the arguments used to propose one or the other set of diagnostic criteria. Gillberg's (1991) criteria require the presence of motor control problems for a diagnosis of AS, but not for HFA. Thus, a diagnosis of AS would entail more motor control problems than would a diagnosis of HFA (which would not require such problems). One systematic study that did try to critically evaluate this problem showed more motor control problems in AS than in HFA (Gillberg, 1989), even in AS cases for which no prerequisite for motor control problems had been made for the original AS diagnosis. Motor control problems were certainly an important constituent of Asperger's own gestalt of the syndrome he tried to delineate (Asperger, 1944).

Issue 2 pertaining to cognitive dysfunction is a contentious one. The WHO (1993) research criteria for AS are not compatible with general retardation, and Asperger's *own view* most of the time tended to concur with that of those who would exclude cases from a diagnosis of AS if there were indications of low IQ. Nevertheless, Asperger's *own cases* were not always free of major cognitive deficits (case Ernst K in his original paper). Most published studies of AS include a few cases with considerably or slightly below-average IQ. However, usually it would appear that, at least in clinical practice, a diagnosis of AS is rarely made unless IQ is at or above 70.

Perhaps the most difficult diagnostic issue (3) in the field relates to early language development. ICD-10 (WHO, 1993) and DSM-IV (APA, 1994) both posit that there be no signs of early language retardation or abnormality and say nothing about later speech or language problems. At the opposite end of the spectrum of diagnostic criteria deployed, Gillberg (1991) proposes that some speech and language peculiarity has to be present for a diagnosis of AS to be made. Again, this is in line with Asperger's own view (both Ernst K and Hellmuth L of the original paper had some speech and language delay). Forty-four percent of Wolff's 32 high-functioning schizoid children—most of whom appear otherwise to meet ICD-10 criteria for AS—had "abnormalities of language development." In any case, the specific ICD-10 criteria for normal early speech–language development (see Table 5-1) are very difficult to ascertain in practice (Ehlers & Gillberg, 1993). Most cases of typical AS are brought to the attention of psychiatrists and other doctors only at age 7 years or later (Gillberg, 1989), at a time when parents may have difficulty remembering explicitly whether or not their child's language development showed minor (or even major) signs of abnormality in the early years (Whitmore & Bax, 1986).

With respect to issue 4 of "dual diagnosis" and issue 5 of the distinction of one syndrome from the other, there are several caveats. First, in clinical studies it would not make much sense if HFA and AS were compared on a groupwise basis and both groups contained individuals who also had the "other" diagnosis. This would argue in favor of using diagnostic criteria that would be mutually exclusive for the two diagnoses. This is the position of ICD-10 and DSM-IV. However, at the present time we do not know which (if any) are the distinguishing features. Exclusion criteria would therefore be arbitrary and would tend to reinforce the notion of a difference (e.g., if AS is only diagnosed in cases without language problems and HFA is only diagnosed in the presence of such problems, all comparative studies would find that there are fewer language problems in AS than in HFA). This is a bit like reinventing the wheel. Until large-scale population studies of all aspects of the various problems encountered on the "autism spectrum" are performed, it will not be possible to determine to what extent the two concepts are different (if at all).

We might add here that there may yet be a need for (slightly) different criteria and guidelines for clinical practice as compared with research. In clinical work, one of the most important points must always be to arrive at the diagnosis that, at the time and in the given demographic/cultural circumstances, will be of most help to the individual and his or her family. This diagnosis, of course, has to be rooted in empirically derived knowledge, but should not be used for splitting academic hairs.

PREVALENCE

Autism occurs at a rate of 7–16 per 10,000 children born (Wing, 1993; Gillberg, 1995, Swettenham, 1995). HFA constitutes only a fraction (11–34%) of such cases. Thus, the prevalence is likely to be less than 1 in 2000 children in the general population, at least if defined according to present diagnostic criteria for autistic disorder/childhood autism plus a total IQ of ≥ 65.

Wolff has estimated that 3–5% of a general child psychiatric clientele might be "schizoid" (often equivalent with AS).

The rate of AS, diagnosed on the basis of Gillberg and Gillberg (1989) (or ICD-10) criteria, appears to be much higher. According to the only published population study in the field, it occurs in at least 3.6, and possibly 7.1 in 1000 children aged 7–16 (Ehlers & Gillberg, 1993). Thus, it is at least 10 times more common than HFA as diagnosed according to currently accepted criteria.

If AS is accepted as one variant of the autism spectrum disorders, the general notion that 75% of all children with "autism" (broadly defined) have concomitant mental retardation would have to be revised. If the prevalence for AS found by Ehlers and Gillberg (1993) can be replicated by other groups, then the rate of associated mental retardation in autism spectrum disorders (comprising autistic disorder and AS) drops to about 15%.

SEX RATIOS

The sex ratio is skewed both in HFA and in AS. In a recent review of the 16 population studies of autism meeting rigorous criteria for inclusion in a meta-analysis, both Wing (1993) and Gillberg (1995) found that the increase of males over females was not as great as previously believed, and was closer to 2–3:1 male:female ratios than the often-quoted 4–5:1. However, in HFA, it is likely that males are more strongly overrepresented. For instance, in Wing's study, all of the cases of autism with an IQ above 70 were male (Wing & Gould, 1979). There are also several other studies suggesting that the male:female ratio in autism goes down with decreasing IQ. In AS, clinical studies have suggested a male:female ratio of 10–15:1 (Wing, 1981a; Gillberg, 1989), but the one population study available suggests that the overrepresentation is less marked than previously believed, and may be on the order of 4:1 instead (Ehlers & Gillberg, 1993).

The underlying reasons for skewed sex ratios in HFA and AS have been proposed to be (1) genetic and accounting for increased male over female ratios, (2) brain damage (occurring at about the same rate in boys and girls) in the more severely cognitively disabled accounting for lower male:female ratios (Wing, 1981b) in this subgroup, and (3) differences in overall cognitive and social styles in males and females leading to males having perhaps more often than females a style characterized by lower empathy, and if empathy problems are present, then they would be more likely to be recognized in males because of a relative lack of "social camouflaging" abilities (Gillberg, 1992).

BACKGROUND FACTORS

It is not clear what causes autism or AS. Nevertheless, there is general agreement that brain dysfunction is at the root of autism in all cases. Whether or not it is also a basic feature of AS is not known, even though there appears to be consensus that this condition too is caused by brain variation/dysfunction (Frith, 1991).

Cognitive Peculiarities

HFA is associated with a particular pattern of peaks and troughs at neuropsychological testing (Lockyer & Rutter, 1970; Rumsey & Hamburger, 1988; Frith, 1989; Happé, 1994; Ehlers et al., 1997). Poor performance on the picture arrangement and comprehension (and possibly object assembly and similarities) subtests of the WISC and WAIS in combination with superior or high average results on block design on those same tests may be typical of all cases of autism, whether high-functioning or not (Frith, 1989). It may be that as individuals with autism grow older, they may begin to score better on the comprehension subtest. This is a type of test measuring "crystallized" intelligence, i.e., intelligence dependent on acquired knowledge (Kline, 1991, Happé, 1994), which would be difficult to pass for young people with autism but for which "stereotyped" solutions might be learned in training (with age). Thus, poor results on comprehension appear to be a less sensitive marker for autism in older than in very young individuals.

Only five studies have detailed systematic data on IQ in individuals diagnosed as suffering from AS (Wurst, 1974; Gillberg, 1989; Szatmari, Offord, Siegel, Finlayson, & Tuff, 1990; Fine, Bartolucci, Ginsberg, & Szatmari, 1991; Ehlers *et al.*, 1997). According to these studies, overall IQ tends to be higher than in cases designated as HFA, even when the requirement for inclusion in the study has been an IQ level of 70 or above (Ehlers *et al.*, 1997). Verbal IQ is often higher than performance IQ in cases with AS, and the reverse appears to be more true in cases given a diagnosis of HFA. However, this might be an artifact introduced by the diagnostic criteria applied. Furthermore, it should be noted that "verbal" is not necessarily equivalent with "speech and language," as speech and language problems—particularly in domains of pragmatics/conversation—may be as prevalent in AS as in HFA, once IQ is controlled for (Ramberg *et al.*, 1996).

In summary, it appears that in cases diagnosed as AS, IQ is generally a little/considerably higher than in HFA, verbal IQ and "comprehension" are usually higher in the former condition, and "picture arrangement" is low in both conditions. The performance on block design is more variable in AS, but object assembly appears to be consistently low (Ehlers *et al.*, 1997). Results on both of these subtests tend to be inversely correlated with the degree of associated motor clumsiness.

Theory of mind—or mentalizing—deficits are very common in young children with HFA (Baron-Cohen, Leslie, & Frith, 1985). "Mentalizing" refers to the ability, present in normal children of preschool age, to attribute "mental states" (thoughts, beliefs, feelings) to others and to oneself. Young children with AS also may have problems in this domain (Frith, 1991; Happé, 1994). As they grow older, they tend to pass theory of mind tasks on formal testing (Prior, Dahlström, & Squires, 1990; Ozonoff, Rogers, & Pennington, 1991; Bowler, 1992; Frith, 1994; Ozonoff, 1994), but not necessarily in real-life settings.

The ability to use cohesive links to create a reciprocal conversation was impaired in HFA and, to a much lesser degree, in AS (Fine, Bartolucci, Szatmari, & Ginsberg, 1994). The AS group made more unclear references that were difficult to interpret than a comparison group of children with "nonspecific" social problems. In a small study of three adults (male), the inner experiences of people with AS were characterized by visual images in contrast to more variable experiences in people without the syndrome (Hurlburt, Happé, & Frith, 1994). In another study, using Asch's line judgment, AS subjects were more likely to adopt a consistently conforming or nonconforming strategy in an experimental social situation (Bowler & Worley, 1994).

Frontal lobe dysfunction in AS and HFA has been inferred from neuropsychological studies demonstrating executive function deficits (Rumsey, 1985;

Rumsey & Hamburger, 1988; Prior *et al.*, 1990; Ozonoff *et al.*, 1991; Ozonoff, 1994). McEvoy, Roger, and Pennington (1993) reported a significant relationship between executive function and social communication skills in a group of preschool children with HFA. The provisional conclusion was that frontal lobe dysfunction causes executive function deficits that, in turn, cause disability on social tasks. Ozonoff (1994) found that individuals with AS passed first- and second-order theory of mind tests better than those with HFA, but that both groups had similar executive function deficits.

Developmental/congenital prosopagnosia (the inability to recognize faces) has recently been proposed as one possible underlying neuropsychological core deficit in certain cases of AS (Kracke, 1994). Tantam and his group has suggested that the gaze avoidance in AS may not be an absolute avoidance but may rather be interpreted as a lack of *expected* gaze (such as when another person is talking) (Tantam, Holmes, & Cordess, 1993). The authors suggest that a lifelong absence of gaze response to social cues (including speech) could explain a number of features of the syndrome including decreased joint attention and response to affects of others, and poor discrimination of facial expression.

Brain Dysfunction and Associated Medical Disorders

Few studies have explored specific indices of brain dysfunction in HFA or AS. Wing (1981a) reported that 47% of her AS cases had indications of severe pre- or perinatal distress "that might have caused brain damage." Gillberg (1989) reported 43% of 23 referred AS patients and Rickarby, Carruthers, and Mitchell (1991) found 67% of a referred group of 12 AS patients had some index of major perinatal distress (such as grossly abnormal mode of delivery or major asphyxia). Incidentally, abnormal mode of delivery, although known to be associated with a much increased risk of sustaining brain damage, could be a symptom of some constitutional defect in the fetus rather than being the cause of brain damage reacting to AS. In one study (Gillberg, Steffenburg, & Jakobsson, 1987), a full 75% of young children and adolescents with HFA ($n=17$) or AS ($n=3$) had some index of brain dysfunction and of these 75%, three had an identifiable medical syndrome. Several case reports documenting the co-occurrence of AS and specific medical disorders, including tuberous sclerosis (Gillberg, Gillberg, & Ahlsén, 1994) and the fragile X syndrome (Hagerman, 1989), have appeared in the literature. For instance, Tantam, Evered, and Hersov (1990) described three AS individuals (two girls and one man) who all had a Marfan-like syndrome, and Berthier, Bayes, and Tolosa (1993) described two male adolescents with AS and Kleine–Levin syndrome. Anneren, Dahl, and Janols (1994) recently described a boy with AS (and no family history of the disorder) and a *de novo* translocation: t (17;19)(p13.3;p 11).

Generally, the rate of associated unequivocal brain dysfunction indices appears to be lower in AS than in HFA (e.g., Gillberg, 1989), but the scope and meaning of this difference are unclear. Anyway, at the present time, almost all studies in the field have been on potentially biased samples, and so no general conclusions are warranted.

The rate of epilepsy is lower in HFA and AS as compared with low-functioning autism (Gillberg & Coleman, 1992). However, it may still be considerably increased as compared with individuals without autism. In one study (Gillberg, 1989) on epilepsy prevalence in AS, the rate was 4%, and in another study by the same group, on different subjects (Ehlers *et al.*, 1997) it was 0% in AS and 10% in HFA. There is not enough information to suggest that a particular type of seizure disorder might characterize AS–HFA epilepsy cases.

Studies Using CAT Scan, MRI, PET Scan, and SPECT of the Brain

In comparing the brain CAT scans of 18 AS and 22 HFA children, Gillberg (1989) found some cerebral atrophy in 17% of the former and 22% of the latter group. One recent study (Berthier *et al.*, 1993) found MRI abnormalities (cortical, mostly right-sided and ventricular enlargement) in the brains of 5 out of 7 young adult males with AS. These patients had Tourette's syndrome in addition to AS. In one study by Piven's group, males with HFA had larger midsagittal brain areas than age- and IQ-comparable-matched controls and a control group of males comparable for age and socioeconomic status. Cerebellar vermal hypoplasia was not more common in the HFA than in the IQ-comparable group, and the pons and fourth ventricle were of the same size in all three groups (HFA and controls) (Piven *et al.*, 1992). At least two studies have looked at PET scan findings in autism (Herold, Frackowiak, Le Couteur, Rutter, & Howlin, 1988; Horwitz, Rumsey, Grady, & Rapoport, 1988). In one of these, 14 HFA men were compared with 14 healthy controls. In the HFA group, there was impairment of interactions between frontal/parietal regions and the neostriatum and the thalamus (Horwitz *et al.*, 1988). The other PET study yielded no significant differences between an HFA and a normal group of adults. A SPECT study of 12 HFA children without epilepsy and 10 children with low-functioning autism and epilepsy showed left and bilateral temporal hypoperfusion in all cases and some frontal hypoperfusion in 36% of the cases (Gillberg, Bjure, Uvebrandt, & Gillberg, 1993). The overall pattern was completely different than for Rett's syndrome, in which brainstem and frontal hypoperfusion were seen.

Studies Using EEG, ABR, and Oculomotor Function Assessment

No specific findings appear to have emerged from EEG, ABR, and oculomotor studies of HFA and AS. However, several studies have reported similar abnormal findings in HFA and AS as have been reported in low-functioning autism (e.g., Gillberg *et al.*, 1987; Gillberg, 1989).

Studies of Neurochemistry

Less than a handful of studies have considered the neurochemistry of HFA and AS. The ratio of homovanillic acid—the breakdown product of dopamine—to hydroxymethoxyphenylglycol the breakdown product of no-repinephrine—was increased over control levels and equal to levels in low-functioning autism in one study including a small number of children with HFA (Gillberg *et al.*, 1987). One boy and one girl with AS (out of 13) and one girl with HFA (out of 17) had raised CSF albumin (Gillberg, 1989). In a study of CSF glial fibrillary acidic protein (GFA-p), a small group of children with AS ($n=4$) had contents of this glial/synapse marker that were in between those of a normal group ($n=10$) and an autism group [which included an HFA subsample ($n=14$) with high GFA-p levels equal to those of the low-functioning cases] (Ahlsén *et al.*, 1993).

Genetic Factors

It now seems likely that many cases of autism are caused by genetic factors (Bolton & Rutter, 1990). However, even though twin studies show a striking concordance for autism in monozygotic twins and discordance in dizygotic twins, it is much too early to conclude that almost all autism cases are caused by genetic factors (alone or acting in conjunction with other factors). For instance, findings obtained in twins are not necessarily generalizable to the general population of nontwin autism cases. Also, the twin studies performed to date have excluded twinpairs in which there was a known medical disorder associated with autism.

It is not clear whether HFA and AS differ from more severe variants on the autism spectrum in this respect, but it has been hypothesized that genetic factors might be particularly important in the high-functioning cases given that these show less clear-cut associations with indices of brain damage (see above) and the conspicuously high male:female ratio in this subgroup (Wing, 1981b). Nevertheless, familial loading was most pronounced in cases with "severe" autism in one study reported by Rutter (1994).

It is likely that the severity of autism correlates to some degree with the severity of intellectual handicap. There have been several case reports (Burgoine & Wing, 1983; Bowman, 1988; Gillberg, 1991; Ghaziuddin, Metler, Ghaziuddin, Tsai, & Giordani, 1993) and at least two formal studies (DeLong & Dwyer, 1988; Gillberg, 1989) that all suggest the importance of familial transmission of AS. In the studies by Szatmari *et al.* (1989), and Gillberg (1989) there was a suggestion of more "AS-like" pathology in the close family members of children diagnosed with AS as compared with those receiving a diagnosis of HFA. In addition, Wolff's study of schizoid children found a high proportion (more than half) of the parents to be themselves schizoid (Wolff, 1991). Again, this would support the notion of AS possibly being a predominantly genetic disorder and HFA being either a genetic disorder with a different inheritance pattern or more often caused by brain damage. Studies by Folstein and Piven (1991) also support the possibility that a broader/milder autism phenotype might be present in many first-degree relatives of children with classic (including low-functioning) autism. However, it appears that in these studies, family members with such milder problems do not meet full criteria for AS or HFA. Pragmatic language deficits in autism parents may be another expression of the same genetic liability as for autism in some families (Landa et al., 1992). DeLong (DeLong & Dwyer, 1988; DeLong & Nohria, 1994) has recently presented preliminary evidence that children with HFA/AS often have close relatives with bipolar and unipolar affective disorders. He proposes the intriguing hypothesis that HFA/AS sometimes represents the earliest and most severe variant of an affective disorder. Gillberg (1985) described the case of an adolescent boy with HFA and bipolar psychosis. Gillberg (1992) suggested that empathy (roughly equivalent to mentalizing/theory of mind skills) might be a normally distributed "trait" in the general population. Hypothetically being born to parents functioning at the lower end of the normal distribution of empathy would increase the statistical risk of empathy skills poor enough to warrant a diagnosis of AS. Perhaps with the addition of brain damage, such cases might present as "classical" autism, or brain damage could act alone to cause AS ("mild" damage) or HFA ("more severe"). This general hypothesis is close to the model suggested by Van Krevelen (1971), and, in fact, implicitly, by Asperger himself in his original writings (e.g., Asperger, 1944). However, again, only population studies will allow generalizable conclusions regarding the proportion of all AS cases that have a predominantly genetic background.

In summary, there is currently widespread agreement that AS is probably a genetic disorder/variant in a majority of all cases. Nevertheless, studies reporting on series of clinical cases (Wing, 1981a, Gillberg, 1989, Rickarby et al., 1991) have all found a high index of perinatal distress, and one of these studies (Rickarby et al., 1991) reported no indication of familial loading. Thus, any generalized conclusion in this respect would seem premature. The same line of reasoning appears reasonable in HFA also.

Social Factors

Autism does not appear to be correlated with social class (Schopler, Andrew, & Strupp, 1979; Wing, 1980, 1993; Gillberg & Schaumann, 1982;

Gillberg, 1995). Kanner's original propositions were suggested on the basis of a referral-biased sample, and Lotter's (1966) finding of high social class in a community survey of young children with autism, now stands out as atypical.

Nevertheless, HFA and AS might be associated with high social class (e.g., Gillberg et al., 1987; Gillberg, 1989). However, this may be no more exciting news than saying that intellectually high-functioning parents (likely to be of higher social class) are more likely to have high-functioning children, than are low-functioning parents (more likely to be of lower social class).

So far, no published studies specifically of HFA or AS have inferred any particular type of social/family dysfunction in these conditions.

Migration from geographically distant cultures has been suggested as a risk factor for the development of autism. So far, there have been no studies implicating such migration as a potential contributory factor in the development of HFA or AS. In the Swedish population study by Gillberg (1991), out of 35 DSM-III-R autism cases, 5 were "HFA" in the sense that they had full scale IQ over 70. Of these, 2 (40%) had at least one immigrant parent. This figure was similar to that obtained in the remaining group of 30 "lower-functioning" cases (13/30=43%).

The finding of a high proportion of parents of children with HFA and AS themselves having autism-associated features begs the question of "parenting skills" in such individuals. It would not be unreasonable to assume that poor empathy in the parent might contribute to some behavioral/psychological problem in the child, quite apart from any genetic influence. However, one might equally argue that a parent with similar but milder problems would be better able to understand and cope with some of the child's problems because these may be perceived as "traits," "personality style," and the like, rather than "disorder." In any case, future studies should seek to explore these issues also and try to sensibly and sensitively avoid the mistakes of the past, so that the scapegoating of parents that plagued the whole of the autism field from 1943 to the early 1980s not be repeated.

DIFFERENTIAL DIAGNOSIS AND COMORBIDITY

The differential diagnosis in HFA/AS involves a lot of differently named psychiatric disorders listed in the DSM-III-R, DSM-IV, and ICD-10. In addition, the boundaries vis-à-vis some learning and language disorders are still blurred.

It is of some interest that many of the behaviorally defined disorders in these diagnostic manuals appear not to have been discussed across the different task forces for the various groups of diagnoses. For instance, several of the criteria for Obsessive-Compulsive-Personality Disorder (OCPD) overlap (albeit slightly differently worded) with those of autistic disorder and AS. This is to be expected, given that many psychiatric disorders lead to restriction of social functioning and this is a "symptom" included in both OCPD and AS. However, few clinicians (and researchers) appear to be aware that an individual with AS often meets full or almost full criteria for OCPD. This is but one instance in which diagnostic boundaries are blurred. Similar cases could be made for obsessive-compulsive disorder (OCD), schizotypal personality disorder, and paranoid personality disorder. Sometimes this is not just a question of a lack of semantic distinction, but an issue of true comorbidity (Caron & Rutter, 1991).

In a population study of AS, Tourette's syndrome was found in one of five school-age children with AS. Tics were demonstrated in another three (Ehlers & Gillberg, 1993).

In a population study of anorexia nervosa (Råstam, Gillberg, & Garton, 1989), AS was diagnosed in 12% of the cases in early adulthood (Gillberg, Råstam, & Gillberg, 1994).

Children with deficits in attention, motor control, and perception (DAMP)—children who also meet criteria for attention deficit hyperactivity disorder (ADHD)—sometimes meet full criteria for AS. In one study, 21% of children with a severe problem of this kind also met full criteria for AS (Gillberg & Gillberg, 1989) and a further 36% had some autistic traits (Gillberg, 1983). Many children with AS are overactive and aggressive (Eaves, Ho, & Eaves, 1994). The diagnostic overlap is illustrated in Figure 5-1. In most of these "conditions," it is likely that some kind of common brain dysfunction/functional variability constitutes the "core," rather than the clinical syndromes being distinctive and clearly separable in all cases. One problem common to the children in which there is a considerable overlap of diagnoses is in the field of empathy. Gillberg (1992) launched the concept of "disorders of empathy" to comprise all of the groups of clinical syndromes in which reciprocal social interaction in real-life settings is severely impaired.

Elective mutism has been described in the near relatives of children with AS (Gillberg & Forsell, 1984; Gillberg, 1989) and in several "schizoid" (AS?) children examined by Wolff (1991).

The possibility of diagnostic overlap of AS/HFA with childhood-onset schizophrenia has been mentioned by Rapoport's group (Gordon et al., 1994).

Shea and Mesibov (1985) highlighted the convergence of high-functioning autism, AS and some forms of learning disability. Children with DAMP usually have some mild–moderate learning problems. Their neurophysiological test profile often infers a "right-hemisphere dysfunction syndrome" (Rourke, 1988, Ellis, Ellis, Fraser, & Deb, 1994)—such a syndrome is sometimes referred to as nonverbal learning disability. It is not clear to what extent such a syndrome is equivalent to, overlapping with, or different from AS/HFA. The same holds for so-called semantic–pragmatic disorders (Bishop, 1989; Lister-Brook & Bowler, 1992).

Wing (Wing & Shah, 1994) recently drew attention to the possibility that some young adolescents with AS/HFA develop catatonic features, raising the

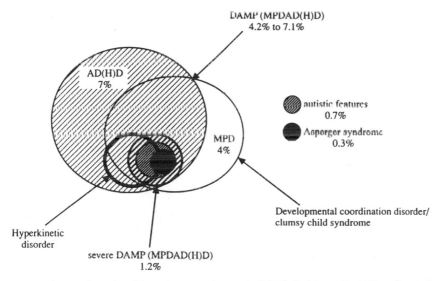

Fig. 5-1. The overlap of (mild–moderate and severe) DAMP [MPD + AD(H)D] and autistic features/Asperger syndrome in the general population of 7-year-olds (data from Gillberg, 1983, Gillberg & Gillberg, 1989a) and the possible overlap with hyperkinetic syndrome and developmental coordination-clumsy child syndrome.

possibility that in some instances of catatonia in adult psychiatry, AS/HFA may be an "antecedent"/comorbid problem.

Scragg and Shah (1994) examining the important hypothesis that AS may be associated with violent behavior, screened the male population at a maximum security hospital. They found a rate of 1.5% AS using Gillberg and Gillberg criteria, and concluded that this might mean a considerable increase in the prevalence of AS in a very violent population of males as compared with males in the general population. The inclusion of equivocal cases raised the rate to 2.3%. The authors proposed that individuals examined in forensic psychiatric services should be examined with a view to diagnosing AS/HFA more often than is currently the case.

WORKUP IN AS AND HFA

All people with HFA/AS should have a neuropsychological/medical workup. This will need, of course, to be tailored to the age and general functioning of the individual. All children (but not all adolescents and adults) with any of these diagnoses will need all of the following: (1) at the very least testing with the WISC-III (or the WAIS-R in adults) (these are currently the most widely used and best validated IQ tests) and (2) a medical workup comprising a meticulous physical examination (looking for possible signs of neurocutaneous disorders and syndromes associated with particular physical phenotypes), a chromosomal culture, and a PCR (polymerase chain reaction) analysis for the fragile-X-gene, and, in cases with IQ under about 90, or if there is a clinical suspicion for other reasons, a neuroimaging examination of the brain, plus any other laboratory workup considered to be appropriate (depending on possible additional problems such as epilepsy, motor deficits, and metabolic or neurological symptoms).

The neuropsychological profile in HFA/AS tends to be slightly different than that shown by lower-functioning individuals. Both performance IQ and, particularly, verbal IQ are higher than in low-functioning cases (Ehlers *et al.*, 1997). In AS, the full-scale IQ levels are often higher than for non-AS individuals in the general population (Ramberg *et al.*, 1996). Although the score for picture arrangement will be low in most cases (just as it is in low-functioning autism), block design (typically high in the low-functioning cases), because of motor and/or attentional deficits, is usually on par with/lower than overall IQ levels. Comprehension is usually low in low-functioning autism cases. In HFA/AS, it may not be deficient, for as individuals grow older, some with HFA/AS learn "by heart" the correct responses to everyday commonsense questions.

The medical workup has a relatively low specific yield (probably under 15% have an associated medical condition). Nevertheless, in those HFA/AS cases who do have an underlying medical disorder/organic condition (the fragile X syndrome, tuberous sclerosis, neurofibromatosis, hypomelanosis of Ito), it is essential to know about them. Specific genetic counseling pertains to some of these disorders, certain treatments (such as stimulants in the fragile X syndrome) are likely to be more beneficial, and the outcome tends to vary considerably depending on which specific disorder is involved. There is usually no way of making the diagnosis of such a disorder without a workup of the kind outlined.

OUTCOME

Very little is known about the long-term outcome of HFA or AS, although it is clear that in many respects it is better than for other autism cases. The fact that, in all of the outcome studies of autism, the strongest predictor of poor outcome has been low IQ, indicates that higher IQ (roughly to be equated with HFA) would be associated with good (or at least relatively good) outcome. However, in all of the autism outcome studies published through 1990 (reviewed in Gillberg, 1991), the absolute numbers of autism cases have been low in each individual study, precluding all definite conclusions with respect to the highest-functioning group. Furthermore, no study to date has systematically studied outcome in AS. This "condition" is probably considerably more common than

HFA, and the indications regarding outcome gained in studies of autism may not generalize at all to this population.

There is some evidence (mostly anecdotal) that AS in childhood can be associated with excellent outcome in adulthood (at least in terms of self-care and academic progress) (e.g., Gillberg, 1991). There are data indicating that about half of the total population of AS cases are not referred to doctors or psychologists in schoolage, even when problems are well recognized by teachers (Ehlers & Gillberg, 1993). Thus, unlike "autism," which usually would prompt referral to some kind of specialist before school age, AS may well remain completely undiagnosed well into adult age. Even then, it is currently more likely that, if referral is made, the diagnosis will not be AS, but may come out as "schizoid" or "schizotypal" personality disorder, "type II schizophrenia," "atypical depression," "paranoid disorder," or "OCD."

One outcome population study that did include cases with AS (Hellgren, Gillberg, Bågenholm, & Gillberg, 1994) has been published. Of three AS cases in that study, two had severe alcohol problems already at age 16.

Rumsey, Rapoport, and Sceery (1985) described the progress of 10 HFA males from childhood through a mean age of 26 (range 18–39) years. Four of these men had been diagnosed by Leo Kanner. The authors found persistent deficiencies on WAIS-R testing (low results on the comprehension, and picture arrangement subtests), typical of young children with autism. Pragmatic language dysfunction and speech dysprosody were common persisting problems. The men were all socially and behaviorally impaired but 9 had completed high school and 2 had completed at least 1 year at a junior college. All had full-scale IQ over 80.

Szatmari (1989) described the outcome of a group of 16 relatively high-functioning individuals with autism (12 males, 4 females) at a mean age of 26 years. IQs ranged from 68 to 110. Twenty-five percent were considered "recovered" and the remainder functioned poorly in terms of occupational–social outcome and psychiatric symptoms. Good nonverbal problem-solving skills correlated with good outcome. The severity of early autistic behavior had no effect on outcome. Both of these studies may have been biased in terms of sample selection, one way or the other, and so generalized conclusions cannot be drawn regarding outcome in HFA.

The retrospective studies by Tantam (1991) of an adult psychiatric in-patient clientele of "eccentrics" and other individuals showing social oddities, indirectly infer that quite a large proportion of adult psychiatric patients may have qualified for a diagnosis of AS in childhood and adolescence. Similar conclusions obtained in a Swedish study by Beier (1993).

The studies by Wolff (e.g., Wolff & Chick 1980; Wolff et al., 1991) on schizoid children and by Sparrow et al. (1986) on "schizoid" and "atypical" children several of whom have AS, suggest that the diagnosis often remains stable over time and that impairments in socialization and communication persist over a number of years. Nevertheless, many change in a positive way, even though others develop "additional" psychiatric symptoms in adolescence and adult age.

These findings should not be taken to mean that the person with AS is likely to become basically very "different" over time, but rather that similar or identical underlying problems show in different ways and are perceived and diagnosed differently in adult age versus childhood.

INTERVENTION

No currently available treatment provides a "cure" for most individuals suffering from HFA or AS. Certainly, in the case of AS in some young children, it is questionable whether a complete "cure" should be sought. If, as has been implied by Gillberg (1991) and Sacks (1995), some individuals with AS, without extreme personal suffering, go on to become adults who are (albeit in a very limited area) creative and contribute to development in their field, then it might even be unethical to be speaking of "treatment" (i.e., an intervention that will turn the individual into someone "normal"). However, in many cases, at least from school age and adolescence, individual and family suffering is such that some kind of management strategy (short of "treatments" and "cures") will need to be considered.

In general, many of the management guidelines suggested for individuals with autism by Rutter (1985) and Gillberg (1989) would seem to apply in HFA and AS as well. These are outlined in Table 5-2.

Clomipramine (Gordon, State, Nelson, Hamburger, & Rapoport, 1993) was found to be effective in reducing rituals, obsessions, and compulsions in a double-blind placebo-controlled study of 24 relatively high-functioning individuals with autism. However, in an open study of preschool children with autism (mostly low-functioning), Sanchez (1994) found so many severe side effects of this drug that she felt it could not be recommended for general use even in ritualistic, high-functioning individuals with autism. Some individuals with AS have severe attention problems and it is possible that, in this subgroup, unlike in lower-functioning cases, central stimulants could be helpful in the treatment of attention problems (Strayhorn, 1989). In those few cases with the combination of HFA/AS and epilepsy, pharmacological treatment may be problematic, in that side effects of some drugs can be especially difficult to evaluate properly.

In our view, in most cases, neither psychotherapy nor pharmacological treatment is indicated in HFA or AS. Nevertheless, occasionally, both have been clinically useful, singly or in combination. Psychological and pharmacological interventions should always be managed by clinicians well informed about the nature of the underlying handicaps.

Table 5-2. Management Guidelines for HFA and AS: Essential Features

1. The first evaluation: appropriate assessment and correct diagnosis essential for optimal understanding and service
2. Neuropsychiatric workup: psychological evaluation including IQ, psychiatric evaluation for comorbidity, medical and laboratory workup for possible associated medical conditions (e.g., fragile X, tuberous sclerosis, hypomelanosis of Ito)
3. Information to and education of all family members (including siblings and grandparents) on helpful coping strategies (educational and behavioral) plus involvement with support groups (if possible)
4. Work with the family
5. Practical and financial support for the family (including respite care)
6. Education for the patient (including special education classrooms for some individuals and "HFA/AS consultants" in normal classrooms for others)
7. Physical education (focusing on social motor skills and "general exercise")
8. Social skills groups for some adolescents and adults
9. Pharmacotherapy in a minority
10. Psychotherapy in a minority (should only be provided by therapist well informed about HFA/AS)
11. Behavior modification in a minority
12. Long-term perspective
13. Integration of approaches: the habilitation team

In addition to the general guidelines, there is a special need to take account of the neuropsychological peaks and troughs. First, in the past, all too often, only the troughs have been highlighted, leading to a pessimistic view with respect to management and outcome. We have had the experience that most children with HFA/AS benefit from an approach acknowledging the difficulty while also realizing that, for most problems, there is another side of the coin. Most deficits/symptoms can be turned into an asset if thoughtfully reconsidered. For instance, the "overfocus" on a narrow interest, which is, indeed, often a severe problem, alternatively might be viewed as an exceptional ability to concentrate, if only the right settings and tasks are provided. The inability to relate normally in a social setting requiring reciprocal interaction could also be seen to represent an ability to shut out "irrelevant" social stimuli and might, in an optimal situation, provide the framework for an unusual capacity for hard, rigorous work. I know, for instance, of a grandfather of a girl with AS, who, despite meeting all criteria for AS himself, has been a highly appreciated medical radiologist for many years. Turning the problems into assets is the key to many of the abnormalities encountered in HFA/AS. Twachtman (1994) and Gray (1994), in their contributions in this book, describe helpful ways of identifying areas of interest and good skills that can be used for teaching other skills. We believe that Gray's approach of using "social stories" to identify problem behaviors and teaching coping strategies could hold particular promise here.

Second, even though an optimistic attitude should be retained in the encounter with families who have young children with HFA/AS, realism also needs to pervade the planning of management. To this end, in some respects, the troughs need to be seen for what they are: handicapping problems in the domains of social interaction, communication, and behavioral adjustment. Thus, for instance, an extremely bright young boy/man with AS might not be able to head a company or a department, even if his overall IQ would seem to predict an extremely bright future. And a young woman with HFA/AS with very good artistic skills but an overall IQ of about 90 might not be expected to cope with the simplest social interactions and will have to be accommodated in sheltered housing and vocation in adult life.

CONCLUSIONS

HFA occurs in fewer than 1 in 2000 children, whereas AS is at an almost 10-fold higher rate. It is unclear to what extent they represent separate or overlapping (or, indeed, sometimes identical) conditions. There is a great need for continued research in all relevant areas of AS and related disorders, perhaps most importantly in epidemiology, differential diagnosis, neuropsychology, neurobiology, and outcome. It is already clear that AS has a better outcome than lower-functioning autism. However, some individuals with AS have persistent severe problems in adult age and consult adult psychiatrists for them. There is a need to train adult psychiatrists in this field so that they will be better able to recognize HFA and AS in their patients currently receiving a plethora of diagnoses, ranging from atypical schizophrenia and atypical depression to paranoid disorder and schizoid/schizotypal personality disorder.

ACKNOWLEDGMENTS

This work was completed with the support of grants from the Wilhelm and Martina Lundgren Foundation for C. Gillberg and S. Ehlers. Portions of this paper were presented at the 15th Annual TEACCH Conference, May 19–20, 1994, at the William and Ida Friday Continuing Education Center, Chapel Hill, North Carolina.

REFERENCES

Ahlsén, G., Rosengren, L., Belfrage, M., Palm, A., Haglid, K., Hamberger, A., & Gillberg, C. (1993). Glial fibrillary acidic protein in the cerebrospinal fluid of children with autism and other neuropsychiatric disorders. *Biological Psychiatry, 33,* 734–743.

American Psychiatric Association. (1987). *Diagnostic and statistical manual of mental disorders*. (3rd ed. rev.). Washington, DC: Author.

American Psychiatric Association. (1994). *Diagnostic and statistical manual of mental disorders*. (4th ed.). Washington, DC: Author.

Annerén, G., Dahl, N., & Janols, L.-O. (1994). Asperger syndrome in a boy with a balanced *de novo* translocation. t(17,19)(p13. 3,p11). *American Journal of Medical Genetics*, 56, 1–8.

Asperger, H. (1944). Die "autistischen Psychopathen" im Kindesalter. *Archiv für Psychiatrie und Nervenkrankheiten*, 117, 76–136.

Asperger, H. (1950). Bild und soziale Wertigkeit der autistischen Psychopathen. *Proceedings of the 2nd International Congress on Orthopedagogics*. Keesing, Amsterdam: Publ. Systemen.

Asperger, H. (1952). *Heilpädagogik*. Berlin: Springer.

Baron-Cohen, S., Leslie, A. M., & Frith, U. (1985). Does the autistic child have a theory of mind? *Cognition*, 21, 37–46.

Beier, H. (1993). Autistiska syndrom. En angelägenhet även inom vuxenpsykiatrin. Autistic syndromes. A concern also in adult psychiatry. *Läkartidningen*, 90, 4360–4364.

Berthier, M. L., Bayes, A., & Tolosa, E. S. (1993). Magnetic resonance imaging in patients with concurrent Tourette's disorder and Asperger's syndrome. *Journal of the American Academy of Child and Adolescent Psychiatry*, 32, 633–639.

Berthier, M. L., Santamaria, J., Encabo, H., & Tolosa, E. S. (1992). Case study: Recurrent hypersomnia in two adolescent males with Asperger's syndrome. *Journal of the American Academy of Child and Adolescent Psychiatry*, 31, 735–738.

Bishop, D. V. M. (1989). Autism, Asperger's syndrome and semantic-pragmatic disorders. Where are the boundaries? *British Journal of Disorders of Communication*, 24, 107–121.

Bolton, P., & Rutter, M. (1990). Genetic influences in autism. *International Review of Psychiatry*, 2, 67–80.

Bowler, D. M. (1992). "Theory of mind" in Asperger's syndrome. *Journal of Child Psychology and Psychiatry*, 33, 877–893.

Bowler, D. M., & Worley, K. (1994). Suspectibility to social influence in adults with Asperger's syndrome: A research note. *Journal of Child Psychology and Psychiatry*, 35, 689–697.

Bowman, E. P. (1988). Asperger's syndrome and autism. The case for a connection. *British Journal of Psychiatry*, 152, 377–382.

Burgoine, E., & Wing, L. (1983). Identical triplets with Asperger's syndrome. *British Journal of Psychiatry*, 143, 261–265.

Caron, C., & Rutter, M. (1991). Comorbidity in child psychopathology: Concepts, issues and research strategies. *Journal of Child Psychology and Psychiatry*, 32, 1063–1080.

Dauner, I., & Martin, M. (1978). Autismus Asperger oder Frühschizophrenic? Zur nosologischen Abgrenzung beider Krankheitsbilder. *Paediatrische Paedologie*, 13, 31–38.

DeLong, G. R., & Dwyer, J. T. (1988). Correlation of family history with specific autistic subgroups: Asperger's syndrome and bipolar affective disease. *Journal of Autism and Developmental Disorders*, 18, 593–600.

DeLong, R., & Nohria, C. (1994). Psychiatric family history and neurological disease in autism spectrum disorders. *Developmental Medicine and Child Neurology*, 36, 441–448.

DeMyer, M., Hingtgen, J. M., & Jackson, R. K. (1981). Infantile autism reviewed: A decade of research. *Schizophrenic Bulletin*, 7, 388–451.

Eaves, L. C., Ho, H. H., & Eaves, D. M. (1994). Subtypes of autism by cluster analysis. *Journal of Autism and Developmental Disorders*, 24, 3–22.

Ehlers, S., & Gillberg, C. (1993). The epidemiology of Asperger syndrome. A total population study. *Journal of Child Psychology and Psychiatry*, 34, 1327–1350.

Ehlers, S., Nydén, A., Gillberg, C., Dahlgren Sandberg, A., Dahlgren, S.-O., Hjelmquist, E., & Oden, A. (1997). Asperger syndrome, autism and attention disorders: A comparative study of the cognitive profiles of 120 children. *Journal of Child Psychology and Psychiatry*, 37, 207–217.

Ellis, H. D., Ellis, D. M., Fraser, W., & Deb, S. (1994). A preliminary study of right hemisphere cognitive deficits and impaired social judgements among young people with Asperger syndrome. *European Child and Adolescent Psychiatry, 3,* 255–266.

Fine, J., Bartolucci, G., Ginsberg, G., & Szatmari, P. (1991). The use of intonation to communicate in pervasive developmental disorders. *Journal of Child Psychology and Psychiatry, 32,* 771–782.

Fine, J., Bartolucci, G., Szatmari, P., & Ginsberg, G. (1994). Cohesive discourse in pervasive developmental disorders. *Journal of Autism and Developmental Disorders, 24,* 315–329.

Folstein, S. E., & Piven, J. (1991). Etiology of autism: Genetic influences. *Paediatrics, 87,* 767–773.

Frith, U. (1989). Autism and "theory of mind." In C. Gillberg (Ed.), *Diagnosis and treatment of autism* (pp. 33–52). New York: Plenum Press.

Frith, U. (1991). 'Autistic psychopathy' in childhood. In U. Frith (Ed.), *Autism and Asperger syndrome* (pp. 37–92). Cambridge: Cambridge University Press.

Frith, U. (1994). *Understanding the mind in autism and Asperger syndrome.* Autism Conference, Olso, Norway.

Ghaziuddin, M., Butler, E., Tsai, L., & Ghaziuddin, N. (1994). Is clumsiness a marker for Asperger syndrome? *Journal of Intellectual Disability Research, 38,* 519–527.

Ghaziuddin, M., Tsai, L. Y., & Ghaziuddin, N. (1992). Brief report: A reappraisal of clumsiness as a diagnostic feature of Asperger syndrome. *Journal of Autism and Developmental Disorders, 22,* 651–656.

Ghaziuddin, N., Metler, L., Ghaziuddin, M., Tsai, L., & Giordani, B. (1993). Three siblings with Asperger syndrome: A family case history. *European Child and Adolescent Psychiatry, 2,* 44–49.

Gillberg, C. (1983). Psychotic behaviour in children and young adults in a mental handicap hostel. *Acta Psychiatrica Scandinavica, 68,* 351–358.

Gillberg, C. (1985). Asperger's syndrome and recurrent psychosis—a case study. *Journal of Autism and Developmental Disorders, 15,* 389–397.

Gillberg, C. (1989). Asperger syndrome in 23 Swedish children. *Developmental Medicine and Child Neurology, 31,* 520–531.

Gillberg, C. (1991). Clinical and neurobiological aspects of Asperger syndrome in six family studies. In U. Frith (Ed.), *Autism and Asperger syndrome* (pp. 122–146). Cambridge: Cambridge University Press.

Gillberg, C. (1992). The Emanuel Miller Memorial Lecture 1991: Autism and autistic-like conditions: subclasses among disorders of empathy. *Journal of Child Psychology and Psychiatry, 33,* 813–842.

Gillberg, C. (1995). The prevalence of autism and autism spectrum disorders. In F. C. Verhulst & H. M. Koot (Eds.), *The epidemiology of child and adolescent psychopathology* (pp. 227–257). London: Oxford University Press.

Gillberg, C., & Coleman, M. (1992). *The biology of the autistic syndromes* (2nd ed.). London: Mac Keith Press.

Gillberg, C., & Forsell, C. (1984). Childhood psychosis and neurofibromatosis—more than a coincidence? *Journal of Autism and Developmental Disorders, 14,* 1–8.

Gillberg, C., & Schaumann, H. (1982). Social class and infantile autism. *Journal of Autism and Developmental Disorders, 12,* 223–228.

Gillberg, C., Steffenburg, S., & Jakobsson, G. (1987). Neurobiological findings in 20 relatively gifted children with Kanner-type autism or Asperger syndrome. *Developmental Medicine and Child Neurology, 29,* 641–649.

Gillberg, C., Steffenburg, S., & Schaumann, H. (1991). Is autism more common now than 10 years ago? *British Journal of Psychiatry, 158,* 403–409.

Gillberg, I. C., Bjure, J., Uvebrandt, P., & Gillberg, C. (1993). SPECT (single photon emission computed tomography) in 31 children and adolescents with autism and autistic-like conditions. *European Child and Adolescent Psychiatry, 2,* 50–59.

Gillberg, I. C., & Gillberg, C. (1989). Asperger syndrome—some epidemiological considerations: A research note. *Journal of Child Psychology and Psychiatry, 30,* 631–638.

Gillberg, I. C., Gillberg, C., & Ahlsén, G. (1994). Autistic behaviour and attention deficits in tuberous sclerosis. A population-based study. *Developmental Medicine and Child Neurology, 36,* 50–56.

Gillberg, I. C., Råstam, M., & Gillberg, C. (1994). Anorexia nervosa outcome: Six year controlled longitudinal study of 51 cases including a population cohort. *Journal of the American Academy of Child and Adolescent Psychiatry, 33,* 729–739.

Gordon, C. T., Frazier, J. A., McKenna, K., Giedd, J., Zametkin, A., Zahn, T., Hommer, D., Hong, W., Kaysen, D., Albus, K. E., & Rapoport, J. L. (1994). Childhood onset schizophrenia: An NIMH study in progress. *Schizophrenia Bulletin, 20,* 697–712.

Gordon, C. T., State, R. C., Nelson, J. E., Hamburger, S. D., & Rapoport, J. L. (1993). A double-blind comparison of clomipramine, desipramine, and placebo in the treatment of autistic disorder. *Archives of General Psychiatry, 50,* 441–447.

Gray, C. (1994). *Social interventions with high functioning people with autism.* Paper read at the 15th Annual TEACCH Conference on High-Functioning Autism and Asperger Syndrome, Chapel Hill.

Hagerman, R. J. (1989). Chromosomes, genes and autism. In C. Gillberg (Ed.), *Diagnosis and treatment of autism* (pp. 105–132). New York: Plenum Press.

Happé, F. G. E. (1994). Current psychological theories of autism: The "theory of mind" account and rival theories. *Journal of Child Psychology and Psychiatry, 35,* 215–229.

Hellgren, L., Gillberg, I. C., Bågenholm, A., & Gillberg, C. (1994). Children with deficits in attention, motor control and perception (DAMP) almost grown up: Psychiatric and personality disorders at age 16 years. *Journal of Child Psychology and Psychiatry, 35,* 1255–1271.

Herold, S., Frackowiak, R. S. J., Le Couteur, A., Rutter, M., & Howlin, P. (1988). Cerebral blood flow and metabolism of oxygen and glucose in young autistic adults. *Psychological Medicine, 18,* 823–831.

Horwitz, B., Rumsey, J. M., Grady, C. L., & Rapoport, S. I. (1988). The cerebral metabolic landscape in autism. Intercorrelations of regional glucose utilization. *Archives of Neurology, 45,* 749–755.

Hurlburt, R. T., Happé, F., & Frith, U. (1994). Sampling the form of inner experience in three adults with Asperger syndrome. *Psychological Medicine, 24,* 385–395.

Kanner, L. (1954). To what extent is early childhood autism determined by constitutional inadequacies? *Proceedings of the Association for Research in Nervous and Mental Diseases, 33,* 378–385.

Klin, A. (1993). Listening preferences in regard to speech in four children with developmental disabilities. *Journal of Child Psychology and Psychiatry, 34,* 763–769.

Kline, P. (1991). *Intelligence. The psychometric review.* London: Routledge.

Kracke, I. (1994). Developmental prosopagnosia in Asperger syndrome: Presentation and discussion of an individual case. *Developmental Medicine and Child Neurology, 36,* 873–886.

Kretschmer, E. (1925). *Physique and character.* London: Kegan Paul, Trench, Trübner (original work published 1924).

Landa, R., Piven, J., Wzorek, M. M., Gayle, J. O., Chase, G. A., & Folstein, S. E. (1992). Social language in parents of autistic individuals. *Psychological Medicine, 22,* 245–254.

Lister-Brook, S., & Bowler, D. M. (1992). Autism by another name? Semantic and pragmatic impairments in children. *Journal of Autism and Developmental Disorders, 22,* 61–81.

Lockyer, L., & Rutter, M. (1970). A five- to fifteen-year follow-up study of infantile psychosis. IV: Patterns of cognitive ability. *British Journal of Social and Cognitive Ability, 9,* 152–163.

Lotter, V. (1966). Epidemiology of autistic conditions in young children. I. Prevalence. *Social Psychiatry, 1,* 124–137.

Marriage, K., Miles, T., Stokes, D., & Davey, M. (1993). Clinical and research implications of the co-occurrence of Asperger's and Tourette syndrome. *Australian and New Zealand Journal of Psychiatry, 27,* 666–672.

McEvoy, R. E., Roger, S. J., & Pennington, B. F. (1993). Executive function and social communication deficits in young autistic children. *Journal of Child Psychology and Psychiatry, 34,* 563–578.

Newson, J., & Newson, E. (1979). The handicapped child: What is an autistic child. *Nursing Times, 75,* Suppl. 4–5.

Ozonoff, S. (1994). *Neuropsychological abilities in high-functioning autism and Asperger syndrome.* Paper read at the 15th Annual TEACCH Conference on High-Functioning Autism and Asperger's Syndrome.

Ozonoff, S., Rogers, S. J., & Pennington, B. F. (1991). Asperger's syndrome: Evidence of an empirical distinction from high-functioning autism. *Journal of Child Psychology and Psychiatry, 32,* 1107–1122.

Piven, J., Nehme, E., Simon, J., Barta, P., Pearlson, G., & Folstein, S. E. (1992). Magnetic resonance imaging in autism: Measurement of the cerebellum. *Biological Psychiatry, 31,* 491–504.

Prior, M., Dahlstrom, B., & Squires, T.-L. (1990). Autistic children's knowledge of thinking and feeling states in other people. *Journal of Child Psychology and Psychiatry, 31,* 587–601.

Ramberg, C., Ehlers, S., Nydén, A., Gillberg, C., & Johansson, M. (1996). Language and pragmatic functions in school-age children on the autism spectrum. *European Journal of Disorders of Communication 31,* 387–414.

Råstam, M., Gillberg, C., & Garton, M. (1989). Anorexia nervosa in a Swedish urban region. A population-based study. *British Journal of Psychiatry, 155,* 642–646.

Rickarby, G., Carruthers, A., & Mitchell, M. (1991). Brief report: Biological factors associated with Asperger syndrome. *Journal of Autism and Developmental Disorders, 21,* 341–348.

Robinson, J. F., & Vitale, L. J. (1954). *Children with circumscribed interest patterns.* Paper presented at the 1953 Annual Meeting. Children's Service Center of Wyoming Valley, Wilkes-Barre, PA.

Rourke, B. P. (1988). The syndrome of non-verbal learning disabled children: Developmental manifestations of neurological disease. *The Clinical Neuropsychologist, 2,* 293–330.

Rumsey, J. M. (1985). Conceptual problem-solving in highly verbal, nonretarded, autistic men. *Journal of Autism and Developmental Disorders, 15,* 23–36.

Rumsey, J. M., & Hamburger, S. D. (1988). Neuropsychological findings in high-functioning men with infantile autism, residual state. *Journal of Clinical and Experimental Neuropsychology, 10,* 201–221.

Rumsey, J. M., Rapoport, J. L., & Sceery, W. R. (1985). Autistic children as adults: Psychiatric and behavioral outcomes. *Journal of The American Academy of Child Psychiatry, 24,* 465–473.

Rutter, M. (1985). Diagnosis and definition. In M. Rutter & L. Hersov (Eds.), *Child and adolescent psychiatry: Modern approaches* (pp. 1–25). Oxford: Blackwell Scientific.

Rutter, M. (1994). *Genetic aspects of autism.* Paper read at the Autism on the Agenda Conference, Leeds.

Sacks, O. (1995). *An anthropologist on Mars.* New York: Knopf.

Sanchez, L. (1994). *Clomipramine in child neuropsychiatry.* Paper read at Recent Advances in Child Neuropsychiatry Research Seminar, Göteborg, Sweden.

Schopler, E., Andrew, C. E., & Strupp, K. (1979). Do autistic children come from upper-class parents? *Journal of Autism and Developmental Disorders, 9,* 139–152.

Schopler, E., Reichler, R. J., & Renner, B. R. (1988). *The Childhood Autism Rating Scale (CARS). Revised.* Los Angeles: Western Psychological Services.

Scragg, P., & Shah, A. (1994). Prevalence of Asperger's syndrome in a secure hospital. *British Journal of Psychiatry, 165,* 679–682.

Shea, V., & Mesibov, G. B. (1985). Brief report: The relationship of learning disabilities and higher-level autism. *Journal of Autism and Developmental Disorders, 15,* 425–435.

Sparrow, S. S., Rescorla, L. A., Provence, S., Condon, S. O., Goudreau, D., & Cicchetti, D. V. (1986). Follow-up of "atypical" children—a brief report. *Journal of the American Academy of Child and Adolescent Psychiatry, 25,* 181–185.

Ssucharewa, G. E. (1926). Die Schizoiden Psychopathien im Kindesalter. *Monatsschrift für Psychiatrie und Neurologie, 60,* 235–261.

Strayhorn, J. (1989). More on methylphenidate in autism [letter]. *Journal of the American Academy of Child and Adolescent Psychiatry, 28,* 299.

Szatmari, P. (1989). The diagnosis of Asperger's syndrome and autistic disorder using DSM-III-R. Unpublished manuscript (Report to DSM-IV committee).

Szatmari, P., Bartolucci, G., & Bremner, R. (1989). Asperger's syndrome and autism: Comparisons on early history and outcome. *Developmental Medicine and Child Neurology, 31,* 709–720.

Szatmari, P., Offord, D. R., Siegel, L. S., Finlayson, M. A. J., & Tuff, L. (1990). The clinical significance of neurocognitive impairments among children with psychiatric disorders: Diagnosis and situational specificity. *Journal of Child Psychology and Psychiatry, 31,* 287–299.

Swettenham, J. (1995, April 27). *Detection of autism in primary care.* Paper presented at the ACPP–Midlands Branch Research Day—Advances in the Assessment of Autism, Birmingham, England.

Tantam, D. (1988). Asperger's syndrome. *Journal of Child Psychology and Psychiatry, 29,* 245–255.

Tantam, D. (1991). Asperger syndrome in adulthood. In U. Frith (Ed.), *Autism and Asperger syndrome* (pp. 147–183). Cambridge: Cambridge University Press.

Tantam, D., Evered, C., & Hersov, L. (1990). Asperger's syndrome and ligamentus laxity. *Journal of the American Academy of Child and Adolescent Psychiatry, 29,* 892–896.

Tantam, D., Holmes, D., & Cordess, C. (1993). Nonverbal expression in autism of Asperger type. *Journal of Autism and Developmental Disorders, 23,* 111–133.

Twachtman, D. (1994). *Social and communication needs in Asperger syndrome: Variations on the theme of autism.* Paper read at the 15th Annual TEACCH Conference on Asperger Syndrome and High-Functioning Autism, Chapel Hill.

Van Krevelen, D. A. (1971). Early infantile autism and autistic psychopathy. *Journal of Autism and Childhood Schizophrenia, 1,* 82–86.

Van Krevelen, D. A., & Kuipers, C. (1962). The psychopathology of autistic psychopathy. *Acta Paedopsychiatrica, 29,* 22–31.

Whitmore, K., & Bax, M. (1986). The school entry medical examination. *Archives of Diseases in Childhood, 61,* 807–817.

Wing, L. (1980). Childhood autism and social class: A question of selection. *British Journal of Psychiatry, 137,* 410–417.

Wing, L. (1981a). Asperger's syndrome: A clinical account. *Psychological Medicine, 11,* 115–129.

Wing, L. (1981b). Sex ratios in early childhood autism and related conditions. *Psychiatry Research, 5,* 129–137.

Wing, L. (1993). The definition and prevalence of autism: A review. *European Child and Adolescent Psychiatry, 2,* 61–74.

Wing, L., & Gould, J. (1979). Severe impairments of social interaction and associated abnormalities in children: Epidemiology and classification. *Journal of Autism and Developmental Disorders, 9,* 11–29.

Wing, L., & Shah, A. (1994, April 8–10). *Catatonic features in autism.* Paper read at the Autism on the Agenda Conference, Leeds.

Wolff, S. (1991). Schizoid personality in childhood and adult life. I: The vagaries of diagnostic labelling. *British Journal of Psychiatry, 159,* 615–620.

Wolff, S. (1996). The first account of the syndrome Asperger described? *European Child & Adolescent Psychiatry, 5,* 119–132.

Wolff, S., & Chick, J. (1980). Schizoid personality in childhood: A controlled follow-up study. *Psychological Medicine, 10,* 85–100.

Wolff, S., Townsend, R., McGuire, R. J., & Weeks, D. J. (1991). Schizoid personality in childhood and adult life. II: Adult adjustment and the continuity with schizotypal personality disorder. *British Journal of Psychiatry, 159,* 620–629.

World Health Organization. (1992). *The ICD-10 classification of mental and behavioural disorders. Clinical descriptions and guidelines.* Geneva: Author.

World Health Organization. (1993). *The ICD-10 classification of mental and behavioural disorders. Diagnostic criteria for research.* Geneva: Author.

Wurst, E. (1974). Lernstörungen aus der Sicht des Arztes. *Paediatrische Paedologie, 9,* 329–335.

6

Asperger Syndrome and Nonverbal Learning Disabilities

FRED R. VOLKMAR and AMI KLIN

INTRODUCTION

The year after Leo Kanner's report (1943) of the syndrome of early infantile autism, Hans Asperger, a Viennese physician, reported on a series of cases in which a major disability also involved interpersonal relationships. He coined the term *autistic psychopathy* (Asperger, 1944) to describe this condition. Asperger had not been aware of Kanner's earlier work; the use of the word *autistic* reflected an awareness on the part of both Asperger and Kanner that major aspects of social development were disturbed in the conditions they described. This apparent point of agreement has, however, led to major controversy about the validity of the conditions apart from each other. Diagnostic confusion and inconsistency has abounded surrounding the concept of Asperger syndrome (AS), as it is now termed. This confusion has related not only to the possible overlap of AS and autism, but also between AS and a series of other conditions or diagnostic concepts, many of which are described elsewhere in this volume. This confusion and the plethora of diagnostic concepts is a testament to the fact that the difficulties of many individuals with problems in social interaction have not fallen so neatly into the more well-established diagnostic categories.

FRED R. VOLKMAR and AMI KLIN • Child Study Center, Yale University School of Medicine, New Haven, Connecticut 06520.

Asperger Syndrome or High-Functioning Autism?, edited by Schopler *et al.* Plenum Press, New York, 1998.

Although the validity of AS remains to be firmly established, the research stimulated by the inclusion of the concept in DSM-IV (APA, 1994) and ICD-10 (WHO, 1990) has already been considerable. Such research is clearly needed to help clarify the diagnostic concept and its continuity, or discontinuity, with autism and with other conditions. In this chapter we note the areas of phenomenological overlap and divergence between what is termed in DSM-IV Asperger disorder and Higher Functioning Autism (HFA). The development of the current (DSM-IV) definition of AS is summarized. We also note areas of overlap between AS and other diagnostic concepts focusing, in particular, on what appears to us to be a very promising lead in this area: the convergence of AS (but not of HFA) with nonverbal learning disability (NLD).

ASPERGER SYNDROME: HISTORICAL BACKGROUND

The evolution of AS as a diagnostic concept has several parallels to the evolution of the concept of autism. Like Kanner's description of autism, Asperger's original report (1944, translated and annotated by Frith, 1991) provides a very lucid and atheoretical description that, in many ways, remains remarkably accurate.

Asperger's 1944 report described four boys who had marked problems in social interaction. The marked social disability and the implications for social adjustment led him to use the term *autistic psychopathy* for the condition; this was a major point of similarity to Kanner's (1943) description of autism. Both authors echoed Bleuler's (1916/1951) use of the term *autism* to signify extreme egocentrism or the shutting off of relations between the person affected and other people. However, Asperger's original description contained some important differences from Kanner's account, e.g., speech was less commonly delayed, cognitive abilities were more preserved, motor deficits were common, the onset appeared to be somewhat later, and all of the initial cases occurred only in boys. While Kanner had noted that his cases exhibited unusual responses to the environment, Asperger emphasized that in his group of cases circumscribed interests were common; these interests were pursued with such intensity that they became all-encompassing and interfered with other aspects of the child's functioning. Asperger originally suggested that similar problems could be observed in family members, particularly fathers.

Asperger's original report met with little interest for many years. Interestingly, reports of cases with many features suggestive of AS did appear in the English language literature; e.g., Robinson and Vitale (1954) described three children with patterns of circumscribed interests. Van Krevelen (1963, 1971) attempted to distinguish Asperger's cases (and syndrome) from Kanner's autism, suggesting that, in contrast to autism, the disability of individuals with AS was not detected until after age 3, early language skills were preserved, and the prognosis was rather good. It was, however, Wing's review and case series (1981) that attracted much greater interest to the diagnostic concept.

In her 1981 review, Wing suggested that some modifications of Asperger's original description were warranted; for example, that it could be observed in girls, that it was sometimes associated with mild degrees of mental handicap and language delays, and that patterns of genetic transmission were more complex than Asperger originally thought. Features of the condition were thought to include: problems related to difficulties with empathy and with a social style characterized by naive, inappropriate, one-sided social interaction with consequent social isolation; pedantic and monotonic speech; poor nonverbal communication; intense absorption in circumscribed topics typically learned in a rote fashion; and poor motor coordination with clumsiness and odd posture (Wing, 1981). Following Wing's report, interest in the condition has gradually, and progressively, increased with both clinical reports and research studies appearing with greater frequency (e.g., Frith, 1991; Gillberg & Gillberg, 1989; Tantam, 1988).

Issues In Syndrome Definition

Although interest in the condition markedly increased, two related sets of problems were the source of much confusion. In the absence, at least until very recently, of "official" definitions, the concept was both used in markedly different ways and overlapped in important ways with other diagnostic concepts. Much of the early controversy centered, and still centers, on the relationship of AS and autism. Essentially four different models of the syndrome developed: (1) AS was equated with higher-functioning autism or (2) equated with the "subthreshold" pervasive developmental disorder [Pervasive Developmental Disorder Not Otherwise Specified (PDD-NOS)] or (3) was sometimes thought to describe adults with autism. None of these conventions is of particular interest from the point of view of classification in that they simply provide alternative terms and not a truly new diagnostic concept. The fourth model, the one adopted in both DSM-IV (APA, 1994) and ICD-10 (WHO, 1990), attempts to delineate the two conditions as separate diagnostic entities, with a view to encourage validation research.

Another source of confusion stemmed from the development of other diagnostic concepts derived from diverse disciplines that shared at least some of the phenomenological features of AS. On the one hand, this is a testament to the complex problems for diagnosis that such cases present and the struggle of clinical investigators, working within different disciplines, to understand them. On the other hand, it has presented a major problem for research and has discouraged the development of broader and interdisciplinary perspectives. Other chapters in this volume provide summaries of some of these concepts, which include Schizoid Personality Disorder (Wolff & Barlow, 1979; Wolff &

Chick, 1980), Semantic–Pragmatic Disorder (Bishop, 1989), and Developmental Learning Disability of the Right Hemisphere (Denckla, 1983; Weintraub & Mesulam, 1983). Work on the concept of Nonverbal Learning Disabilities (Rourke, 1989) is described later in this chapter.

CURRENT DEFINITIONS

The absence of "official" definitions of AS contributed to the confusion surrounding the validity of the diagnostic concept (see Ghaziuddin, Tsai, & Ghaziuddin, 1992; Pomeroy, Friedman, & Stephens, 1991; Szatmari, 1992a,b; Szatmari, Tuff, Finlayson, & Bartolucci, 1990; Rutter and Schopler, 1992; Wing, 1991). AS was not included as an official diagnostic concept in DSM-III (APA, 1980) or DSM-III-R (APA, 1987), nor had it been included in ICD-9 (WHO, 1978). A draft definition of the condition was included in ICD-10 (WHO, 1990). The issue of whether or not to include AS as an "official" category in DSM-IV (APA, 1994) was controversial. Data from the large multisite DSM-IV field trial for autism (Volkmar et al., 1994) were helpful in the decision to include it as an official diagnostic category within the PDD class.

The DSM-IV field trial for autism was undertaken primarily for purposes of developing the definition of autism. The issue of compatibility between the two major official diagnostic systems, i.e., DSM and ICD, was a serious concern in that major inconsistencies in categories and criteria might further complicate interpretation of research. In the field trial, nearly 1000 cases were evaluated at over 20 sites in the United States and abroad. Raters used a standard coding system to record information about cases; in addition to ratings of various criteria for autism, raters also responded to a series of items relevant to the definition of AS, as it was then defined in the draft ICD-10. The definitions of AS and autism in ICD-10 were similar in their definition of the social deficits but differed in that in AS there should be no clinically significant general delay in language or cognitive development in the first 3 years of life. In ICD-10, for a diagnosis of AS the case also had to meet the criteria for restricted, repetitive, and stereotyped patterns of behavior, interests, and activities of the type observed in autism. The text of the ICD-10 draft definition emphasized that the validity of AS apart from higher-functioning autism remained controversial. ICD-10 also noted that motor delays/motor clumsiness were frequently associated features and that isolated special skills (often related to abnormal preoccupations) might be present.

In the DSM-IV field trial, 48 cases were submitted in which the rater felt that the primary clinical diagnosis (i.e., independent of formal diagnostic criteria) was most consistent with AS. In addition there were 3 additional cases in which criteria for the condition were apparently met. A series of analyses addressed aspects of the validity of AS apart from high-functioning autism (HFA) (this being the major comparison relevant to DSM-IV). The cases that appeared either by clinical diagnosis or ICD-10 criteria to have AS were indeed unlikely to exhibit delay in the development of spoken language. Although it might be argued that this is simply circular reasoning, the ICD-10 definition of AS stated only that early language should develop normally and not, necessarily, that it subsequently be normal in form or use (i.e., early language might appear on schedule but monotonic voice, pedantic speech, or other unusual features might be observed somewhat later). Accordingly, it was of interest that cases with apparent AS were significantly less likely than cases with a clinical diagnosis of autism or with an ICD-10 diagnosis of autism and IQ>85 to exhibit other associated language/communication deviance (χ^2=29.15, df=1, p<.001). In contrast to HFA cases, AS cases were significantly more likely to exhibit Verbal IQ scores greater than Performance IQ scores, a pattern not seen for HFA cases. Consistent with the ICD-10 definition, motor delays were more variable in AS than in HFA cases (χ^2=0.536, df=1, NS) (see Ghaziuddin et al., 1992). Isolated special skills, often related to abnormal preoccupations, were, however, more common in the group with a clinical diagnosis of AS (χ^2=3.917, df=1, p<.05). In an additional series of comparisons, apparent AS was compared with HFA as to the total number of criteria exhibited in various areas. Cases with either a clinical diagnosis of AS or, in three instances, a retrospective diagnosis of AS based on ICD-10 criteria, were noted to have significantly fewer total social symptoms, significantly fewer problems in communication, and significantly fewer resistance to change criteria. In addition, apparent AS was compared with clinical diagnoses of either atypical autism or PDD-NOS that did not meet criteria for autism. These comparisons are particularly relevant to the question of whether AS is simply a variant of PDD-NOS/atypical autism. In these comparisons, AS cases exhibited significantly more social and resistance to change criteria. The groups did not differ in terms of the total number of language/communication criteria, but if the analysis was restricted only to those items related to aspects of communication (as opposed to language per se), the AS group exhibited significantly fewer such symptoms.

Based on these findings, a decision was made to include AS in DSM IV. The definitions of AS in DSM-IV and ICD-10 are similar but not identical (see Klin, Sparrow, Volkmar, Cicchetti, & Rourke, 1995, for a discussion). In both diagnostic systems, motor clumsiness and unusual circumscribed interests can be associated with the condition but are not required for the diagnosis. The failure to include these features as central in the definition is somewhat problematic, given that these symptoms have sometimes been thought to be specific markers of the condition. Starting with Asperger's original description (1944), and continuing to the present (Tantam, 1991), delays in the acquisition of motor milestones and the presence of motor clumsiness have frequently been mentioned. In our experience in clinical work with such individuals, it is typical for parents to report delays in activities such as learning to ride a bicycle, catching a ball, using the hands for fine motor activities, and so on. Activities that require visual-motor coordination are usually not an area of strength; this is in contrast to autism where motor abilities, at least early in life, are relatively preserved (Volkmar *et al.*, 1987). In DSM-IV there is a requirement that adaptive skills (other than in social interaction) not be significantly delayed; in fact, this criterion is poorly worded. The essential issue here, not adequately captured by the final wording of the criterion, is that *early* adaptive skills are generally within normal limits; i.e., consistent with Asperger's original report, parents are not usually concerned about the child's development until after age 3. It is the case that later in life multiple deficits in the development of various adaptive skills are, in fact, observed.

It also appears that individuals with AS have a much more narrowly defined deficit in the area of restricted interests and activities relative to persons with autism. In autism, skills that involve object manipulation, and visual-spatial or musical skills, are sometimes relatively well preserved, and, occasionally, represent areas of peak performance. In contrast, in AS it is much more common for the individual to be geared toward amassing tremendous amounts of factual detail about some all-absorbing, circumscribed topic (Gillberg, 1989; Wing, 1991). Although the particular topic may change over time, it usually dominates essentially all social interaction between individuals with AS and others. This symptom can be difficult, at times, to identify in younger children, i.e., when interests in dinosaurs or similar topics are so ubiquitous. However, with time, the interest usually does differ either in terms of its unusual focus (e.g., in deep-fat fryers, telegraph pole insulators) or the intensity with which it is pursued. In general, extraordinary amounts of factual information relative to the person's developmental level are learned about the topic with surprisingly little conceptual understanding of the basic phenomena involved.

Although the availability of compatible official definitions of the conditions will undoubtedly help to stimulate further and more consistent research, it must be noted that the validity status of the concept remains controversial and that the current definitions of the condition will surely be further refined in years to come. In particular, the issues of whether or not motor clumsiness and/or circumscribed interests should be essential diagnostic features of AS will need to be clarified. The lack of truly operational definitions for motor clumsiness is problematic. A developmental and longitudinal perspective will clearly be needed as it appears that symptoms change over time, and may have more or less discriminative power depending on the developmental period examined (see Klin & Volkmar, 1997, for a discussion).

VALIDITY OF ASPERGER SYNDROME APART FROM AUTISM

As noted, the validity of AS relative to autism has been the focus of considerable controversy. In establishing that the two conditions are indeed distinctive, several issues are important. The use of explicit and operational definitions is critical. Also, potential validating features should not arise in a circular fashion from the definitions employed.

There is little disagreement that AS is on a continuum with autism, particularly in relation to the problems in the areas of social functioning. For example, using DSM-III-R (APA, 1987), about 50% of persons with what we now recognize as AS would have met criteria for autistic disorder (Volkmar et al., 1994). What is less clear is whether the condition is qualitatively different from HFA. A handful of studies (e.g., Klin, Volkmar, Sparrow, Cicchetti, & Rourke, 1995; Ozonoff, Rogers, & Pennington, 1991; Szatmari et al., 1990) have addressed this issue with mixed results. Differences have been observed with regard to aspects of AS such as its apparent later onset, association with better language abilities, motor clumsiness, special interests, and so forth.However, Wing (1981) noted that a few individuals in her series of cases appeared to exhibit autism early in life but then had a presentation in adolescence more suggestive of AS. The lack of systematic longitudinal studies complicates the interpretation of such case reports; it does appear to us that a diagnosis of AS can be made more confidently for older children, when the most conspicuous symptoms — verbosity and circumscribed areas of interest — become more apparent.

On the other hand, a number of studies have supported Asperger's (1979) observation of much better outcome in AS relative to HFA (Howlin, in press; Rutter & Schopler, 1987). Other studies have also supported Asperger's original (1944) observation of much higher rates of the condition in first-degree relatives (e.g., Burgoine & Wing, 1983; Gillberg & Gillberg, 1989). There is, however, a growing appreciation of the role of genetic factors in autism as well (Rutter, 1992).

A final area of work has focused on differences in neurocognitive profiles associated with AS and HFA. This work is of particular interest given the earlier observation, in the DSM-IV autism/PDD field trial (Volkmar et al., 1994), that the patterns of strength/weakness in cognitive ability significantly differed in the two conditions, at least in regard to profiles in IQ testing. This observation has led us to undertake a program of research in which the potential convergence of AS and the nonverbal learning disabilities (NLD) profile is being systematically examined.

NONVERBAL LEARNING DISABILITIES

The concept of NLD was originally proposed by Johnson and Myklebust (Myklebust, 1975) and, subsequently, has been extensively studied by Rourke and colleagues (see Rourke, 1989). NLD refers to a profile of neuropsychological assets and deficits that impact negatively on the person's capacity for social interaction and produce characteristic styles of communication and social interaction. As outlined by Rourke (1989), characteristics of NLD include deficits in tactile perception, psychomotor coordination, visual-spatial organization, non-verbal problem-solving, and appreciation of incongruities and humor. Persons with NLD typically exhibit relatively well-developed rote verbal capacities and verbal memory skills. They also typically have difficulty in adapting to novel and complex situations; in such situations, they tend to overly rely on their rote memory skills rather than adjusting to and compensating for novelty. Typically, poor pragmatics and prosody in speech are observed.

The social deficits associated with the NLD profile are significant and include problems in social perception as well as in social judgment. Difficulties with social interaction stem from difficulties in adjusting to novelty and in the failure to appreciate subtle but important nuances in nonverbal communication. As a result, Rourke has suggested that persons with the NLD profile are likely to experience much frustration in social situations and in establishing relationships, and are at a high risk for mood disorders (Rourke, Young, & Leenaars, 1989).

A major contribution of work on the NLD concept has been the attempt to understand, in a truly developmental sense, the interplay of children's social and emotional development with a unique profile of neuropsychological assets and deficits. Many of the clinical features associated with the NLD profile have also been described in the neurological literature in relation to the concepts of Developmental Learning Disability of the Right Hemisphere or Social-Emotional Learning Disabilities (Denckla, 1983; Voeller, 1991; Weintraub & Mesulam, 1983). Children presenting with this condition exhibit profound disturbances in interpretation and expression of affect and other basic interpersonal skills that are thought to relate to underlying right-hemisphere dysfunction and the central role of that brain area in processing social-emotional information (Voeller, 1986, 1991). This observation is particularly interesting, as neuropsychologists have typically speculated that left-hemisphere dysfunction is more characteristic of autism (e.g., Dawson, Finley, Phillips, & Galpert, 1986). The potential for an empirical distinction of HFA and AS on the basis of neuropsychological profiles, independent of diagnostic criteria, avoids the problem of circularity and may provide much stronger evidence for distinctions between the two conditions.

Neuropsychological Studies

Several studies have examined aspects of neurocognitive profiles that might differentiate individuals with AS from those with HFA (Klin, Sparrow, et al., 1995; Klin, Volkmar, et al., 1995; Ozonoff et al., 1991; Szatmari et al., 1990). Unfortunately, various problems complicate the interpretation of this work. Szatmari et al. (1990) administered a battery of tests to groups of subjects thought to have AS and HFA. The groups were similar in terms of IQ but differed in chronological age. Group differences were minimal but the AS group did have a significantly higher score on one subtest of the WISC-R (Similarities), and the HFA group exhibited better performance on a test of motor coordination and speed and were slightly more likely to engage in perseveration. Ozonoff *et al.* (1991) administered an extensive test battery to 13 subjects with HFA and 10 with AS. The two groups differed in terms of verbal IQ (VIQ) but did not differ on full-scale IQ, performance IQ (PIQ), or chronological age. Differences between the groups were minimal, except for better verbal memory in the AS subjects, which likely reflected the better verbal abilities of the AS group.

In contrast to these two studies, we (Klin, Volkmar, *et al.*, 1995) found major differences between groups of very stringently defined AS and HFA cases. This study was inspired by the observation of marked differences in patterns of VIQ–PIQ noted in the DSM-IV field trial. In light of the ambiguities in diagnosis that we observed, even with the DSM-IV and ICD-10 criteria, we made the explicit decision to employ a particularly stringent definition of AS. For this study, to be included in the AS group, the case had to meet ICD-10 criteria and had to exhibit motor clumsiness and a circumscribed interest (i.e., two features that have consistently been reported in AS but are not technically required in the DSM-IV/ICD-10 definitions of AS). It appeared to us that an appropriate research strategy would be to look for group differences with the most stringent definition, i.e., if group differences were not observed with a stringent definition, it was unlikely that they would be observed in less stringently defined groups. Also, the definition of AS employed was probably much closer to Aperger's original (1944) diagnostic concept.

Nineteen individuals with HFA (as established using ICD-10 draft research criteria) and 21 with AS (using ICD-10 research criteria and the requirement of delayed motor milestones/motor clumsiness and an isolated special interest or skill) were examined. Cases were evaluated either at Yale or elsewhere (cases in the latter group had contacted us through the Learning Disabilities Association of America). To be selected for either group, the case had to have a full-scale IQ of over 70. The mean full-scale IQ of the HFA group was 95.6 and that of the AS group was 96.7; the groups did not differ in terms of chronological age or sex distribution. Diagnoses were assigned independently of IQ by two experienced clinicians. Twenty-two items were abstracted from Rourke's (1989) description of NLD and rated independently by two neuropsychologists. Items assessed predicted areas of strength/weakness as described in Rourke's model of NLD. Reliability of clinical diagnosis, diagnostic criteria, and the NLD items were fair to excellent.

Although the two groups did not differ in terms of their full-scale IQ, the AS group exhibited a pattern of significantly higher VIQ and lower PIQ in comparison with the HFA group, for which VIQs and PIQs were not significantly different. There was a high degree of correspondence between the NLD profile

Table 6-1. Frequency of Subjects Exhibiting Deficits on the
22 NLD Items

Item	HFA	AS	Fisher's p
Fine motor skills	6/19	19/21	.001[c]
Gross motor skills	12/19	21/21	.003[b]
Visual-motor integration	8/19	19/21	.002[b]
Visual-spatial perception	5/19	16/21	.004[b]
Auditory perception	10/19	1/21	.001[b]
Novel material	11/19	15/21	.510
Rote material	2/19	0/21	.219
Verbal memory	11/19	5/21	.049[a]
Visual memory	9/19	19/21	.005[b]
Verbal concept formation	10/19	10/21	1.000
Nonverbal concept formation	5/19	16/21	.004[b]
Articulation	11/19	1/21	.001[c]
Vocabulary	8/19	0/21	.001[b]
Verbal output	11/19	1/21	.001[c]
Verbal content	18/19	20/21	1.000
Prosody	17/19	19/21	1.000
Pragmatics	16/19	20/21	.331
Word decoding	7/19	2/21	.060
Reading/comprehension	10/19	10/21	1.000
Arithmetic	8/19	9/21	1.000
Social competence	19/19	21/21	1.000
Emotional	19/19	21/21	1.000

[a] $p < .05$, [b] $p < .01$, [c] $p < .001$.
From Klin, A., Volkmar, F. R., Sparrow, S. S., Cicchetti, D. V., & Rourke, B. P. (1995).
Validity and neuropsychological characterization of Asperger syndrome. *Journal of
Child Psychology and Psychiatry, 36*, 1127–1140. Adapted by permission.

and AS (21 cases) whereas only 1 of the 19 HFA cases appeared to exhibit the
NLD profile ($p<.001$). Of 22 items related to NLD, significant differences were
observed in 11 comparisons (see Table 6-1). Six areas of deficit were associated
with AS (deficits in fine and gross motor skills, visual-motor integration, visual-
spatial perception, nonverbal concept formation, and visual memory); con-
versely, five areas of deficit were predictive of a diagnosis of "not-AS"
(articulation, verbal output, auditory perception, vocabulary, and verbal memory). In summary, this study indicated a marked overlap of NLD with AS, but
not with HFA; this suggests an important empirical distinction between AS and
HFA based on neurocognitive profiles independent of diagnostic criteria. The
results obtained regarding the pattern of neuropsychological ability observed are
consistent with previous case reports of AS (Gillberg, 1989; Wing, 1981) and
HFA (e.g., Dawson, 1983; Lincoln, Courchesne, Kilman, Elmasian, & Allen,
1988).

How are the differences from this study and the two earlier studies to be
reconciled? It seems very likely that the differences in the neuropsychological

studies reported to date are a function of different approaches to diagnosis, i.e., the definition of AS subjects has differed from study to study and results have varied accordingly. In our study, we explicitly adopted what we thought would be the most stringent diagnostic approach. This approach produced results very similar to the pattern obtained in the DSM-IV field trial (Volkmar *et al.*, 1994). The definition employed by Szatmari *et al.* (1990) was much less stringent, whereas that employed by Ozonoff *et al.* (1991) was based on ICD-10 but excluded the onset criteria and did not include any additional requirement regarding special interests or motor clumsiness; future studies should strive to adopt similar definitions in order to make possible direct comparisons.

NLD as a Neuropsychological Model of AS

From a developmental viewpoint, the overlap of NLD and AS (but not of HFA) could suggest two different pathogenic courses and consequent profiles of adjustment in AS and HFA (Klin *et al.*, 1996). Autism is typically marked by a profound lack of interest in social stimuli beginning very early in life (Lord, 1993), expressed in the lack of acquisition of basic social skills such as reacting differentially to speech sounds (Klin, 1991), appreciating the salience of faces (Volkmar, 1987), acquiring very basic social adaptive skills typically seen in normatively developing infants (Klin, Volkmar, & Sparrow, 1992), and develop ing the typical patterns of attachment normatively seen in babies (Kasari, Sigman, Mundy, & Yirmiya, 1990). The developmental path that follows takes place alongside and shows little interaction with the social realm, as emotional, cognitive, language, and play skills unfold in a manner that is both rigid and lacking in symbolic content; a sense of self is diminished as a result of a poor conception of others, their feelings and motivations (Klin, 1989). In other words, a constitutional lack of mechanisms of sociability, yet to be fully understood (Brothers, 1989), sets the limitations on social adjustment irrespective of cognitive endowment.

In contrast, AS is marked by a cluster of neuropsychological deficits (as well as assets) that are captured by the NLD profile (see Table 6-2). This profile limits the children's ability to make full use of intact sociability mechanisms because it affects their capacity to process a wide range of nonverbal stimuli in the various modalities (tactile, visual, auditory). As the context of social inter-actions is conveyed primarily through nonverbal means (tone and melody of voice, facial and body gestures, social touch), individuals with AS may miss the value and meaning of the interaction, resorting to the more explicit, and verbal, aspects of the contact. As a consequence, they may hold on to the explicit and literal value of communications, which can only approximate (and may often mislead, e.g., in teasing, humor) the actual valence of the social interchange. Devoid of nonverbal and intuitive social understanding, the emotions, motiva-

Table 6-2. The NLD Profile of Deficits and Assets

Deficits	Assets
Tactile and visual-spatial perception	Auditory perception
Visual-motor integration	Verbal skills
Visual memory	Verbal memory
Novel learning	Rote learning
Prosody	Articulation
Verbal content	Vocabulary
Pragmatics	Verbal output

tions, and intentions of other people may present individuals with AS with an ongoing puzzle, leading them to take charge of the interaction by talking incessantly and one-sidedly about a topic that they know well as a result of their drive to amass factual information (see Table 6-3). By so doing, they may adjust to the reciprocity demands inherent in social conversation by presenting with a semblance of competent communication. This strategy is only partially success-ful, as this eccentricity and one-sidedness often alienate others, leading to repeated experiences of social failure and the resultant feelings of despondency and negativism. In other words, the neuropsychological disability prevents them from fulfilling their wish to establish relationships.

Although these models are certainly too simplistic to capture the wide range of phenotypic expression in both AS and HFA, they may have heuristic value insofar as they delineate different pathogenic courses for the two condi-tions. If supported by research into the onset patterns and early life of individuals with AS and HFA, they could help focus future studies and help us understand potential differences in course and associated clinical features. In this respect, preliminary data pertaining to these issues appear to support the general predic-tions made by this model (Klin *et al.*, 1996). Models such as these could also provide some guidelines for developmental, psychopathological research into

Table 6-3. Phenotypic Illustrations of Developmental
Implications of NLD Profile

- Talkative but often fails to convey coherent message
- Insensitive to nonverbal cues
- Conformity to rules and poor ability to cope with novel situation when intuition and/or improvisation are needed
- Difficulty with nonliteral language
- Empathy may be formal and explicit but not spontaneous and implicit
- Rigidity in regard to social conventions
- Social approaches are based on explicit verbal, one-sided communication about narrow interest
- Insight into self and condition is limited

other social disabilities that do not fall neatly into any of the current categorical definitions. It is very likely that there may be multiple pathways to severe social disabilities other than the one known to characterize individuals with classic autism.

SUMMARY

Interest in AS has markedly increased in recent years. This reflects an awareness that many individuals with marked social problems do not seem to exhibit autism as the latter is usually defined. The plethora of diagnostic concepts attests to the fact that individuals from diverse disciplines deal with this group of cases in different, but also convergent, ways. The current interest in AS as a diagnostic concept is reflected both in research and in the growing use, often ill-considered, of the term in clinical practice.

Another, and more fundamental, reason for the current upsurge of interest in AS is the increasing appreciation that the study of this condition, and of autism, may help us understand more about the neurobiological bases of socialization. In this regard, work from a neuropsychological and developmental perspective on the NLD syndrome has particular interest. The convergence of this profile of deficits and assets with AS suggests particular strategies for intervention and diagnosis as well as a broader line of research inquiry into the neurobiological correlates of the condition. Finally, a review of the studies completed over the last several years underscores the need to adopt explicit, and whenever possible, consensual, definitions of the condition to facilitate both comparability of research and clinical service.

REFERENCES

American Psychiatric Association. (1980). *Diagnostic and statistical manual of mental disorders* (3rd ed.). Washington, DC: Author.

American Psychiatric Association. (1987). *Diagnostic and statistical manual of mental disorders* (3rd ed. rev.). Washington, DC: Author.

American Psychiatric Association. (1994). *Diagnostic and statistical manual of mental disorders* (4th ed.). Washington, DC: Author.

Asperger, H. (1944). Die "Autistischen Psychopathen" im Kindesalter. *Archiv für Psychiatrie und Nervenkrankheiten, 117*, 76–136.

Asperger, H. (1979). Problems of infantile autism. *Communication, 13*, 45–52.

Bishop, D. V. M. (1989). Autism, Asperger's syndrome and semantic-pragmatic disorder: Where are the boundaries? *British Journal of Disorders of Communication, 24*, 107–121.

Bleuler, E. (1951). *Textbook of psychiatry*. (A. A. Brill, Trans.). New York: Dover. (Original work published 1916).

Brothers, L. (1989). A biological perspective on empathy. *American Journal of Psychiatry, 146*, 10–19.

Burgoine, E., & Wing, L. (1983). Identical triplets with Asperger's syndrome. *British Journal of Psychiatry, 143*, 261–265.

Dawson, G. (1983). Lateralized brain dysfunction in autism: Evidence from the Halstead–Reitan Neuropsychological Battery. *Journal of Autism and Developmental Disorders, 13*, 269–286.

Dawson, G., Finley, C., Phillips, S., & Galpert, L. (1986). Hemispheric specialization and the language abilities of autistic children. *Child Development, 57*(6), 1440–1453.

Denckla, M. B. (1983). The neuropsychology of social-emotional learning disabilities. *Archives of Neurology, 40*, 461–462.

Frith, U. (Ed.). (1991). *Autism and Asperger syndrome*. Cambridge: Cambridge University Press.

Ghaziuddin, M., Tsai, L. Y., & Ghaziuddin, N. (1992). A reappraisal of clumsiness as a diagnostic feature of Asperger syndrome. *Journal of Autism and Developmental Disorders, 22*, 651–656.

Gillberg, C. (1989). Asperger syndrome in 23 Swedish children. *Developmental Medicine and Child Neurology, 31*, 520–531.

Gillberg, I. C., & Gillberg, C. (1989). Asperger syndrome — some epidemiological considerations: A research note. *Journal of Child Psychology and Psychiatry, 30*, 631–638.

Kanner, L. (1943). Autistic disturbances of affective contact. *Nervous Child, 2*, 217–250.

Kasari, C., Sigman, M., Mundy, P., & Yirmiya, N. (1990). Affective sharing in the context of joint attention interactions of normal, autistic, and mentally retarded children. *Journal of Autism and Developmental Disorders, 20*, 87–100.

Klin, A. (1989). Understanding early infantile autism: An application of G. H. Mead's theory of the emergence of mind. *L.S.E. Quarterly, 4*(3), 336–356.

Klin, A., Sparrow, S. S., Volkmar, F. R., Cicchetti, D. V., & Rourke, B. P. (1995). Asperger syndrome. In B. P. Rourke (Ed.), *Syndrome of nonverbal learning disabilities: Neurodevelopmental manifestations* (pp. 93–118). New York: Guilford Press.

Klin, A., & Volkmar, F. R. (1997). Asperger's syndrome. In D. J. Cohen & F. R. Volkmar (Eds.), *Handbook of autism and pervasive developmental disorders*. New York: Wiley.

Klin, A., Volkmar, F. R., & Sparrow, S. S. (1992). Autistic social dysfunction: Some limitations of the theory of mind hypothesis. *Journal of Child Psychology and Psychiatry, 33*, 861–876.

Klin, A., Volkmar, F. R., Sparrow, S. S., Cicchetti, D. V., & Rourke, B. P. (1995). Validity and neuropsychological characterization of Asperger syndrome. *Journal of Child Psychology and Psychiatry, 36*, 1127–1140.

Klin, A., Volkmar, F. R., Sparrow, S. S., Rourke, B. P., & Cicchetti, D. V. (1996, June). *A developmental psychopathological model of Asperger syndrome*. Paper presented at the 19th Annual Mid-Year Meeting of the International Neuropsychological Society. Veldhoven, Netherlands.

Lincoln, A. J., Courchesne, E., Kilman, B. A., Elmasian, R., & Allen, M. (1988). A study of intellectual abilities in high-functioning people with autism. *Journal of Autism and Developmental Disorders, 18*, 505–524.

Lord, C. (1993). Early social development in autism. In E. Schopler, M. E. Van Bourgondien, & M. M. Bristol (Eds.), *Preschool issues in autism* (pp. 61–94). New York: Plenum Press.

Myklebust, H. R. (1975). Nonverbal learning disabilities: Assessment and intervention. In H. R. Myklebust (Ed.), *Progress in learning disabilities* (Vol. 3, pp. 281–301). New York: Grune & Stratton.

Ozonoff, S., Rogers, S. J., & Pennington, B. F. (1991). Asperger's syndrome: Evidence of an empirical distinction from high-functioning autism. *Journal of Child Psychology and Psychiatry, 32*, 1107–1122.

Pomeroy, J. C., Friedman, C., & Stephens, L. (1991). Autism and Asperger's: Same or different? *Journal of the American Academy of Child and Adolescent Psychiatry, 30*, 152–153.

Robinson, J. F., & Vitale, L. J. (1954). Children with circumscribed interests. *American Journal of Orthopsychiatry, 24*, 755–764.

Rourke, B. (1989). *Nonverbal learning disabilities: The syndrome and the model*. New York: Guilford Press.

Rourke, B., Young, G. C., & Leenaars, A. A. (1989). A childhood learning disability that predisposes those afflicted to adolescent and adult depression and suicide risk. *Journal of Learning Disabilities, 22*, 169–185.

Rutter, M. (1992, May). *Autism: Genetic aspects*. Paper presented at the 4th Congress, Autism Europe, Den Haag, Holland.

Rutter, M., & Schopler, E. (1987). Autism and pervasive developmental disorders: Concepts and diagnostic issues. *Journal of Autism and Developmental Disorders, 17,* 159–186.

Rutter, M., & Schopler, E. (1992). Classification of pervasive developmental disorders: Some concepts and practical considerations. *Journal of Autism and Developmental Disorders, 22,* 459–482.

Szatmari, P. (1992a). A review of the DSM-III-R criteria for autistic disorder. *Journal of Autism and Developmental Disorders, 22,* 507–524.

Szatmari, P. (1992b). The validity of autistic spectrum disorders: A literature review. *Journal of Autism and Developmental Disorders, 22,* 583–600.

Szatmari, P., Tuff, L., Finlayson, M. A. J., & Bartolucci, G. (1990). Asperger's syndrome and autism: Neurocognitive aspects. *Journal of the American Academy of Child and Adolescent Psychiatry, 29,* 130–136.

Tantam, D. (1988). Annotation: Asperger's syndrome. *Journal of Child Psychology and Psychiatry, 29,* 245–255.

Tantam, D. (1991). Asperger syndrome in adulthood. In U. Frith (Ed.), *Autism and Asperger syndrome* (pp.147–183). Cambridge: Cambridge University Press.

Van Krevelen, D. A. (1963). On the relationship between early infantile autism and autistic psychopathy. *Acta Paedopsychiatrica, 30,* 303–323.

Van Krevelen, D. A. (1971). Early infantile autism and autistic psychopathy. *Journal of Autism and Childhood Schizophrenia, 1,* 82–86.

Voeller, K. K. S. (1986). Right-hemisphere deficit syndrome in children. *American Journal of Psychiatry, 143,* 1004–1009.

Voeller, K. K. S. (1991). Social-emotional learning disabilities. *Psychiatric Annals, 21*(12), 735–741.

Volkmar, F. R. (1987). Social development. In D. J. Cohen & A. M. Donnellan (Eds.), *Handbook of autism and pervasive developmental disorders* (pp. 41–60). New York: Wiley

Volkmar, F. R., Klin, A., Siegel, B., Szatmari, P., Lord, C., Campbell, M., Freeman, B. J., Cicchetti, D. V., Rutter, M., Kline, W., Buitelaar, J., Hattab, Y., Fombonne, E., Fuentes, J., Werry, J., Stone, W., Kerbeshian, J., Hoshino, Y., Bregman, J., Loveland, K., Szymanski, L., & Towbin, K. (1994). DSM-IV autism/pervasive developmental disorder field trial. *American Journal of Psychiatry, 151,* 1361–1367.

Volkmar, F. R., Sparrow, S. S., Goudreau, D., Cicchetti, D. V., Paul, R., & Cohen, D. J. (1987). Social deficits in autism: An operational approach using the Vineland Adaptive Behavior Scales. *Journal of the American Academy of Child and Adolescent Psychiatry, 26,* 156–161.

Weintraub, S., & Mesulam, M. M. (1983). Developmental learning disabilities of the right hemisphere: Emotional, interpersonal, and cognitive components. *Archives of Neurology, 40,* 463–468.

Wing, L. (1981). Asperger's syndrome: A clinical account. *Psychological Medicine, 11,* 115–129.

Wing, L. (1991). The relationship between Asperger's syndrome and Kanner's autism. In U. Frith (Ed.), *Autism and Asperger syndrome* (pp. 93–121). Cambridge: Cambridge University Press.

Wolff, S., & Barlow, A. (1979). Schizoid personality in childhood: A comparative study of schizoid, autistic and normal children. *Journal of Child Psychology and Psychiatry, 20,* 19–46.

Wolff, S., & Chick, J. (1980). Schizoid personality in childhood: A controlled follow-up study. *Psychological Medicine, 10,* 85–100.

World Health Organization. (1978). *Mental disorders: Glossary and guide to their classification in accordance with the ninth revision of the international classification of diseases*. Geneva: Author.

World Health Organization. (1990, May). *International classification of diseases: Tenth revision. Chapter V. Mental and behavioral disorders (including disorders of psychological development). Diagnostic criteria for research*. Geneva: Author.

7

Schizoid Personality in Childhood

The Links with Asperger Syndrome, Schizophrenia
Spectrum Disorders, and Elective Mutism

SULA WOLFF

INTRODUCTION

The aim of this chapter is to draw attention to a group of patients, not uncom-
monly seen in child psychiatric practice, who were diagnosed as having a
schizoid personality disorder. They appear to be quite similar to the patients
Asperger described (1944), but do not entirely fulfill current diagnostic criteria
for Asperger syndrome (AS) (WHO, 1992, 1993; APA, 1994). The children's
impairments are less severe and their future outlook is much better than those of
patients now given a diagnosis of AS. In addition, a few did have significant
early language delays. In clinical practice it is important to recognise schizoid
children so that their treatment and educational needs can be adequately met.
The condition raises important questions about etiology and classification.

The chapter starts with an account of the main features of the condition and
of a prognostic validation study. The multiple diagnostic labels that have been
applied to affected children will be mentioned, and the similarity of the syndrome
to Asperger's original description of autistic psychopathy pointed out. Next, the link
between schizoid personality of childhood and the schizophrenia spectrum will be
described. The relationship between schizoid personality and childhood autism will

SULA WOLFF • Formerly of the Department of Psychiatry, Royal Hospital for Sick Children and
the University of Edinburgh, Edinburgh EH9 1RL, Scotland.

Asperger Syndrome or High-Functioning Autism?, edited by Schopler *et al.* Plenum Press, New York,
1998.

be clarified in terms of the similarities and differences of symptoms and of psychological functioning, and in terms of a possible common genetic factor. Current concepts of AS as defined in ICD-10 and DSM-IV will be reviewed in relation to our own outcome studies of schizoid children. Treatment needs will then be discussed. A note on the association with developmental language disorders and elective mutism follows. The chapter ends with some conclusions.

SCHIZOID PERSONALITY IN CHILDHOOD AND ITS RELATIONSHIP TO ASPERGER'S AUTISTIC PSYCHOPATHY

The Core Features and Their Persistence over Time

In the 1960s, before DSM-III categories of personality disorders were available, we found that about 4% of children referred to a general child psychiatric department had an unusual clinical picture with persistent social isolation and idiosyncratic behavior (Wolff, 1964, 1995; Chick, 1978; Wolff & Chick, 1980). The children often presented with common child psychiatric symptoms such as conduct disorders or school refusal, but their difficulties could not be explained by adverse life experiences. Exploratory approaches failed to illuminate the problems and sometimes made matters worse. Over half the children were outgoing but a few were withdrawn and uncommunicative, and occasionally they had elective mutism. They often caused enormous difficulties for parents and teachers because they could not conform socially, reacting with outbursts of weeping, rage, or aggression if pressed to do so. More boys than girls were affected, at a ratio later found to be 3.4:1 (Wolff & McGuire, 1995). Intelligence was within the normal range but upwardly skewed in the boys who, unlike affected girls, also came from an upwardly skewed social class background (Wolff & McGuire, 1995).

In a prognostic validation study of the syndrome (Wolff & Chick, 1980) we operationalized what seemed to be its core features: solitariness (the children were "loners"); lack of empathy for the feelings and thoughts of others, with emotional detachment; increased sensitivity, at times with paranoid ideation; rigidity of mental set, especially the single-minded pursuit of special interests (such as electronics, architectural drawings, antiques, astronomy, dinosaurs, politics); and unusual styles of communicating such as odd use of metaphor, over- or undertalkativeness. In a 10-year follow-up study by a "blind" interviewer, using a semistructured and reliable interview, these core features distinguished significantly between a group of schizoid boys and a matched control group of boys who had been referred to the same clinic with other diagnoses, as did one further characteristic: an unusual fantasy life (Chick, 1978; Wolff & Chick, 1980). Moreover, the interviewer identified 18 of the 22 schizoid young men and only 1 of the 22 controls as "definitely schizoid." The syndrome was clearly very long lasting, as one would expect from a personality disorder.

Why We Chose the Label Schizoid Personality

We used the diagnostic label *schizoid personality* before we were aware of Asperger's seminal paper, because the children resembled accounts of patients with this personality disorder in the older psychiatric literature. The term was then used for a constellation of personality traits found to excess premorbidly in a proportion of schizophrenic patients and in their biological relatives (Wolff & Chick, 1980; see also Ssucharewa, 1926; Heston & Denney, 1968; Bleuler, 1978).

A Confusion of Diagnostic Terms

What appears to be the same childhood condition has been described under a variety of different diagnostic terms. Psychoanalysts reported on children with "benign psychoses," "ego" disturbances, and "borderline states" (Mahler, Ross, & De Fries, 1949; Weil, 1953; Geleert, 1967); others on children with "circum-scribed interest patterns" (Robinson & Vitale, 1954), or young people with "right hemisphere deficits" (Weintraub & Mesulam, 1983; Voeller, 1986). Yet another label, "multiplex developmental disorder," has been applied (Cohen, Paul, & Volkmar, 1986), sometimes to rather more seriously impaired children who would generally now be diagnosed as having AS (van der Gaag, 1993).

Perhaps the first account of the condition, under the label *schizoid personality disorder*, appeared in 1926. This is a report of six cases of "schizoid psychopathy of childhood" from the hospital school of the Moscow psychoneurological children's in-patient department (Ssucharewa, 1926; Wolff, 1996). All were boys, aged 10 to 14 years. They had been different from other children since early childhood: They were solitary; adapted poorly to the demands of their environment; and, although themselves excessively sensitive, their responses to other people were superficial. They showed limited facial expressions of emotion, and had oddities of speech and voice as well as thinking, with a tendency to abstract, ruminative thought processes. Motor clumsiness was striking and obsessionality a frequent feature. Three of the six boys were musical, one was interested in politics and social issues, and two had literary gifts. Five were of above-average intelligence, several came from gifted families, and their parents often had similar personality traits. Dr. Ssucharewa thought the children resembled Kretschmer's schizoid types: that they had an inborn predisposition to an unusual personality that had some but not all of the features of schizophrenia, but that their course was quite different from that of patients with schizophrenia because there was no deterioration with age.

The Links with Asperger's Autistic Psychopathy

As soon as Asperger's 1944 paper on autistic psychopathy of childhood became familiar to English readers (Van Krevelen, 1971; Wing, 1976; Everard, 1976), we recognized the resemblance of our children to those he had described (see chapter 2 of this volume), except that we found a number of girls to be affected also. Asperger himself never saw the full syndrome in girls before puberty in the absence of brain damage (Asperger, 1944; Wolff & Chick, 1980).

A Systematic Look at the Childhood Picture

In order to put the childhood symptomatology on a firmer basis, we undertook an analysis of the clinical case records of 32 matched pairs of schizoid and control boys and 33 matched pairs of girls, all of whom had been referred to a child psychiatric department (Wolff, 1991; Wolff & McGuire, 1995). Although the main rater was not "blind" to the diagnoses, agreement with a "blind," independent rater was satisfactory (mean weighted kappa 0.73). We found that being a "loner" and having "unusual fantasies" significantly differentiated schizoid girls and boys from their matched controls with other diagnoses. The third feature that could be rated, special interest patterns, differentiated highly between schizoid and control boys, but was rare among the girls in childhood and did not significantly distinguish between the two groups. The other core features we had found for schizoid personality—impaired empathy, excessive sensitivity, and odd styles of communication—were rarely recorded in the case notes particularly of the control children.

The case note analysis established high rates of comorbidity, especially conduct disorder, as also reported for AS by Szatmari et al. (1989). These workers stressed the diagnostic difficulties this can pose. Conduct disorders were particularly striking among our schizoid girls. Pure emotional disorders were rare. A further finding was the high rate of specific developmental delays affecting not only motor and educational functioning but language development too. Asperger (1944) himself had described frequently associated educational difficulties. Specific developmental delays in children diagnosed as having AS have also been recorded (see, e.g., Wing, 1981; Ehlers & Gillberg, 1993). In these children, as in our schizoid children, both motor and language development were affected, so that the exclusion criterion, of clinically significant general delay of spoken or receptive language, in the ICD-10 definition for AS (WHO, 1993), was not upheld.

In the case note study of 32 matched pairs of schizoid and control boys and 33 matched pairs of girls (Wolff, Townshend, McGuire, & Weeks, 1991; Wolff & McGuire, 1995) we also found that three of the schizoid boys but no schizoid girls and no controls had had earlier symptoms suggestive of autism, but never the full syndrome of abnormal and/or impaired development of communication; and social interaction; with restricted, repetitive behavior, beginning before the age of 3 years (WHO, 1992). Three schizoid boys and three schizoid girls had been electively mute (see below).

SCHIZOID PERSONALITY AS PART OF THE SCHIZOPHRENIA SPECTRUM

Asperger had thought the condition he described to be a lifelong, genetically based, personality disorder, different from preschizophrenic states (Asperger, 1961). Although he did not carry out systematic follow-up studies, apparently only 2 of 200 patients he saw developed schizophrenia in later life.

In ICD-9 (WHO, 1978), schizoid personality disorder is still defined in a broad way, as in the older psychiatric literature referred to above, and this is how we too had used the term (Wolff, 1995). DSM-III divided the schizoid category into schizotypal (the commonest and most strongly linked genetically to schizophrenia); paranoid; and schizoid personality disorders. Our use of the term *schizoid* is thus equivalent to the current Type A personality disorders. It needs to be stressed that these are not as distinct as is sometimes thought. They often occur together in the biological relatives of schizophrenic patients (Parnas *et al.*, 1993; Kendler *et al.*, 1993) and in the premorbid histories of both adults (Foerster, Lewis, Owen, & Murray, 1991; McCreadie, Connolly, Williamson, Atthawes, & Tilak-Sing, 1994) and children (Werry, 1992) with schizophrenia. A recent study found an excess of premorbid social withdrawal, aloofness, and detachment as well as developmental disorders of speech, language and motor functioning in children with juvenile schizophrenia (Hollis, 1995, 1996). Moreover, "high-risk" children, the offspring of parents with schizophrenia, are distinguished from their controls in later life only by the incidence of *all* cluster A personality disorders, not by each separate disorder (Erlenmeyer-Kimling *et al.*, 1995).

A second follow-up study done in Edinburgh (Wolff *et al.*, 1991; Wolff & McGuire, 1995) was prompted both by the definitions of Type A personality disorders in DSM-III (APA, 1980) and by Nagy and Szatmari's (1986) account of a group of schizotypal children who, apart from their slightly lower intelligence, exactly resembled our schizoid children. [Szatmari rarely referred to this paper in later years and now believes these children to belong to the AS group (personal communication)]. In this second follow-up, in which the Baron Schedule for Schizotypal Personalities (see Benishay and Lencz, 1995) was incorporated into the research interview, we found that over three-quarters of schizoid boys and girls in adult life fulfilled the criteria for DSM-III schizotypal personality disorder. Five of the ten Baron scales differentiated significantly between schizoid and control subjects: ideas of reference; magical thinking; impaired rapport; odd communications; and social isolation. Five did not: illusions; depersonalization; suspiciousness; social anxiety; and transient delusions or hallucinations (Wolff *et al.*, 1991).

Furthermore, a psychiatric records search established that in our total cohort of 109 schizoid boys and 32 schizoid girls then over the age of 16, 7 (4 men and 3 women) had developed schizophrenic illnesses by a mean age of 26.5 years, compared with a single case among the matched control group of other referred children grown-up (Wolff, 1995). This represents an overall prevalence of 5.0% compared with 0.7% in the control group, when the estimated prevalence for a British national birth cohort by the age of 27 years is 0.31–0.49% (Done, Johnstone, Frith, Golding, & Shepherd, 1991). Thus, although the risk for later schizophrenia in our schizoid group is increased above that expected for the general population and is congruent with a genetic link between schizoid personality and schizophrenia, it is still sufficiently low for the clinician to be able to reassure anxious families of schizoid children that a psychotic development in later life is unlikely.

THE LINKS WITH AUTISM

Asperger himself thought that the syndrome he described and Kanner's autism were similar in many ways, but "concerned basically different types" (Asperger, 1979, p.47). The children he described are not so seriously disturbed, have a much better social prognosis, and may find their way into highly specialized scientific or artistic careers, occasionally with an ability bordering on genius. Asperger thought that for success in original endeavor, a necessary ingredient may be the ability to turn away from the everyday world and rethink a subject with originality, creating a new "untrodden" path. [For an example of a schizoid genius, see the analysis of Ludwig Wittgenstein's life and personality (Wolff, 1995)].

Similarity and Differences of Symptoms

From the start we realized that the symptoms of schizoid personality, as indeed those of Asperger's autistic psychopathy (Asperger, 1944), resembled but also differed from those of childhood autism. In both conditions there are qualitative abnormalities of reciprocal social interactions; unusually intense circumscribed interests and repetitive activities; and abnormalities in verbal and nonverbal communication. Moreover, in a few cases of high-functioning autism (HFA) and of severe schizoid disorder associated with a low normal IQ [where a diagnosis of AS (Wing, 1981, 1991; WHO, 1992, 1993) could as readily have been made], it may be difficult to decide which diagnosis is the more appropriate. But, although the features of our children *resembled* those of autism, they were not the same. The deficits in social interaction usually became apparent only on school entry and did not markedly affect the children's attachments to their parents. Peer relationships were the most impaired. The children's special interest patterns were often sophisticated, quite unlike the simple, repetitive, stereotyped behaviors and utterances of autistic children. And their unusual modes of communication were not gross and immediately apparent to everyone, like those of autistic children (e.g., echolalia, pronomial reversals, even mutism) but had to be carefully looked for. In addition, the schizoid children were not, like autistic children, deficient in imaginative play capacities. On the contrary, a number engaged in unusual imagination and much fantasy, even (successful) pathological lying (Wolff, 1995).

Yet the concept of an autistic spectrum is valid. Well-functioning autistic people and severely impaired people with schizoid personality disorder and AS as defined in ICD-10, have much in common. But whether the term *autistic spectrum disorder* should be applied to the full range of allied conditions, from autism and AS to schizoid personality disorder, which in mildly affected children can later manifest merely as schizoid features in otherwise normal, even highly gifted, people, is more problematical. Certainly, the treatment and educational needs of most children with schizoid personality are different from those of children with even HFA and of children with AS as currently defined. And from a research point of view too, it may be more illuminating to use narrower rather than wider syndrome definitions (Rutter & Schopler, 1992).

Similarity of Psychological Functioning

An early experimental validation study, in which schizoid, autistic, and normal children were compared (Wolff & Barlow, 1978), showed the children diagnosed as schizoid to resemble autistic children in many of their psychological functioning, but to be even more impaired in their capacity to attribute emotions to other people. The problem with this study was that, in order to achieve matching between the comparison groups, neither the autistic nor the schizoid children were representative of the clinical cohorts fom which they had been drawn: The children with autism were more high functioning; those with schizoid disorders much more intellectually limited than the rest.

One psychological deficit of autistic people and of some people currently diagnosed as having AS affects the development of mentalizing capacity or theory of mind (Frith, 1991a; Happé, 1994), that is, the capacity to imagine what other people think and feel. We found "lack of empathy" to be a cardinal feature of schizoid personality, a key question in our follow-up interview, the basis for a self-rating of empathy, being "Would you say you are someone who is good at putting yourself into other people's shoes? ... quite sensitive to what other people are feeling or thinking? ... or do you find it difficult to guess what goes on inside them?" (Chick, 1978). Moreover, our interviewer's overall rating of empathy correlated significantly with our test for "psychological construing," that is, for attributing emotions and motivations to people in photographs (Wolff & Barlow, 1978; Chick, Waterhouse, & Wolff, 1979). Although tests for theory of mind deficits have focused on cognitive processes, the case has been made that from a developmental viewpoint, affective and cognitive aspects of human relatedness develop together (Hobson, 1993). Frith's concept of mentalizing ability comprises both cognitive and emotional capacities. And it has been found that in nonretarded autistic children, cognitive and affective understanding are even more highly associated than in normal children (Yirmiya, Sigman, Kasari, & Mundy, 1992).

People with HFA and with AS as currently defined, are less impaired in theory of mind tests than lower-functioning autistic people, but have deficiencies, as have schizophrenic patients, in tests of executive functions (Ozonoff, Pennington, & Rogers, 1991; Bishop, 1993; Ozonoff & McEwey, 1994). Sadly, such tests had not been systematically incorporated into our follow-up interviews.

Another hypothesized deficit in autistic children is a lack of "central coherence" (Frith, 1989; Happé, 1994). From middle childhood onwards, normal children can extract essential meanings from their experiences without being distracted by detail. They have better recall for meaningful than for jumbled material. Autistic children, in contrast, are often supernormally good at embedded figures and at block design tests, not being distracted by whole configurations from finding the parts. The more severely affected of our schizoid children, who participated in our experimental validation study (Wolff & Barlow, 1978), resembled autistic children but differed from normals in their lack of improvement in remembering word sequences when these consisted of meaningful sentences rather than random words.

A Possible Link between Schizoid Personality and Autism

In a blind, controlled study, we found an excess of schizoid personality traits in the parents of autistic children (Wolff, Narayan, & Moyes, 1988; Narayan, Moyes, & Wolff, 1990). Our findings are congruent with those of Piven et al. (1990) that parents of autistic children are more aloof, untactful, and unresponsive.

Twin and family studies have established that a "lesser variant of autism" occurs to excess among the siblings and monozygotic twin partners of children with autism (Folstein & Rutter, 1988; Bolton et al., 1994; Bailey et al., 1996).

This "lesser variant" consisted of subtle impairments of social interaction (with lack of friendships and reciprocity, impaired conversation, and social disinhibition); of communication (including language delay, articulation disorder, reading retardation, and spelling difficulties); together with repetitive, stereotyped behavior (circumscribed interests), all of which were features of our schizoid children. The "lesser variant" did not fulfill current diagnostic criteria for Asperger syndrome, presumbably because it involved language delays and, while resembling our own picture of schizoid personality disorder, affected people seemed to be more seriously impaired (Le Couteur *et al.*, 1996).

IS THERE A COMMON GENETIC FACTOR FOR AUTISM AND SCHIZOPHRENIA?

I have argued that the clinical picture of our schizoid children was that of the Type A personality disorders and that the children had a mild predisposition to schizophrenia (Wolff, 1995). I have also argued that their symptomatology and psychological functioning were similar to but not the same as those of children even with HFA, and that among biological relatives of autistic children there is an excess of people with schizoid features. How can we reconcile this with the fact that autism and schizophrenia do not aggregate in the same families and only very rarely occur in the same patient? If the same genetic factor, manifesting phenotypically as schizoid personality traits, predisposes to both autism and schizophrenia, one would need to postulate that for autism, now thought to be the result of several interacting genes (Bailey *et al.*, 1996; Piven & Palmer, 1997), as well as for schizophrenia, thought to be caused by groups of interacting genes as well as environmental factors (Owen & McGuffen, 1996), a further gene (or genes), different for each condition, is also among the necessary causes.

PERSONALITY OR PERVASIVE DEVELOPMENTAL DISORDER?

Whether to call a schizoid symptomatology a personality or a developmental disorder is a matter of choice so long as it is clear that schizoid children, Asperger's original cases, adults with DSM-IV Type A personality disorders, and biological relatives of autistic children have common features. The situation has become less frought now that schizophrenia itself is regarded as a neurodevelopmental disorder (Murray & Lewis, 1987; Weinberger, 1995), a view already current but without scientific foundation, when the syndrome of schizoid personality disorder in childhood was first described (Ssucharewa, 1926).

THE FEATURES OF SCHIZOID PERSONALITY IN RELATION TO CURRENT CONCEPTS OF ASPERGER SYNDROME

The label of AS seems to be used for children at the more severe end of the range of cases Asperger himself reported, so that in more mildly affected children the constitutional basis of their difficulties may go unrecognized.

From the start, a group of British workers considered the children Asperger described to have HFA but with good verbal abilities, in contrast to other autistic children who have good visuospatial skills but are linguistically impaired (Everard, 1976; Wing, 1976, 1981). This distinction has been questioned more recently (Gillberg & Coleman, 1992; Manjiviona & Prior, 1995).

Current diagnostic criteria for AS in ICD-10 (WHO, 1992, 1993) and Asperger's disorder in DSM-IV (APA, 1994) were developed largely on the basis of work stimulated by Wing's seminal paper that introduced Asperger's work to a wider readership (Wing, 1981). This paper suggested that Wing's patients were more impaired than Asperger's own cases, and Wing wrote later: "The majority need help and guidance in sheltered settings for all their lives" (Wing, 1991, p. 118). Wing developed the concept of an autistic continuum for children with what is now a classic triad of essential features (see chapter 2, this volume, and Wing, 1991, 1992).

As a result of this work, much research into the psychological functioning of affected people has treated the diagnosis of AS as equivalent to HFA (Frith, 1991a; Happé, 1994); the suggestion has been made that the syndromes described by Asperger and Kanner were equivalent; and doubt has been cast on Asperger's own accounts of the giftedness and later occupational achievements of some of his patients (Frith, 1991b).

Tantam's work strengthened these ideas. He examined a series of adult psychiatric patients with "lifelong eccentricity and social isolation" and found that among those who fulfilled Asperger's diagnostic criteria, many had had clear features of autism either beginning in very early life or of later onset (Tantam, 1986, 1988a,b, 1991). His studies too suggested a gloomy prognosis. Over one-half of his patients required sheltered care in adult life; only 2 out of 60 were living independently; less than 1 in 10 were working; and only 2 out of 60 had ever married. It should be noted that among these cases, a few had affective psychoses, 14 had at one time been diagnosed as having schizophrenia and, as a group, they had high scores for schizoid and schizotypal personality traits (Tantam, 1988b).

Although the diagnostic criteria for AS developed by Gillberg (Ehlers & Gillberg, 1993) and Szatmari (Szatmari, Bartolucci, & Bremner, 1989) were somewhat different from ICD-10 and DSM-IV criteria, both groups of workers, in their epidemiological and clinical studies of the syndrome, appear to have selected subjects who were quite seriously impaired. And the relationship, if any, between AS and schizotypal personality disorder, as described by Nagy and Szatmari (1986), has never been clarified. None of these 20 schizotypal children had fulfilled the criteria for autistic disorder in early childhood, and two later developed schizophrenia, resembling our own series in both respects (Wolff & Chick, 1980; Wolff, 1992).

In a recent study, using ICD-10 criteria, adolescents with AS were compared with matched groups of HFA and conduct-disordered children (Gilchrist, 1995). One finding was that the AS children were much more impaired in self-care and daily living skills than children with conduct disorders, quite unlike our own schizoid children, and another was that their early developmental impairments, despite the lack of early language delay, were as great as those of autistic children, again in contrast to our own series.

THE PSYCHOSOCIAL ADJUSTMENT OF SCHIZOID CHILDREN GROWN-UP

Our studies (Wolff et al., 1991; Wolff, 1995; Wolff & McGuire, 1995) revealed a different prognostic picture from that suggested by Wing (1991) and Tantam (1986, 1988a, 1991) for AS. Schizoid children did have increased rates of treatment for psychiatric disorder in adult life compared with the control group of other referred children grown-up, and their rate of working harmoniously at their expected level of occupation and, in boys, the rate of having had an intimate sexual relationship were reduced. But their rates of independent living, of marriage, and stability of employment were not statistically different from those of their matched clinic controls. By the age of 26.5 years, 20 out of 32 schizoid men personally followed-up had left the parental home, compared with 19 out of 32 controls; 10 schizoid men were married or cohabiting, compared with 15 controls; and only 9 out of 32 schizoid men, compared with 6 of the controls, had ever been unemployed for over 12 months (Wolff et al., 1991). Among the 17 schizoid women personally followed-up, 14 had left the parental home; 9 were married or cohabiting; but 9 had been unemployed for over 12 months, the working lives of young women being of course different from those of men (Wolff & McGuire, 1995). Only 1 of the 49 schizoid children personally followed-up was in residential care: a young woman who had developed a schizophrenic illness with intellectual deterioration.

A few of our children, those with low average IQ and/or evidence of brain damage, functioned like children currently given an AS diagnosis. Yet neither clinical analysis of symptoms and life histories, nor factor analyses were able to discern any clearly demarcated subgroups within the total cohort of our schizoid cases (Wolff, 1995). None of the schizoid children, again unlike Tantam's cases, had had the full symptomatic picture of early childhood autism.

It is of great clinical importance that our children in later life were far less impaired than children currently diagnosed as having Asperger syndrome and that their personal relationships too had often improved once they had left school and were no longer exposed to the pressures for conformity imposed by school life (Wolff, 1995). Like Asperger, we had a few gifted children in our group: Two of our 32 young men personally followed-up, a musician and an astrophysicist, were able to translate their exceptional gifts and special interests into satisfactory careers, and several others were successful in professional occupations, just as in Asperger's own series. As in his cases, social adaptation tended to improve with age, although intimate relationships often remained impaired.

Although a few of our former child patients functioned like people fulfilling current diagnostic criteria for AS, and had similar needs for special education in childhood, and for sheltered training and occupation in later life, the majority required help of a different kind.

Two conclusions for the clinician follow from Asperger's work and from our own: (1) There is a group of children, not as clearly handicapped as are children with HFA or Asperger syndrome or disorder, as currently defined (WHO, 1992, 1993; APA, 1994), who have more subtle and very long-lasting underlying difficulties, and who need to be diagnosed because their treatment calls for a different approach from that for children whose disturbances are mainly due to adverse life experiences; and (2) the overall prognosis for such children is reasonably good.

THE TREATMENT NEEDS OF SCHIZOID CHILDREN

There have been no controlled trials of treatment for these children. Asperger himself (1979) had reservations about behavior therapy for his group of intelligent children who value their freedom. Many of our schizoid children needed remedial education for their associated, developmental learning difficulties; many benefited from small group teaching in a setting in which their social difficulties could more readily be tolerated, and their idiosyncratic interests could be used as a basis for education. A few responded to social skills training; to a behavioral approach for secondary psychiatric symptoms such as aggressive outburst; and to medication for transient psychotic symptoms, or associated hyperkinesis.

What they had in common was a need to have their difficulties correctly diagnosed as stemming from their inherent personality makeup, neither parent engendered nor related to ill-will on their part. This is particularly important for these more mildly affected children who, unlike children currently given an Asperger diagnosis, are not obviously impaired, and are easily misdiagnosed as having experientially engendered psychiatric disorders. Parents, teachers, and the children themselves need to know that they have not caused the problems and that their personality characteristics are likely to endure. Treatment should not aim to turn a solitary child into a sociable one, nor insist on social conformity at all cost, with the inevitable disappointment at failure. Instead, family and school should be prepared to accommodate to the children's needs for privacy and the pursuit of their special interests. The psychiatrist or psychologist is most helpful by adopting a nonintrusive, supportive role over many years as the family's advocate, helping to smooth the child's path through his or her school career, into further education, and a working life. When antisocial behavior brings schizoid children into contact with the law, as it sometimes does, help is needed to explain the constitutional nature of the child's difficulties, and to avoid, if at all possible, custodial settings that involve noisy and aggressive group living (see Wolff, 1995, pp. 136–149).

THE ASSOCIATION WITH LANGUAGE DISORDERS AND ELECTIVE MUTISM

The association between the developmental dysphasias and personality features in adulthood which resemble those of our schizoid children grown-up, has been repeatedly described (Cantwell, Baker, Rutter, & Mawhood, 1989; Rutter & Mawhood, 1991; Bishop, 1994). And Bishop (1989) suggested the possibility of a continuum between autism, AS, and semantic–pragmatic language disorders. Moreover, Rutter and Mawhood (1991) found that 3 out of 25 men with a severe receptive language disorder in childhood, had developed paranoid psychoses in later life.

Language Disorders and Elective Mutism in Schizoid Children

We found specific developmental disorders of all kinds to be highly associated with schizoid personality in childhood (Wolff, 1991; Wolff & McGuire, 1995). Among 32 schizoid boys, 15 had serious or multiple developmental delays. Of these, 8 had had language disorders including language delay, dyslalia, and expressive language disorder; 1 had had serious expressive and receptive difficulties; and 1 had had elective mutism. In addition, 2 other boys without serious or multiple developmental delays had presented with elective mutism. In the control group of 32 boys, only 4 had had serious or multiple developmental delays, none affecting language.

Among 13 out of 33 schizoid girls with serious or multiple developmental delays, 7 had delays of language, including 1 with a serious expressive language disorder and elective mutism. Two other schizoid girls without serious or multiple developmental delays had also had elective mutism. Among the 33 controls, only 1 girl had had multiple or severe developmental disorders, not affecting language development.

Of the 6 electively mute children, follow-up information was available for all 3 boys but for only 2 of the 3 girls. In addition, among 6 boys who took part in the first follow-up study (Wolff & Chick, 1980) but who could not be contacted in the second, and whose case notes were not included among those systematically analyzed, were 2 further boys who had been electively mute. Elective mutism was thus very much more common in our schizoid children (8 out of 71) than in the general population (0.8 per 1000 seven-year-olds [Kolvin & Fundudis, 1981]; 1.8 per 1000 7- to 15-year-olds [Kopp & Gillberg, 1997]) or even among psychiatrically referred children (around 0.5% [Sternhausen & Juzi, 1996]).

Constitutional Shyness as a Possible Common Factor

All eight electively mute, schizoid children (but not all schizoid children) were recorded as excessively shy and socially withdrawn in childhood (Wolff, unpublished data). Of the seven with some follow-up data, five were rated as oversensitive in adult life. Three had had a delayed onset of speech, one had stammered, and four had been enuretic. A family history of language abnormalities was present in three cases. In one of these, both mother and father had been late talkers, the mother and her younger brother had been excessively shy, the patient's sister had had elective mutism and speech delay, and the patient's young son also had late onset of speech. In another case, a sister and a paternal cousin had been dyslalic and the father excessively shy. In the third case, the mother had been excessively shy and electively mute in childhood and a brother had been a late talker.

In persistently elective mute children, speech difficulties were found in 50% and constitutional shyness in over 80% (Kolvin & Fundudis, 1981). Excessive shyness and social isolation have been observed in electively mute children by others (e.g., Baker & Cantwell, 1991; Sternhausen & Juzi, 1996). Social phobia and avoidant disorder have also been described in such children (Dummit et al., 1997). And excessive shyness, social isolation, and social phobia, as well as elective mutism itself, have, as in our own small series, been found in the biological relatives of those affected (Krolin et al., 1992; Black & Uhde, 1995).

The preponderance of girls among electively mute children, repeatedly described (Wilkins, 1985; Baker & Cantwell, 1991; Tancer, 1992; Black & Uhde, 1995), can perhaps be explained by the greater persistence into middle childhood of extreme temperamental shyness, fearfulness, and social inhibition in girls than boys (Kagan, 1994). The sex ratio of electively mute children makes it likely that the majority suffer from constitutional shyness rather than schizoid disorder.

The excess of girls among socially withdrawn children is borne out even in our own small series of schizoid children without elective mutism and their matched controls. Only some of our schizoid children had been socially withdrawn. Seven out of 32 schizoid boys and 14 out of 33 schizoid girls without elective mutism had been so rated, compared with 3 out of 32 control boys and 8 out of 33 control girls with other childhood diagnoses (Wolff, unpublished data).

Yet it is possible that schizoid personality as an explanation for social withdrawal may be overlooked in a minority of electively mute children. At least one case associated with elective mutism is recorded in the literature: of the two children reported by Tramer (1934), who coined the term *elective mutism*, one whose mutism began after an operation, had definite schizoid features (emotional deficits, autism, stereotypies, and obstinacy); the other, with a family history of shyness and mutism, did not.

It is also relevant that elective mutism has been recorded in children with AS (Fine *et al.*, 1991) and in their biological relatives (Gillberg, 1989); and that the "silent twins" described by Wallace (1986) appeared to fulfill the criteria for schizoid personality disorder, perhaps even for AS. These identical twins were electively mute, solitary, and aggressive, and engaged in creative and imaginative writing from childhood. They were admitted to a secure hospital in their late teens because of fire raising and subsequently developed schizophrenic illnesses (Wolff, 1995).

What Can We Conclude?

The numbers of children with language disorders and/or elective mutism among our schizoid subjects were far too small for definite conclusions to be drawn, and our research methods had not been designed to clarify the association between schizoid personality and elective mutism. All that can be said is that elective mutism and developmental language delays overlapped and were found to excess in our schizoid children; that *all* schizoid electively mute children were shy and socially withdrawn unlike the rest of the schizoid children without mutism; and that even in our small groups of schizoid and control children the predominance of girls among the socially withdrawn was confirmed. The literature suggests that many children with elective mutism have developmental language delays but that even more of them are excessively shy and socially withdrawn. We might speculate that this could explain their unusual sex ratio. What we do not yet know is how many children with elective mutism have schizoid personality traits, although in their population-based study, Kopp and Gillberg (1997) found as many as half the electively mute children personally interviewed to fulfill the diagnostic criteria for Asperger syndrome.

CONCLUDING REMARKS

It is important, both clinically and for research purposes, to be clear that current diagnostic conventions identify only the more seriously impaired cases of the groups described by Asperger (1944), Ssucharewa (1926), and ourselves. More mildly affected children, some of whom are gifted, require recognition of the constitutional nature of their difficulties so that their secondary behavioral and emotional disorders are not erroneously attributed to faulty upbringing. Their associated specific developmental disorders may need special educational provisions; care is needed to preserve and foster special interests and gifts; and the children and their families often need psychiatric or psychological help for many years. It may be difficult to diagnose these children because of their high rates of comorbidity and because they are not as clearly impaired as children currently given an AS diagnosis. Yet the problems they pose to their families and schools can be formidable.

Epidemiological studies are now needed to shed light on the prevalence of schizoid personality disorders in the community, on the overlap with developmental disorders including disorders of language and elective mutism, and on the association of schizoid personality with giftedness.

From a classificatory viewpoint, it may be difficult to reconcile the fact that schizoid personality disorder in childhood lies at one extreme of the autistic spectrum, where it shades into normal personality variation, while at the same time there is evidence for its relatedness to the schizophrenia spectrum. Yet etiologically the problem may be less serious. Both schizophrenia and autism are now regarded as neurodevelopmental disorders with a partially genetic basis involving several genes. And schizophrenic and autistic patients are now thought to have some psychological and language deficits in common (Frith & Frith, 1991; Baltaxe & Simmons, 1992). Family history studies of the less seriously affected, schizoid, children should help to clarify whether or not there is genetic overlap between schizoid personality, AS, and autism on the one hand, and schizophrenia on the other.

REFERENCES

American Psychiatric Association (1980). *Diagnostic and statistical manual of mental disorders* (3rd ed.). Washington, DC: Author.
American Psychiatric Association (1994). *Diagnostic and statistical manual of mental disorders* (4th ed.). Washington, DC: Author.
Asperger, H. (1944). Die "autistischen Psychopathen" im Kindesalter. *Archiv für Psychiatrie und Nervenkrankheiten, 117,* 76–136.
Asperger, H. (1961). *Heilpaedagogik* (3rd ed., pp. 200–205). Berlin: Springer.
Asperger, H. (1979). Problems of infantile autism. *Communication, 13,* 45–52.

Asperger, H. (1991). 'Autistic psychopathy' in childhood (U. Frith, Trans.). In U. Frith (Ed.), *Autism and Asperger syndrome* (pp. 37–92). Cambridge: Cambridge University Press.

Bailey, A., Phillips, W., & Rutter, M. (1996). Autism: Towards and integration of clinical, genetic, neuropsychological and neurobiological perspectives. *Journal of Child Psychology and Psychiatry 37* 89–126.

Baker, L., & Cantwell, D. P. (1991). Disorders of language, speech and communication. In M. Lewis (Ed.), *Child and adolescent psychiatry: A comprehensive textbook* (pp. 516–521). Baltimore: Williams & Wilkins.

Baltaxe, C. A. M., & Simmons, J. Q. (1992). A comparison of language issues in high-functioning autism and related disorders with onset in childhood and adolescence. In E. Schopler & G. B. Mesibov (Eds.), *High-functioning individuals with autism* (pp. 201–225). New York: Plenum Press.

Benishay, D. S., & Lencz, T. (1995).Semistructured interviews for the measurement of schizotypal personality. In A. Raine, T. Lencz, & S. A. Mednick (eds.), *Schizotypal Personality* (pp. 463–479). Cambridg: Cambridge University Press.

Bishop, D. V. M. (1989). Autism, Asperger's syndrome and semantic–pragmatic disorder: Where are the boundaries? *British Journal of Disorders of Communication, 24,* 107–121.

Bishop, D. V. M. (1993). Annotation: Autism, executive functions, and theory of mind: A neuropsychological perspective. *Journal of Child Psychology and Psychiatry, 34,* 279–293.

Bishop, D. V. M. (1994). Speech and language disorders. In M. Rutter, E. Taylor, & L. Hersov (Eds.), *Child and adolescent psychiatry: Modern approaches* (3rd ed., pp. 546–568). Oxford: Blackwell.

Black, B., & Uhde, T. W. (1995). Psychiatric characteristics of children with selective mutism. *Journal of the American Academy of Child and Adolescent Psychiatry, 34,* 847–856.

Bleuler, M. (1978). *The schizophrenic disorders* (p. 434). New Haven: Yale University Press.

Bolton, P., MacDonald, H., Pickles, A., Rios, P., Goode, S., Crowson, M., Bailey, A., & Rutter, M. (1994). A case–control family history study of autism. *Journal of Child Psychology and Psychiatry, 35,* 877–900.

Cantwell, D. P., Baker, L., Rutter, M., & Mawhood, L. (1989). Infantile autism and developmental receptive dysphasia: A comparative follow-up into middle childhood. *Journal of Autism and Developmental Disorders, 19,* 19–31.

Chick, J. (1978). *Schizoid personality in childhood: A follow-up study.* M.Phil. thesis, University of Edinburgh.

Chick, J., Waterhouse, L., & Wolff, S. (1979). Psychological construing in schizoid children grown-up. *British Journal of Psychiatry, 135,* 425–430.

Cohen, D. J., Paul, R., & Volkmar, F. R. (1986). Issues in the classification of pervasive developmental disorders: Towards DSM-IV. *Journal of the American Academy of Child Psychiatry, 25,* 213–220.

Done, D. J., Johnstone, E. C., Frith, C. D., Golding, J., & Shepherd, P. M. (1991). Complications of pregnancy and delivery in relation to psychosis in adult life: Data from the British perinatal mortality survey sample. *British Medical Journal, 302,* 1576–1580.

Dummit III, E. S., Klein, R. G., Tancer, N. K., Asche, B., Martin, J., & Fairbanks, J. A. (1997). Systematic assessment of 50 children with selective mutism. *Journal of the American Academy for Child and Adolescent Psychiatry, 36,* 653–660.

Ehlers, S., & Gillberg, C. (1993). The epidemiology of Asperger syndrome. A total population study. *Journal of Child Psychology and Psychiatry, 34,* 1327–1350.

Erlenmeyer-Kimling, L., Squire-Wheeler, E., Hilldoff, U., Bassett, A. S., Cornblatt, B. A., Kestenbaum, C. J., Rock, D., Roberts, S. A., & Gottesman, I. I. (1995). The New York High-Risk Project: Psychoses and cluster A personality disorders in offspring of schizophrenic patients at 23 year of follow-up. *Archives of General Psychiatry, 52,* 857–865.

Everard, M. P. (1976). *Mildly autistic young people and their problems.* Paper presented at International Symposium on Childhood Autism, St. Gall, Switzerland.

Fine, J., Bartolucci, G., Ginsberg, G., & Szatmari, P. (1991). The use of intonation to communicate in pervasive developmental disorders. *Journal of Child Psychology and Psychiatry, 32*, 771–782.

Foerster, A., Lewis, S. W., Owen, M. J., & Murray, R. M. (1991). Premorbid adjustment and personality in psychosis: Effects of sex and diagnosis. *British Journal of Psychiatry, 158*, 171–176.

Folstein, S., & Rutter, M. (1988). Autism: Familial aggregation and genetic implications. *Journal of Autism and Developmental Disorders, 18*, 297–331.

Frith, C. D., & Frith, U. (1991). Elective affinities in schizophrenia and childhood autism. In P. E. Bebbington (Ed.), *Social psychiatry: Theory, methodology and practice* (pp. 65–88). London: Transaction.

Frith, U. (1989). *Autism: Explaining the enigma*. Oxford: Blackwell.

Frith, U. (Ed.). (1991a). *Autism and Asperger syndrome*. Cambridge: Cambridge University Press.

Frith, U. (1991b). Asperger and his syndrome. In U. Frith (Ed.), *Autism and Asperger syndrome* (pp. 1–36). Cambridge: Cambridge University Press.

Geleert, E. R. (1967). Borderline states in childhood and adolescence. *Psychoanalytic Study of the Child, 13*, 279–295.

Gilchrist, A. (1995). *Clinical features of Asperger syndrome*. Paper presented at the 10th International Congress of the European Society for Child and Adolescent Psychiatry, Utrecht, Netherlands.

Gillberg, C. (1989). Asperger syndrome in 23 Swedish children. *Developmental Medicine and Child Neurology, 31*, 520–531.

Gillberg, C., & Coleman, M. (1992). *The biology of the autistic syndromes* (2nd ed.). Oxford: Blackwell.

Happé, F. (1994). *Autism: An introduction to psychological theory*. London: UCL Press.

Heston, L., & Denney, D. (1968). Interaction between early life experience and biological factors in schizophrenia. In D. Rosenthal & S. Kety (Eds.), *The transmission of schizophrenia* (pp. 363–376). Oxford: Pergamon.

Hobson, R. P. (1993). *Autism and the development of mind*. Hillsdale, NJ: Erlbaum.

Hollis, C. (1995). Child and adolescent (juvenile onset) schizophrenia. A case control study of premorbid developmental impairments. *British Journal of Psychiatry, 166*, 489–495.

Hollis, C. (1996). Childhood antecedents of schizophrenia. *Schizophrenia Monitor, 6*(4). 1–5.

Kagan, J. (1994). *Galen's prophesy: Temperament in human nature*. New York: Basic Books.

Kendler, K. S., McGuire, M., Gruenberg, A. M., O'Hare, A., Spellman, M., & Walsh, D. (1993). The Roscommon family study: III. Schizophrenia-related personality disorders in relatives. *Archives of General Psychiatry, 59*, 781–788.

Kolvin, I., & Fundudis, T. (1981). Elective mute children: Psychological development and background factors. *Journal of Child Psychology and Psychiatry, 22*, 219–232.

Kopp, S. & Gillberg, C. (1997). Selective mutism: A population-based study: A research note. *Journal of Child Psychology and Psychiatry, 38*, 257–262.

Krohn, D. D., Weckstein, S. M., & Wright, H. L. (1992). A study of the effectiveness of a specific treatment for elective mutism. *Journal of the American Academy of Child and Adolescent Psychiatry, 31*, 711–718.

Le Couteur, A., Bailey, A., Goode, S., Pickles, A., Loeber, R., & Eaves, L. (1996). A broader phenotype of autism: The clinical spectrum in twins. *Journal of Child Psychology and Psychiatry, 37*, 785–801.

MacGregor, R., Pullar, A., & Cundall, D. (1994). Silent at school: Elective mutism and abuse. *Archives of Disease in Childhood, 70*, 540–541.

Mahler, M. S., Ross, J. R., & De Fries, Z. (1949). Clinical studies in benign and malignant cases of childhood psychoses. *American Journal of Orthopsychiatry, 19*, 295–305.

Manjiviona, J., & Prior, M. (1995). Comparison of Asperger syndrome and high-functioning autistic children on a test of motor impairment. *Journal of Autism and Developmental Disorders, 25*, 23–39.

McCreadie, R. G., Connolly, M. A., Williamson, D. J., Atthawes, R. W. B., & Tilak-Sing, D. (1994). The Nithsdale schizophrenia surveys XII. 'Neurodevelopmental' schizophrenia: A search for clinical correlates and putative aetiological factors. *British Journal of Psychiatry, 165,* 340–346.

Murray, R. M., & Lewis, S. W. (1987). Is schizophrenia a neurodevelopmental disorder? *British Medical Journal, 295,* 681–682.

Nagy, J., & Szatmari, P. (1986). A chart review of schizotypal personality disorders in children. *Journal of Autism and Developmental Disorders, 16,* 351–367.

Narayan, S., Moyes, B., & Wolff, S. (1990). Family characteristics of autistic children: A further report. *Journal of Autism and Developmental Disorders, 20,* 523–535.

Owen, M. & McGuffin, P. (1996). The genetics of schizophrenia: Future directions. *Schizophrenia Monitor, 6*(1), 1–5.

Ozonoff, S., & McEwey, R. F. (1994). A longitudinal study of executive function and theory of mind development in autism. *Development and Psychopathology, 6,* 415–431.

Ozonoff, S., Pennington, B. F., & Rogers, S. J. (1991). Executive function deficits in high-functioning autistic individuals: Relationship to theory of mind. *Journal of Child Psychology and Psychiatry, 32,* 1081–1105.

Parnas, J., Cannon, T. D., Jacobsen, B., Schulsinger, H., Schulsinger, F., & Mednick, S. A. (1993). Lifetime DSM-III-R diagnostic outcomes in the offspring of schizophrenic mothers: Results from the Copenhagen high-risk study. *Archives of General Psychiatry, 50,* 707–714.

Piven, J., Gayle, J., Chase, G., Fink, B., Landa, R., Wzorek, M., & Folstein, S. (1990). A family history study of neuropsychiatric disorders in the adult siblings of autistic individuals. *Journal of the American Academy of Child and Adolescent Psychiatry, 29,* 177–184.

Piven, J. & Palmer, P. (1997). Cognitive deficits in parents from multiple-incidence autism families. *Journal of Child Psychology and Psychiatry, 38,* 1011–1021.

Robinson, J. F., & Vitale, L. J. (1954). Children with circumscribed interest patterns. *American Journal of Psychiatry, 24,* 755–767.

Rutter, M., & Mawhood, L. (1991). The long-term psychosocial sequelae of specific developmental disorders of speech and language. In M. Rutter & P. Casaer (Eds.), *Biological risk factors for psychosocial disorders* (pp. 233–259). Cambridge: Cambridge University Press.

Rutter, M., & Schopler, E. (1992). Classification of pervasive developmental disorders: Some concepts and practical considerations. *Journal of Autism and Developmental Disorders, 22,* 459–482.

Ssucharewa, G. E. (1926). Die schizoiden Psychopathien im Kindesalter. *Monatschrift für Psychiatrie und Neurologie, 60,* 235–261.

Steinhausen, H.-C., & Juzi, C. (1996). Elective mutism: An analysis of 100 cases. *Journal of the American Academy for Child and Adolescent Psychiatry, 35,* 606–614.

Szatmari, P., Bartolucci, G., & Bremner, R. (1989). Asperger's syndrome and autism: Comparisons on early history and outcome. *Developmental Medicine and Child Neurology, 31,* 709–720.

Tancer, N. K. (1992). Elective mutism: A review of the literature. In B. B. Lahey & A. E. Kazdin (Eds.), *Advances in Clinical Psychology, 14,* 265–288.

Tantam, D. (1986). *Eccentricity and autism.* Ph.D. thesis, University of London.

Tantam, D. (1988a). Lifelong eccentricity and social isolation I: Psychiatric, social and forensic aspects. *British Journal of Psychiatry, 153,* 777–782.

Tantam, D. (1988b). Lifelong eccentricity and social isolation II: Asperger's syndrome or schizoid personality disorder? *British Journal of Psychiatry, 153,* 783–791.

Tantam, D. (1991). Asperger's syndrome in adulthood. In U. Frith (Ed.), *Autism and Asperger syndrome* (pp. 147–183). Cambridge: Cambridge University Press.

Tramer, M. (1934). Elektiver Mutismus bei Kindern. *Zeitschrift für Kinderpsychiatrie, 1,* 30–35.

van der Gaag, R. J. (1993). *Multiplex development disorder: An exploration of borderlines on the autistic spectrum.* M.D. thesis, University of Utrecht.

Van Krevelen, D. A. (1971). Early infantile autism and autistic psychopathy. *Journal of Childhood Autism and Schizophrenia, 1*, 82–86.

Voeller, K. K. S. (1986). Right hemisphere deficit syndrome in children. *American Journal of Psychiatry, 143*, 1004–1009.

Wallace, M. (1986). *The silent twins*. Harmondsworth, Middlesex: Penguin.

Weil, A. P. (1953). Certain severe disturbances of ego development in childhood. *Psychoanalytic Study of the Child, 8*, 271–287.

Weinberger, D. R. (1995). Schizophrenia as a neurodevelopmental disorder. In S. R. Hirsch & D. R. Weinberger (Eds.), *Schizophrenia* (pp. 293–323). Oxford: Blackwell.

Weintraub, S., & Mesulam, M. M. (1983). Developmental learning disabilities of the right hemisphere: Emotional, interpersonal, and cognitive components. *Archives of Neurology, 40*, 463–468.

Werry, J. S. (1992). Child and adolescent (early onset) schizophrenia: A review in the light of DSM-III-R. *Journal of Autism and Developmental Disorders, 22*, 601–624.

Wilkins, R. (1985). A comparison of elective mutism and emotional disorders in children. *British Journal of Psychiatry, 146*, 198–203.

Wing, L. (Ed.). (1976). *Early infantile autism* (2nd ed.). Oxford: Pergamon.

Wing, L. (1981). Asperger's syndrome: A clinical account. *Psychological Medicine, 11*, 115–129.

Wing, L. (1991). The relationship between Asperger's syndrome and Kanner's autism. In U. Frith (Ed.), *Autism and Asperger syndrome* (pp. 93–121). Cambridge: Cambridge University Press.

Wing, L. (1992). Manifestations of social problems in high-functioning autistic people. In E. Schopler & G. B. Mesibov (Eds.), *High-functioning people with autism* (pp. 129–142). New York: Plenum Press.

Wolff, S. (1964). Schizoid personality disorder in childhood. Unpublished paper presented at the Sixth International Congress of Psychotherapy, London.

Wolff, S. (1991). 'Schizoid' personality in childhood and adult life III: The childhood picture. *British Journal of Psychiatry, 159*, 629–635.

Wolff, S. (1992). Psychiatric morbidity and criminality in 'schizoid' children grown-up: A records survey. *European Child and Adolescent Psychiatry, 1*, 214–221.

Wolff, S. (1995). *Loners: The life path of unusual children*. London: Routledge.

Wolff, S. (1996). The first account of the syndrome Asperger described? *European Child and Adolescent Psychiatry, 5*, 119–132.

Wolff, S., & Barlow, A. (1978). Schizoid personality in childhood: A comparative study of schizoid, autistic and normal children. *Journal of Child Psychology and Psychiatry, 19*, 175–180.

Wolff, S., & Chick, J. (1980). Schizoid personality in childhood: A controlled follow-up study. *Psychological Medicine, 10*, 85–100.

Wolff, S., & McGuire, R. J. (1995). Schizoid personality in girls: A follow-up study — What are the links with Asperger's syndrome? *Journal of Child Psychology and Psychiatry, 36*, 793–817.

Wolff, S., Narayan, S., & Moyes, B. (1988). Personality characteristics of parents of autistic children: A controlled study. *Journal of Child Psychology and Psychiatry, 29*, 143–153.

Wolff, S., Townsend, R., McGuire, R. J., & Weeks, D. J. (1991). 'Schizoid' personality in childhood and adult life II: Adult adjustment and the continuity with schizotypal personality disorder. *British Journal of Psychiatry, 159*, 620–629.

World Health Organization. (1978). *Mental disorders: Glossary and guide to their classification in accordance with the ninth revision of the international classification of diseases*. Geneva: Author.

World Health Organization. (1992). *The ICD-10 classification of mental and behavioural disorders. Clinical descriptions and diagnostic guidelines*. Geneva: Author.

World Health Organization. (1993). *The ICD-10 classification of mental and behavioural disorders. Diagnostic criteria for research*. Geneva: Author.

Yirmiya, N., Sigman, M. D., Kasari, C., & Mundy, P. (1992). Empathy and cognition in high-functioning children with autism. *Child Development, 63*, 150–160.

III

Neuropsychological Issues

8

Neurobiology of Asperger Syndrome
Seven Case Studies and Quantitative Magnetic Resonance Imaging Findings

ALAN LINCOLN, ERIC COURCHESNE, MARK ALLEN,
ELLEN HANSON, and MICHAELA ENE

INTRODUCTION

The atypical pattern of development first described by Hans Asperger over 50 years ago (Asperger, 1944, 1968), commonly referred to as Asperger syndrome (AS), has only recently been included by the American Psychiatric Association as one subtype of Pervasive Developmental Disorder (PDD; APA, 1994). It is now believed that all PDD, including AS, are caused by abnormalities of brain development and function. Of the PDD, Autistic Disorder (AD) has been the most extensively studied with respect to abnormal brain development and function (for review see, Courchesne 1995, 1997). Few studies, however, have evaluated brain development and function in persons with AS. This chapter will

ALAN LINCOLN • Laboratory for Research on the Neuroscience of Autism, Children's Hospital and Health Center, La Jolla, and California School of Professional Psychology–San Diego, San Diego, California 92121.   ERIC COURCHESNE • Laboratory for Research on the Neuroscience of Autism, Children's Hospital and Health Center, and Department of Neurosciences, University of California at San Diego, La Jolla, California 92093.   MARK ALLEN • Laboratory for Research on the Neuroscience of Autism, Children's Hospital and Health Center, La Jolla, California 92037. ELLEN HANSON and MICHAELA ENE • California School of Professional Psychology–San Diego, San Diego, California 92121.

Asperger Syndrome or High-Functioning Autism?, edited by Schopler *et al.* Plenum Press, New York, 1998.

review factors related to the neurobiology of AS. In addition, we will describe seven cases of individuals with AS who have had quantitative magnetic resonance imaging (MRI) through our laboratory.

The literature is sparse regarding the neuropsychology and neurobiology of AS. Distinct neuropsychological and neurobiological differences between AS and other PDD spectrum disorders such as AD would provide evidence for the validity of AS as a meaningful syndrome (Schopler, 1996).

Neuropsychology of Intellectual Functions in AD and AS

There has been a good deal written regarding the neuropsychology of intellectual abilities of persons with AD (Freeman, Lucas, Forness, & Ritvo, 1985; Lincoln, Allen, & Kilman, 1995; Lincoln, Courchesne, Kilman, Elmasian, & Allen, 1988; Ohta, 1987; Rumsey & Hamburger, 1988, 1990; Siegel, Minshew, & Goldstein, 1996). However, there is relatively little known about the intellectual abilities of persons with AS. In AD, multiple studies show that specific verbal abilities involving verbal comprehension and expressive vocabulary tend to be more impaired than visual-spatial reasoning skills (see Lincoln et al., 1995, for review). Relative to AD, one would expect that in AS this pattern might be qualitatively different because of the history of more normal early language development and apparently subnormal reported fine and gross motor development. However, evaluating the current literature in order to ascertain whether such differences do exist in the intellectual functioning between the two disorders could prove difficult. First, AS was not recognized in the earlier versions of the American Psychiatric Association's *Diagnostic and Statistical Manual of Mental Disorders* (DSM-III or DSM-III-R). Because of this, and the significant overlap in symptoms between AD and AS individuals, it is likely that AS and AD cases were both represented in many studies examining relatively high-functioning persons with autism. For example, recent studies examining executive functions in persons with AD included AS subjects in the AD sample (Ozonoff, Strayer, McMahon, & Filloux, 1994). Other studies concerned with the intellectual abilities of high-functioning AD individuals describe very young AD children with exceptional verbal skills (Freeman et al., 1985; Siegel et al., 1996). Those studies that relied on DSM-III or DSM-III-R would have had little way to separate AS cases from the AD sample. Interestingly enough, these same studies tended to not show the significant verbal comprehension deficits in their AD samples that are so clearly observed in the meta-analytic review of intellectual characteristics of persons with AD (see Lincoln et al., 1995, and Siegel et al., 1996, for reviews).

In older, nonretarded individuals with AD, there is evidence that verbal abilities improve with age (Kuck, Lincoln, & Heaton, submitted; Lincoln et al., 1995). Thus, there may be less of a marked discrepancy between verbal and nonverbal intellectual abilities in older, nonretarded AD individuals. Because of this improvement in language ability, it is important to recognize that at younger ages AD individuals are more language impaired, and therefore less intellectually competent on tests that require language and verbal reasoning ability.

The significant problems that younger AD individuals experience on intellectual tasks involving vocabulary and verbal reasoning compared to their relatively intact visual-spatial and visual-motor ability are a marked contrast to the abilities demonstrated by AS individuals. Individuals with AS are described as having an opposite pattern of intellectual abilities. Even at young ages, they are typically described as having vocabulary and verbal reasoning abilities that are not only relatively intact, but better than their social or visual-spatial and visual-motor abilities (Szatmari, Archer, Fisman, Streiner, & Wilson, 1995). In a group of 4- to 6-year-olds characterized with PDD and differentiated into AD and AS groups by the presence of significant history of language impairment for AD, but not for AS children, it was found that the AD children performed poorly on the Verbal Reasoning subtests of the Stanford–Binet Intelligence Scale (4th ed.) (Thorndike, Hagen, & Sattler, 1986). The AD children performed better, but not significantly better, than AS children on the Beery Visual-Motor Integration Test and the Motor Skills scale of the Vineland Adaptive Behavior Scales (Sparrow, Balla, & Cicchetti, 1984). Thus, such patterns of performance in AD and AS individuals could suggest that AD is a more severe form of AS with greater language impairment.

We reviewed six recent studies that included separate groups of AS ($N = 110$) and AD individuals ($N = 96$) and added 61 cases of AD from our previous report (Lincoln et al., 1995) as well as the IQ information from the 7 AS cases described in this chapter (see Table 8-3). The Wechsler Performance IQs of each of the groups differed by about 8 points favoring the AS individuals (AD PIQ = 86.5, AS PIQ = 94.6) (Wechsler, 1974, 1981 (Table 8-1). The Verbal IQs of the AD (AD VIQ = 78.2) individuals were substantially lower than those for the AS group (AS VIQ = 95.7). In contrast to the AD group, who demonstrated markedly impaired Verbal IQs relative to their Performance IQs, the AS group had higher Verbal IQ scores than Performance IQ scores. In addition, AS group also tended to have generally higher Verbal, Performance, and Full Scale IQ scores compared with the IQ scores of the AD group. Thus, the AS cases were generally of higher intelligence and less impaired in their verbal intellectual abilities than persons with AD.

It is noteworthy that in two recent reviews of studies evaluating the intellectual characteristics of AD individuals (Lincoln et al., 1995; Siegel et al., 1996) there was evidence to support the relative verbal intellectual impairments in persons with AD. Table 8-2 shows a combined review of those studies of 333 individuals with AD. In this review the mean Verbal IQ of the AD individuals is 76.9 and the mean Performance IQ, 86.2. The latter value is very similar to the mean Performance IQ of the AD individuals shown in Table 8-1. Moreover, the

Table 8-1. IQ Comparisons of 157 Autistic and 117 Asperger Individuals

	Autism				Asperger			
Study	*n*	VIQ	PIQ	FSIQ	*n*	VIQ	PIQ	FSIQ
Szatmari *et al.* (1990)	17	84	81	82	26	85	87	86
Ozonoff *et al.* (1991)	13	76	101	87	10	92	94	93
Fine *et al.* (1994)	18	85	81	82	23	86	88	·87
Klin *et al.* (1995)	19	95	97	96	27	109	85	97
Marjiviona and Prior (1995)	21	86	85	85	12	102	104	104
Ghaziuddin *et al.* (1995)	8	83	89	83	12	102	97	99
Means	**96**	**85.64**	**88.42**	**86.19**	**110**	**95.45**	**90.30**	**92.93**
Lincoln *et al.* (1995)								
WISC-R	34	58.5	83.9	69.0				
WAIS-R	27	76.8	83.0	79.4				
Mean of all	**157**	**78.24**	**86.51**	**81.30**				
Lincoln *et al.* (1995)					7	99.29	80.86	89.43
Mean of all					**117**	**95.68**	**89.72**	**92.72**

Table 8-2. Wechsler Verbal, Performance, and Full
Scale IQs of Persons with Autism

	n	VIQ	PIQ	FSIQ
Venter *et al.* (1992)	52	80	83	79
Minshew *et al.* (1992)	15	99	93	96
Allen *et al.* (1991)	20	57	85	68
Rumsey & Hamburger (1990)	10	96	96	96
Szatmari *et al.* (1990)	17	85	81	82
Lincoln *et al.* (1998)	33	71	83	76
Lincoln *et al.* (1988)	13	60	84	69
Rumsey & Hamburger (1988)	10	103	104	104
Asarnow *et al.* (1987)	23	85	99	91
Narita & Koga (1987)	45	61	78	66
Ohta (1987)	16	65	85	72
Schneider & Asarnow (1987)	15	80	94	86
Freeman *et al.* (1985)	21	90	105	97
Tymchuk *et al.* (1977)	20	90	81	88
Lockyer & Rutter (1970)	19[a]	74	71	75
Wassing (1965)	4	59	88	71
Mean	**333**	**76.92**	**86.19**	**80.23**

Note. Overall means adjusted relative to the number of subjects in each study.
[a]Lowest reported n used to calculate mean.
Adapted from Lincoln *et al.* (1995) and Siegel *et al.* (1996)

Table 8-3. Psychometric Assessment of Seven AS Individuals

Measure	Case 1	Case 2	Case 3	Case 4	Case 5	Case 6	Case 7
VIQ	101	81	106	90	98	110	109
PIQ	96	73	71	83	91	65	87
FSIQ	99	76	87	85	94	86	99
PPVT SS	112	70	88	61	70	[a]	99
VMI SS	103	83	74	88	94	[a]	71
WRAT RSS	97	86	98	110	84	121	114
WRAT SSS	100	86	106	109	78	102	123
WRAT ASS	106	72	133	103	79	99	83
CARS	17	36	27	23	20	29	27

[a]No data available

mean Verbal IQ in Table 8-2 is respectively about 9 and about 18 points lower than for AD and AS individuals in Table 8-1. Thus, the results of these meta-analytic reviews of IQ performance on the Wechsler Verbal and Performance scales provide evidence that in AD there is a relative impairment in verbal intellectual ability and that in AS the verbal intellectual functions appear to be more generally intact. Moreover, there is no evidence of impairment in the less verbal, Performance IQ abilities in either the AS or AD group.

Neurobiology of AS

The literature is sparse regarding the possible causes of biological abnormalities associated with AS. There has been some conjecture that birth trauma, such as hypoxia, might lead to medial temporal lobe pathology in persons with AS (Brown & Brierley, 1973). Slightly over 60% of the AS children studied by Gillberg (1989) revealed abnormal results on ABR, EEG, CAT scans, chromosomal cultures, or cerebrospinal fluid (CSF) analysis, or had a major diagnosis indicating brain abnormality (e.g., epilepsy, cerebral palsy). However, 80% of the individuals with AD also had similar types of abnormal results. There was no pathology specifically associated with AS.

Evidence of brain pathology in persons with AS was reported by Ozbayrak, Kapucu, Erdem, and Aras (1991). Their study found left occipital hypoperfusion that may have included some of the left parietal and superior temporal visual association areas. However, their evaluation of global and regional blood flow, as well as oxygen metabolism, did not differentiate persons with AS from normal controls.

In a study of AS by McKelvey, Lambert, Mottron, and Shevell (1995), all three AS patients showed evidence of abnormal right hemisphere functioning on single photon emission computed tomographic (SPECT) imaging. One patient showed right temporal hypoperfusion, another showed diffusely decreased right hemispheric uptake, and the third showed decreased frontal and occipital uptake. Cerebellar abnormalities were evident in each patient. Two patients showed evidence of abnormal uptake in the right cerebellar hemisphere. In addition, two patients showed decreased uptake in the cerebellar vermis.

Few MRI studies of the brain in AS have been reported and none have employed quantitative measurements of specific brain structures. DeLong and Nohria (1994) reported in their study of 40 children with Autism Spectrum Disorder that 20 probands had evidence of neurological abnormality. However, of the 4 more clearly diagnosed with AS, none showed evidence of neurological or brain MRI abnormality.

Evidence of structural brain abnormality was described in 2 AS cases showing focal areas of cortical polymicrogyria (Berthier, Santamaria, Encabo, & Tolosa, 1992; Berthier, Starkstein, & Leiguarda, 1990). Berthier, Bayes, and Tolosa (1993) reported that 5 of 7 individuals with concurrent Tourette's disorder and AS (TD-AS) had MRI scans revealing structural brain abnormalities. Of their 9 cases of Tourette's disorder, only 1 individual's MRI scan showed evidence of structural brain abnormality. Four of the five TD-AS individuals had MRI scans showing cortical abnormalities. They reported that cortical defects were found in 2 of these patients involving the right central perisylvian area. In their words, "the posterior-inferior frontal gyrus, the inferior precentral gyrus, and the anterior portion of the superior temporal gyrus were incompletely formed that resulted in the widening of the Sylvian fissure and partial exposure of the insular cortex.... One of these patients had hypoplasia of the right temporo-occipital cortex" (p. 635). Two other patients showed evidence of small gyri in the posterior parietal lobe. The fifth TD-AS patient showed evidence of enlargement of the right lateral ventricle, but no evidence of abnormality of brain parenchyma. Subsequent to this report, Berthier (1994) reviewed the MRIs of 19 AS individuals (aged 13–37 years; some are the same patients reported above) and found abnormalities in 10 of the 19. Abnormalities included lateral ventricular enlargement in 3 patients, and small gyri and increased sulcal width in 7 patients. Four of these seven patients showed such cortical abnormalities in the perisylvian region. Two patients showed evidence of cortical abnormality in the posterior superior parietal lobes. In 1 patient, cortical abnormality was observed in the left parieto-occipital junction. The 3 patients with abnormalities in the parietal lobes also showed thinning of the posterior corpus callosum, a finding earlier reported by Courchesne, Press, and Yeung-Courchesne (1993) in patients with infantile autism. Additional evidence of enlargement of the right lateral ventricle was also described in one of the 3 AS cases reported by McKelvey et al. (1995).

A recent case study found similar brain anatomical abnormalities in both a 15- year-old boy with AS and his father, who also demonstrated some AS traits (Volkmar et al., 1996). MRIs of the father and son revealed frontal lobe abnormalities. In the father, there was a "large V-shaped wedge missing tissue just superior to the ascending ramus of the Sylvian fissure, at about where the middle frontal gyrus normally intersects with the precentral sulcus." This abnormality was bilateral, but larger on the left. The son showed a smaller "bilateral dysmorphology in exactly the same area" (p. 121). However, in the son there was also decreased tissue in the anterior-inferior temporal lobe. It is not clear, however, whether the abnormalities reported and shown represent neuropathology specific to AS or are normal variations of gyral patterns (Ono, Kubik, & Abernuthey, 1990, p. 37, panel C).

Methods

Subject Identification

The files of individuals referred to the Laboratory for Research on the Neuroscience of Autism of Children's Hospital and Health Center in San Diego were reviewed by two psychologists (A.L. and M.A.) for potential inclusion as AS cases. Each potential participant was thoroughly evaluated with an NIH-approved diagnostic protocol. That protocol included a phone screen by a clinical psychologist, intake history and Autism Diagnostic Interview (ADI; Le Couteur et al., 1989; Lord, Rutter, & Le Couteur, 1994), psychometric testing, behavior observations (generally employing the Autism Diagnostic Observation Schedule; Lord et al., 1989), completion of the Childhood Autism Rating Scale (Schopler, Reichler, & Renner, 1988), genetic testing (including fragile X testing), EEG, brainstem audiometry, and a structured neurological examination. The diagnosis of AS was made only when a subject met all DSM-IV criteria for AS (APA, 1994). In addition, all participants that we considered to have AS also had to meet ADI algorithm criteria consistent with impairments in social functioning and ritualistic or repetitive behaviors while not meeting ADI algorithm criteria for language impairment. Table 8-3 shows Wechsler IQ scores, receptive vocabulary standard scores, visual-motor standard scores, achievement standard scores, and Childhood Autism Rating Scale scores and Table 8-4 provides pertinent historical information for each of the seven AS cases we studied.

Eight AS individuals between the ages of 8 and 28 were identified and classified as having AS. The 8 year-old had not had an MRI, and was excluded from the study.

MRIs were obtained and quantitative area measurements of specific brain structures were completed for each of the seven AS individuals. The MRI protocols and measurement procedures were identical to those employed by our laboratory for AD and normal control individuals for imaging and measuring the cerebellar vermis (Courchesne et al., 1994), the corpus callosum (Egaas, Courchesne, & Saitoh, 1995), and the hippocampus (Saitoh, Courchesne, Egaas, Lincoln, & Schreibman, 1995). The following MRI anatomical structures were measured for each of the seven AS individuals: the area of the sagittal cerebellar

Table 8-4. Subject Characteristics

	Case 1	Case 2	Case 3	Case 4	Case 5	Case 6	Case 7
Prenatal abnormalities	No	No	Yes	Yes	No	No	No
Perinatal abnormalities	No	Yes	No	No	No	No	Yes
Postnatal abnormalities	No	No	No	No	No	No	No
Abnormal developmental milestones	No	No	No	No	No	No	No
Phrase speech by age 3	Yes	Yes	Yes	Yes	Yes	Yes	Yes
Atypical patterns/social use of expressive speech	Yes	Yes	Yes	Yes	Yes	Yes	Yes
Excessive reference to unusual/highly specific topics	Yes	Yes	Yes	Yes	Yes	Yes	Yes
Abnormal social interactions	Yes	Yes	Yes	Yes	Yes	Yes	Yes
Fine/gross motor abnormalities	No	Yes	Yes	Yes	Yes	Yes	Yes
Family history of learning/neurological/ psychological disorders	Yes	Yes	Yes	Yes	Yes	Yes	Yes
EEG abnormalities	Mild	No	No	No	No	No	No
Brainstem audiometry/chromosome/ fragile X testing/blood/urine assay abnormalities	No	No	No	No	No	No	No

vermal lobules I to V, the area of the sagittal cerebellar vermal lobules VI and VII, the total area of the sagittal corpus callosum, the area of each of the five segments of the sagittal corpus callosum (see Egaas *et al.*, 1995), and the cross-sectional area of the hippocampal body. We then compared these measurements to all of the AD and control subjects of a similar age range (14–28 years) for whom we had the above brain measurements, namely for 49 AD subjects and 70 control subjects, sagittal cerebellar vermal lobules I to V; for 49 AD subjects and 70 controls, vermal lobules VI and VII; for 51 AD and 64 controls, corpus callosum; for 50 of the AD subjects and 64 controls, each of the five corpus callosum subregions (Clark; Clk); and for 31 autistic subjects and 26 controls, cross-sectional area of the hippocampal body.

RESULTS

Figure 8-1 shows the seven AS midsagittal MRIs.

Midsagittal Cerebellar Vermis

Quantitative MRI measurements of the midsagittal cerebellar vermal lobules I to V were similar among the AD, AS, and normal control individuals [means: AD = 438 mm^2, control = 453 mm^2, Asperger = 457 mm^2; F = 1.08 (2, 124), p = .34; see Figure 8-2]. However, the midsagittal areas of vermal lobules

VI and VII differ for the three groups [means: AD = 260 mm^2, control = 286 mm^2, AS = 288 mm^2; F = 4.85 (2,124), p = .0094; see Figure 3]. Planned comparisons showed that only the AD group was statistically smaller than the normal control group [F = 9.31 (1, 124), p = .0031]. Unfortunately, because of the small number of AS participants and limited statistical power, it is difficult to fully evaluate the meaning of not finding a statistically significant difference between AS participants and either AD or normal control participants. It is interesting to note, however, that one of the seven AS cases had midsagittal vermal lobule VI and VII area measurements that were significantly smaller than the mean area measurements for each of the three groups of participants (Case 7, 222 mm^2). Moreover, four of the five remaining AS participants had area

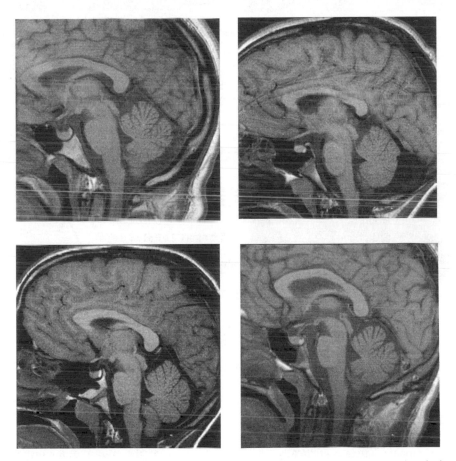

Fig. 8-1. Midsagittal MRI images of each of the seven Asperger cases. The arrows identify the area defined as the corpus callosum and each of the five Clark areas within the corpus callosum.

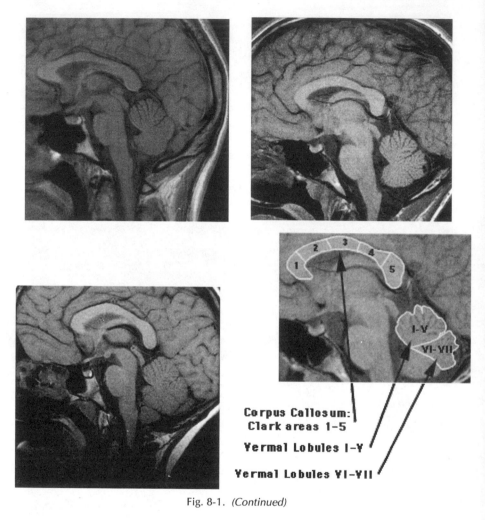

Fig. 8-1. *(Continued)*

measurements that were approximately one-half standard deviation or greater than the normal control participants.

Corpus Callosum

Planned pairwise comparisons among the three groups showed that AD participants had a statistically smaller total area of the midsagittal corpus callosum than AS participants [mean: AD = 579 mm^2, AS = 648 mm^2; F = 3.94 (1, 119), p = .0493; see Figure 8-4], but this was not smaller than for normal

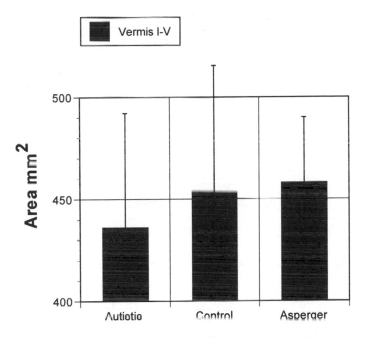

Fig. 8-2. Mean area measurements of midsagittal cerebellar vermal lobules I–V.

control participants [mean: NC = 602 mm^2; F = 1.90 (1, 119), p = .1702]. Pairwise comparisons also showed that the AS participants had significantly larger anterior corpus callosum measurements [Clk 1: AD = 122 mm^2, AS = 137 mm^2; F = 4.08 (1, 119), p = .046; see Figure 8-5] than AD participants, but not normal control participants [F = 2.14 (1, 119), p = .159]. However, the posterior corpus callosum of AD participants was significantly smaller than normal control participants [Clk5: AD = 166.6 mm^2, NC = 176.9 mm^2; F = 3.93 (1, 119), p = .049], but only was close to reaching statistical significance, largely because of insufficient power, when compared with AS participants [Clk5: AS = 181 mm^2; F = 3.25 (1, 119), p = .074].

Hippocampal Body

AD, AS, and normal control participants did not differ as to size of the hippocampal body [AD = 51.2 mm^2, AS = 52.6 mm^2, NC = 51.7 mm^2; F = 0.45 (2, 61), p = .641; see Figure 8-6].

ALAN LINCOLN *et al.*

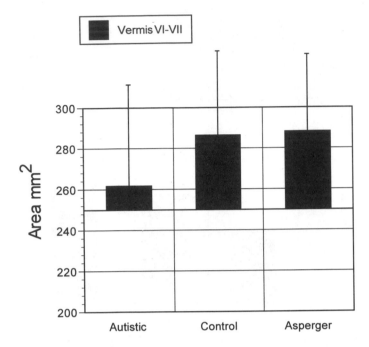

Fig. 8-3. Mean area measurements of midsagittal cerebellar vermal lobules VI and VII.

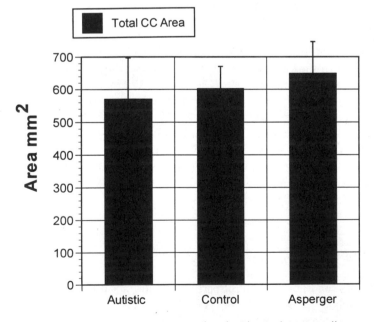

Fig. 8-4. Mean area measurements of total midsagittal corpus callosum.

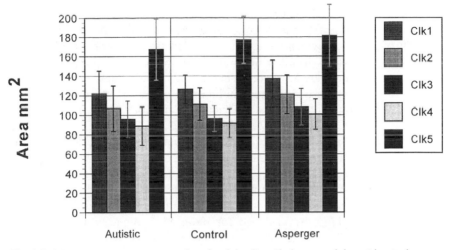

Fig. 8-5. Mean area measurements of each of the five Clark areas of the midsagittal corpus callosum.

DISCUSSION

There is little doubt that AS results from abnormal brain development and function. However, the etiology and nature of the brain pathology that is associated with AS is still unknown. Although genetic and environmental factors are likely to influence abnormal brain development and function in persons with

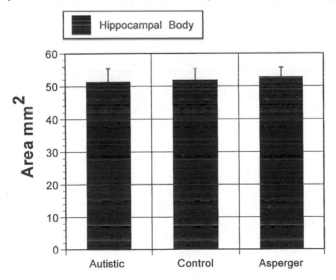

Fig. 8-6. Mean area measurements of the hippocampal body.

AS, there is still no consistent or conclusive evidence of specific factors, either genetic or environmental, that are common to the syndrome. Moreover, there is a paucity of biological evidence that can aid in addressing the problem of whether AS and AD are distinct disorders or are different forms of a single disorder.

Currently, there are 35 reported cases of AS individuals who have had brain MRIs. Twenty-two AS cases, including the 7 cases we are discussing herein, do not show gross neuroradiological evidence of MRI brain abnormality. In 13 of the 35 cases, brain MRI abnormalities have been reported. These include cortical abnormalities of the frontal, temporal, parietal, and occipital lobes, thinning of the posterior corpus callosum, and increased volume of the lateral ventricles (generally the right lateral ventricle). These findings do not suggest a common gross brain abnormality associated with AS, at least not one that can be detected by standard neuroradiological readings of the MRI. However, in weighing the evidence for brain MRI abnormality, there is a growing body of AS cases (13 of 35) consistent with gross, nonspecific neuroradiological brain abnormality.

Ours are the only AS cases in which there is quantitative measurement of specific brain structures using MRI and statistical comparisons to normative data. One of our seven AS cases had relatively small neocerebellar vermal lobule VI and VII midsagittal area measurements versus the other AS cases and normal control cases. Four of the seven AS cases were about one-half standard deviation or greater than the mean of the normal control cases for this brain measurement. Thus, some degree of cerebellar hypoplasia is possible in this one AS case, perhaps similar to those cases we and others have reported in persons with AD (Courchesne, 1995; Courchesne, Yeung-Courchesne, Press, Hesselink, & Jernigan, 1988). However, there are too few AS cases with quantitative MRI measurement of the neocerebellar vermis to draw a meaningful conclusion regarding the significance of these findings.

In addition, the anterior corpus callosum was relatively large in our seven AS cases. We did not find evidence of thinning of the posterior corpus callosum described for three AS cases by Berthier (1994); and unlike AD cases (Egaas *et al.*, 1995), our AS group did *not* have a reduction in the area of subregions of the posterior corpus callosum. The anterior corpus callosum was statistically larger in AS, but more cases are needed to confirm this finding. It is interesting that some AS cases with parietal involvement may show the pattern of thinning reported by Berthier (1994), whereas other AS cases with more anterior hemisphere abnormality may show changes in the size of the anterior corpus callosum. A larger anterior corpus callosum suggests the presence of excessive interhemispheric frontal excitation, which may be consistent with the reported deficits of executive functions described in AS individuals (Ozonoff *et al.*, 1994).

Does the current neurocognitive and neuroradiological evidence suggest that AS and AD are different disorders or fall on some continuum of common pathology? Is AD a more severe form of AS? These questions are still difficult to answer because of the limited case information and because such questions have not been researched in a systematic manner with appropriate methods and controls. However, it is possible to make some early and tentative observations about the current case literature.

The neurocognitive evidence of intellectual abilities observed in persons with AS and AD suggests that AD results in generally more severe neurocognitive and intellectual deficits. These deficits are particularly evident in the verbal intellectual abilities of AD individuals. AS individuals are not as impaired in their verbal intelligence. These observations, however, cannot answer whether the disorders are in fact different. It is possible that AD is simply a more severe form of AS wherein language functions and other intellectual functions are more compromised. The meta-analytic results reported above that compare AS and AD on less verbal, performance measures, show that on the whole, both seem to function in a similar manner (the AD individuals performing slightly worse as a group). There was no evidence of consistent performance deficits characterized by visual-motor or visual-perceptual problems. However, isolated AS cases (our Cases 3 and 6) demonstrated such problems. This is consistent with previous literature that also finds evidence of such visual-motor and visual-perceptual deficits in AS. Thus, there may be a subgroup of AS individuals with greater compromise to visual and motor systems, but such deficits are not characteristic of the AS group as a whole.

The neuroradiological evidence, however, leads to somewhat different conclusions suggesting biological differences between AS and AD. There appears to be more consistent pathology of the cerebellar vermis in AD relative to AS. In addition, the posterior corpus callosum is thin in persons with AD, but not AS. In contrast, the anterior corpus callosum in AS is larger than in AD. Thus, there is a different pattern of anatomy in AD and AS cases. If further research supported such differences in the underlying anatomy of AS and AD cases, then it would be suggestive of each disorder having a different pathological basis.

The only way to determine whether AS is characterized by some form of consistent structural brain abnormality will be to systematically diagnose, complete MRI brain scans, and quantify measurements of brain structures in relatively large samples of AS individuals. Moreover, comparing such findings with analogous studies of AD individuals may shed light on whether abnormalities of structural brain development are common to each disorder.

ACKNOWLEDGMENTS

Thanks to Osamu Saitoh, Brian Egaas, and Heather Chisum for help with anatomical measurements. This research was supported by NINDS grant #2-Rol-NS-19855 awarded to E. Courchesne.

REFERENCES

Allen, M. H., Lincoln, A. J., & Kaufman, A. S. (1991). Sequential and simultaneous processing abilities of high-functioning autistic and language impaired children. *Journal of Autism and Developmental Disorders, 21*, 483–502.

American Psychiatric Association. (1994). *Diagnostic and statistical manual of mental disorders* (4th ed.). Washington, DC: Author.

Asarnow, R. F., Tanguay, P. E., Bott, L., & Freeman, B. J. (1987). Patterns of intellectual functioning in non-retarded autistic and schizophrenic children. *Journal of Child Psychology and Psychiatry, 28*, 273–280.

Asperger, H. (1944). Die "autistischen Psychopathen" im Kindesalter. *Archiv. für Psychiatrie.und Nervenkrankheiten, 117*, 76–136.

Asperger, H. (1968). Zur Differentialdiagnos des kindlichen Autismus. *Acta Paedopsychiatrica, 35*, 136–145.

Berthier, M. L. (1994). Corticocallosal anomalies in Asperger's syndrome. *American Journal of Roentgenology., 162*, 236–237.

Berthier, M. L., Bayes, A., & Tolosa, E. S. (1993). Magnetic resonance imaging in patients with concurrent Tourettes disorder and Asperger's syndrome. *Journal of the American Academy of Child and Adolescent Psychiatry, 32*, 633–639.

Berthier, M. L., Santamaria, J., Encabo, H., & Tolosa, E. S. (1992). Recurrent hypersomnia in two adolescent males with Asperger syndrom. *Journal of the American Academy of Child and Adolescent Psychiatry, 31*(4), 735–738.

Berthier, M., Starkstein, S. E., & Leiguarda, R. (1990). Developmental cortical anomalies in Asperger's syndrome: Neuroradiological findings in two patients. *Journal of Neuropsychiatry and Clinical Neurosciences, 2*, 197–201.

Bowman, E. (1988). Asperger's syndrome and autism: The case for a connection. *British Journal of Psychiatry, 152*, 377–382.

Brown, A., & Brierley, J. (1973). The earliest alterations in rat neurons and astrocytes after anoxia-ischaemia. *Acta Neuropathologica, 23*, 9–22.

Burgoine, E., & Wing, L. (1983). Identical triplets with Asperger's syndrome. *British Journal of Psychiatry, 143*, 261–265.

Courchesne, E. (1995). Infantile autism. Part I: MR imaging abnormalities and their neurobiological correlates. Part II: A new neurodevelopmental model. *International Pediatrics, 10*(2), 141–154.

Courchesne, E., Press, G. A., & Yeung-Courchesne, R. (1993). Parietal lobe abnormalities detected with MR in patients with infantile autism. *American Journal of Roentgenology, 160*, 387–393.

Courchesne, E., Saitoh, O., Yeung-Courchesne, R., Press, G. A., Lincoln, A. J., Haas, R. H., & Schreibman, L. (1994). Abnormality of cerebellar vermian lobules VI and VII in patients with infantile autism: Identification of hypoplastic and hyperplastic subgroups with MR imaging. *American Journal of Roentgenology, 162*, 123–130.

Courchesne, E., Yeung-Courchesne, R., Press, G., Hesselink, J., & Jernigan, T. (1988), Hypoplasia of cerebellar vermal lobules VI and VII in autism. *New England Journal of Medicine, 318*, 1349–1354.

DeLong, G. (1978). A neuropsychologic interpretation of infantile autism. In M. Rutter & E. Schopler (Eds.), *Autism: A reappraisal of concepts and treatment* (pp. 207–218). New York: Plenum Press.

DeLong, G., & Dwyer, J. (1988). Correlation of family history with specific subgroups: Asperger's syndrome and bipolar affective disease. *Journal of Autism and Developmental Disorders, 18*(4), 593–600.

DeLong, R., & Nohria, C. (1994). Psychiatric family history and neurologic disease in autistic spectrum disorders. *Developmental Medicine and Child Neurology, 36*(5), 441–448.

Egaas, B., Courchesne, E., & Saitoh, O. (1995). Reduced size of the corpus callosum in autism. *Archives of Neurology, 45*, 317–324.

Fine, J., Bartolucci, G., Szatmari, P., & Ginsberg, G. (1994). Cohesive discourse in pervasive developmental disorders. *Journal of Autism and Developmental Disorders, 24*, 315–329.

Folstein, S., & Rutter, M. (1977). Infantile autism: A genetic study of 21 twin pairs. *Journal of Child Psychology and Psychiatry, 18*, 297–321.

Fragoso, R., & Cantu, J. (1984). A new psychomotor retardation syndrome with peculiar facies and marfanoid habitus. *Clinical Genetics, 25*, 187 190.

Freeman, B. J., Lucas, J. C., Forness, S. R., & Ritvo, E. R. (1985). Cognitive processing of high-functioning autistic children: Comparing the K-ABC and the WISC-R. *Journal of Psychoeducational Assessment, 4*, 357–362.

Ghaziuddin, M., Leininger, L., & Tsai, L. (1995). Brief report: Thought disorder in Asperger syndrome: Comparison with high-functioning autism. *Journal of Autism and Developmental Disorders, 25*, 311–317.

Gillberg, C. (1989). Asperger syndrome in 23 Swedish children. *Developental Medicine and Child Neurology, 31*, 520–531.

Gillberg, C., & Wahlstrom, J. (1985). Chromosome abnormalities in infantile autism and other childhood psychoses: A population study of 66 cases. *Developmental Medicine and Child Neurology, 27*, 293–304.

Gillberg, I. C., & Gillberg, C. (1989). Asperger syndrome — some epidemiological considerations: A research note. *Journal of Child Psychology and Psychiatry, 30*, 631–638.

Hauser, S., DeLong, G., & Rosmah, N (1975) Pneumographic findings in the infantile autistic syndrome — a correlation with temporal lobe disease. *Brain, 98*, 667–688

Jones, P., & Kerwin, R. (1990). Left temporal lobe damage in Asperger's syndrome. *British Journal of Psychiatry, 156*, 570–572.

Klin, A., Volkmar, F. R., Sparrow, S. S., Cicchetti, D. V., & Rourke, B. P. (1995). Validity and neuropsychological characterization of Asperger syndrome: Convergence with nonverbal learning disabilities syndrome. *Journal of Child Psychology and Psychiatry, 36*, 1127–1140.

Kuck, J., Lincoln, A. J., & Heaton, R. (submitted). Age related changes in intellectual ability among individuals with autistic disorder. *Journal of Developmental Neuropsychology.*

Le Couteur, A., Rutter, M., Lord, C., Rios, P., Robertson, S., Holdgrafer, M., & McLennan, J. D. (1989). Autism Diagnostic Interview: A standardized investigator-based instrument. *Journal of Autism and Developmental Disorders, 19*, 363–387.

Lincoln, A. J., Allen, M., & Kilman, A. (1995). The assessment and interpretation of intellectual abilities in people with autism. In E. Schopler & G. Mesibov (Eds.), *Learning and cognition in autism* (pp. 89–117). New York: Plenum Press.

Lincoln, A. J., Courchesne, E., Kilman, B., Elmasian, R., & Allen, M. (1988). A study of high-functioning people with autism. *Journal of Autism and Developmental Disorders, 18*, 505–524.

Lockyer, L., & Rutter, M. (1970). A five- to fifteen-year follow-up study of infantile psychosis. IV: Patterns of cognitive ability. *British Journal of Social and Clinical Psychology, 9*, 152–163.

Lord, C., Rutter, M., Goode, S., Heemshergen, J., Jordan, H., Mawhood, L., & Schopler, E. (1989). Autism Diagnostic Observation Schedule: A standardized observation of communicative and social behavior. *Journal of Autism and Developmental Disorders, 19*, 185–212.

Lord, C., Rutter, M., & Le Couteur, A. (1994). Autism Diagnostic Interview-Revised: A revised version of diagnostic interview for caregivers of individuals with possible pervasive developmental disorders. *Journal of Autism and Developmental Disorders, 24*, 659–685.

Marjiviona, J., & Prior M. (1995). Comperison of Asperger syndrome and high-functioning autistic children on a test of motor impairment. *Journal of Autism and Developmental Disorders, 25*, 23–39.

McKelvey, J. R., Lambert, R., Mottron, L., & Shevell, M. (1995). Right-hemisphere dysfunction in Asperger's syndrome. *Journal of Child Neurology, 10*, 310–314.

Minshew, N. J., Goldstein, G., Muenz, L. R., & Patyon, J. B. (1992). Neuropsychological functioning in non-mentally retarded autistic individuals. *Journal of Clinical and Experimental Neuropsychology, 14*, 749–761.

Narita, T., & Koga, Y. (1987). Neuropsychological assessment of childhood autism. *Advances in Biological Psychiatry, 26*, 156–170.

Ohta, M. (1987). Cognitive disorders of infantile autism: A study employing the WISC, spatial relationship conceptualization, and gesture imitations. *Journal of Autism and Developmental Disorders, 17*, 45–62.

Ono, M., Kubik, S., & Abernathey, D. (1990). *Atlas of the cerebral sulci.* New York: Thieme Medical.

Ozbayrak, K., Kapucu, O., Erdem, E., & Aras, T. (1991). Left occipital hypoperfusion in a case with the Asperger syndrome. *Brain and Development, 13*(6), 454–456.

Ozonoff, S., Rogers, S. J., & Pennington, B. F. (1991). Executive function deficits in high-functioning autistic individuals: Relationship to theory of mind. *Journal of Child Psychology and Psychiatry, 32*, 1081–1105.

Ozonoff, S., Strayer, D., McMahon, W., & Filloux, F. (1994), Executive function abnormalities in autism: An information processing approach. *Journal of Child Psychology and Psychiatry, 35*, 1015–1031.

Rumsey, J. M., & Hamburger, S. D. (1988). Neuropsychological findings in high-functioning men with infantile autism, residual state. *Journal of Clinical and Experimental Neuropsychology, 10*, 210–221.

Rumsey, J. M., & Hamburger, S. D. (1990). Neuropsychological divergence of high-level autism and severe dyslexia. *Journal of Autism and Developmental Disorders, 20*, 155–168.

Saitoh, O., Courchesne, E., Egaas, B., Lincoln, A. J., & Schreibman, L. (1995). Cross-sectional area of the posterior hippocampus in autistic patients with cerebellar and corpus callosum abnormalities. *Neurology, 45*, 317–324.

Saliba, J., & Griffiths, M. (1990). Brief report: Autism of the Asperger type associated with an autosomal fragile site. *Journal of Autism and Developmental Disorders, 20*, 569–575.

Schneider, S. G., & Asarnow, R. F. (1987). A comparison of cognitive/neuropsychological impairments of nonretarded autistic and schizophrenic children. *Journal of Abnormal Child Psychology, 15*, 29–46.

Schopler, E. (1996). Are autism and Asperger syndrome (AS) different labels or different disabilities? *Journal of Autism and Developmental Disorders, 26*, 109–110.

Schopler, E., Reichler, R. J., & Renner, B. R. (1988). *The Childhood Autism Rating Scale (CARS).* Los Angeles: Western Psychological Corporation.

Siegel, D. J., Minshew, N. J., & Goldstein, G. (1996). Wechsler IQ profiles in diagnosis of high-functioning autism. *Journal of Autism and Developmental Disorders, 26*, 389–406.

Sparrow, S., Balla, D., & Chicchetti, D. (1984). *Vineland Adaptive Behavior Scales.* Circle Pines, MN: American Guidance Service.

Szatmari, P., Archer, L., Fisman, S., Streiner, D., & Wilson, F. (1995). Asperger's syndrome and autism: Differences in behavior, cognition and adaptive functioning. *Journal of the American Academy of Child and Adolescent Psychiatry, 34*, 1662–1671.

Szatmari, P., Tuff, L., Finlayson, A., & Bartolucci, G. (1990). Asperger's syndrome and autism: Neurocognitive aspects. *Journal of the American Academy of Child and Adolescent Psychiatry, 29*, 130–139.

Tantam, D., Evered, C., & Hersov, L. (1990). Asperger's syndrome and ligamentous laxity. *Journal of the American Academy of Child and Adolescent Psychiatry, 29*(6), 892–896.

Thorndike, R., Hagen, E., & Sattler, J. (1986). *Stanford–Binet Intelligence Scale* (4th ed.). Chicago: Riverside.

Tymchuk, A. J., Simmons, J. Q., & Neafsey, S. (1977). Intellectual characteristics of adolescent childhood psychotics with high verbal ability. *Journal of Mental Deficiency Research, 21*, 133–138.

Venter, A., Lord, C., & Schopler, E. (1992). A follow-up study of high functioning autistic children. *Journal of Child Psychology and Psychiatry, 33*, 489–507.

Volkmar, F., Klin, A., Schultz, R., Bronen, R., Maranas, W., Sparrow, S., & Cohen, D. (1996). Asperger syndrome. *Journal of the American Academy of Child and Adolescent Psychiatry, 35*, 118–123.

Wassing, H. E. (1965). Cognitive functioning in early infantile autism: An examination of four cases by means of the Wechsler Intelligence Scale for Children. *Acta Paedopsychiatrica, 32*, 122–135.

Wechsler, D. (1974). *The Wechsler Intelligence Scale for Children — Revised.* San Antonio: Psychological Corporation.

Wechsler, D. (1981). *The Wechsler Adult Intelligence Scale — revised.* San Antonio: Psychological Corporation.

IV

Treatment Issues

9

Social Stories and Comic Strip Conversations with Students with Asperger Syndrome and High-Functioning Autism

CAROL A. GRAY

It is impossible to observe a social interaction, or a social impairment, in a person who is alone. Regardless, the phrase *social impairment in autism* is frequently used to refer to the social challenges associated with disorders identified by Leo Kanner (1943) and Hans Asperger (1944). The words *in autism* in this case may leave a misleading impression that the social impairment lies *solely* within the individual with autism. This is inconsistent with the definition of the word *social*, which requires the involvement of more than one person. Firsthand accounts by people with autism (e.g., Cesaroni & Garber, 1991; Grandin & Scariano, 1986; Volkmar & Cohen, 1985; Williams, 1992), and families of individuals with autism (Hart, 1989; McDonnell, 1993; Moreno, 1992) raise awareness of the frustrations experienced by all parties as they work to understand, communicate, and interact successfully with one another. Confusion and feelings of being overwhelmed and misunderstood are experienced not only by people with high-functioning autism and Asperger syndrome (HFA/AS), but also by parents, professionals, and friends.

CAROL A. GRAY • Jenison Public Schools, Jenison, Michigan 49428.

Asperger Syndrome or High-Functioning Autism?, edited by Schopler *et al.* Plenum Press, New York, 1998.

To improve social interaction, methods and materials must address both sides of the social equation. First, parents and professionals need help understanding the person with HFA/AS. In addition, the person with HFA/AS needs assistance to understand the myriad of daily interactions and events. This chapter describes *social stories*, short stories that describe social situations, and *Comic Strip Conversations*, an instructional process that illustrates shared information with simple drawings, symbols, and color. These social interventions are based on a philosophy of improved social skills through improved social understanding, and a shared responsibility for social success.

RATIONALE

To understand the rationale behind social stories and Comic Strip Conversations, parents and professionals are encouraged to *abandon all assumptions*. People readily make a variety of assumptions to interpret the behavior of others. These assumptions are based on a common social understanding. Applied to a person with HFA/AS, who may perceive events differently, these same assumptions may be in error. The result is a shared social impairment: two parties responding with equally valid but different perceptions of the same event. This makes it difficult to understand one another and interact. Parents may become frustrated when their child responds "inappropriately" or "without apparent reason"; the child with autism may view the actions or statements of others as out of context, illogical, or overwhelming. There are no "bizarre" behaviors, only human responses that originate from an experience that is not fully understood or appreciated. By abandoning the assumptions that are effective in most social situations, parents and professionals have the opportunity to develop social skills interventions that are meaningful to the person with HFA/AS.

Attitudes reflecting acceptance, creativity, and humor are central to social stories and Comic Strip Conversations. Asperger (1944) identified a sense of humor as an important trait for parents and professionals working with children with autistic disorders, stating:

> These children often show a surprising sensitivity to the personality of the teacher. However difficult they are even under optimal conditions, they can be guided and taught, but only by those who give them true understanding and genuine affection, people who show kindness towards them and, yes, humor. (p. 48)

Humor is also valued by people with autism. A survey completed by members of a Social Skills Group for adults with HFA indicated humor was a valued personality trait, a factor determining popularity among group members (Mesibov & Stephens, 1990). Humor may play an important role in teaching social skills. This is especially true when humor is defined as a form of creativity:

a response to typical situations from new, different, and unexpected perspectives. It may be this type of humor — the ability to positively and automatically see things from a different point of view — that is most important for those who work with students with disorders on the autistic spectrum. Specifically, it is this ability that guides the development of each social story and influences each Comic Strip Conversation.

One area of research important to social stories and Comic Strip Conversations is *theory of mind*: the ability to attribute thoughts and feelings to others, and to understand that others have perspectives that are unique and different from our own (Leslie, 1987). Theory of mind has been referred to as the "capacity to mind-read" (Happé & Frith, 1995, p. 177). This ability provides a person with basic information regarding the feelings and thoughts of others. Evidence suggests that there is a significant impairment in theory of mind in individuals with autism (Cohen, 1990), which may impact their ability to pretend (see discussions in Baron-Cohen, 1995, and Harris, 1993; Baron-Cohen, Leslie, & Frith, 1985) with "far reaching implications for social interaction" (Frith, 1991, p. 19). Discussions surrounding theory of mind have increased our awareness that most people are privy to a "secret code": a system of unspoken communication that carries essential information; a system that eludes and frustrates individuals with HFA/AS. As one person with autism stated, "people give each other messages with their eyes, but I do not know what they are saying" (Wing, 1992, p. 131).

Frith (1989) proposed another theory that is based on the ability to derive meaning from diverse pieces of information in context, *central coherence*. Frith proposes that "autism is characterized by a specific imbalance in integration of information at different levels" (Happé, 1995, p. 116). For example, high school students attending a school pep assembly may not be able to recall the details of each cheer or routine, but readily understand the meaning of the event as a whole — to foster enthusiasm for the football team. Other examples of central coherence include the ability to assign the correct meaning to words in conversation based on context, as in "I will meet [not *meat*] you later," or to describe the plot of a story after reading pages of details and conversation between characters (Happé, 1995). Central coherence raises awareness of yet another "secret" that influences the ability to understand and relate meaningfully to daily encounters and activities.

Comic Strip Conversations and social stories translate these "secrets" surrounding social interaction into practical, tangible social information for students with HFA/AS. Recognizing the student may be missing or misperceiving important social information, these approaches establish social understanding as an integral and prerequisite component to teaching social skills. Parents and professionals first learn to consider the student's understanding of a given situation, then try to ensure, beyond all assumptions, that the student has accurate and specific social information.

Each social story and Comic Strip Conversation is designed to bring predictability to a situation that from the perspective of the student with HFA/AS is confusing, frightening, and/or difficult to "read." Recognizing that predictability has been shown to improve social responsivity and play behavior in children with autism (Dawson & Adams, 1984; Dawson & Galpert, 1990; Ferrara & Hill, 1980; Klinger & Dawson, 1992, cited in Klinger & Dawson, 1995), understanding the unknown may be prerequisite to social success for students with HFA/AS.

One premise of social stories and Comic Strip Conversations is that materials and instructional methods used to present social information should be consistent with the visual learning strengths of students with HFA/AS. Temple Grandin (1995a) describes that she has:

> no language-based memory. When I hear the word *over* by itself, I visualize a childhood memory of a dog jumping over a fence. To store material that I have read, I either read it off a page I have photographed in my memory or I translate the written material into visual images. To retrieve the information, I have to replay the "video." (p. 143)

In a discussion of her visual thinking style, Grandin indicates this ability may be expanded to compensate for impairments in language. She advises educators and parents to use visual methods of instruction to enhance learning, suggesting the use of typewriters or word processors at an early age (Grandin, 1995b).

Interventions incorporating the use of visual supports have been effective in the education of children with autistic spectrum disorders (Hodgdon, 1995; Quill, 1995). Visually based strategies provide structure to daily experiences and learning. For example, picture schedules help students understand the sequence and timing of classroom activities (Schopler, Mesibov, & Hearsey, 1995) and changes in routine (Twachtman, 1995). Often, picture schedules have highly individualized formats based on student ability and interest (Dalrymple, 1995). Another approach, Cognitive Picture Rehearsal (Groden & LeVasseur, 1995), uses simple pictures with accompanying scripts to help individuals rehearse a sequence of behaviors. Social stories and Comic Strip Conversations are also "visually dependent" strategies that require parents/professionals and students with HFA/AS to communicate concepts and ideas with the support of written words, simple illustrations, symbols, and color.

Understanding the learning style of individuals with HFA/AS lays the foundation for further modifications based on individual student needs and abilities. Each social story and Comic Strip Conversation presents social information using a writing style, vocabulary, format, materials, and instructional techniques individually tailored to maximize student success.

Finally, parents and professionals who use social stories and Comic Strip Conversations recognize that motivation is critical to learning, and student interests are critical to motivation. A student with HFA/AS may focus on interests that parents/professionals dismiss as irrelevant or unimportant. However, these same interests may be creatively utilized to increase a student's desire to learn new skills. Koegel and Koegel (1995) have reviewed research findings that support the use of individual choice and interest to teach target behaviors. This is consistent with recommendations that even interests regarded as unusual or unconventional should be used in instruction to increase the likelihood of success (Grandin, 1995b; Olley, 1986; Schuler, 1995). The TEACCH program recognizes that students with autism often are not motivated by traditional incentives, and emphasizes the importance of student interest in the selection of reinforcers (Schopler *et al.*, 1995). Individual interests play an important role in both social stories and Comic Strip Conversations, influencing the format and content of instruction.

In summary, parents and professionals are encouraged to abandon all of the typical assumptions used to interpret and explain the behavior of others, as they may be inaccurate if applied to students with HFA/AS. Replacing assumptions with attitudes of acceptance and understanding, and creatively viewing situations from a student's perspective, is central to each social story and Comic Strip Conversation. Recognizing that a student may differently predict, "read," or interpret events or social interactions, the goal of these approaches is to provide students with accurate social information. This information is presented using materials, methods, and instructional techniques that are consistent with the learning characteristics of students with HFA/AS. Comic Strip Conversations and social stories are tailored for each student; incorporating individual needs and abilities, as well as preferences and interests, maximizes a student's understanding of the social environment.

SOCIAL STORIES

A social story is a short story that adheres to a specific format and guidelines to objectively describe a person, skill, event, concept, or social situation. Most social stories are written by parents or professionals. The goal of a social story is to share relevant information. This information often includes (but is not limited to) *where* and *when* a situation takes place, *who* is involved, *what* is occurring, and *why*. Often, the most relevant information may be a factor in a situation that is "obvious" to others, though overwhelming or confusing for the student with HFA/AS. For example, Evan, an adolescent with autism, became upset whenever traffic lights changed color. A social story explaining how traffic lights work immediately eliminated his negative response. This enabled Evan and his teachers to complete community outings more easily. Social stories may also explain concepts that are abstract and difficult to understand, or in some cases, they may explain what other people know, feel, or believe. Derrick, a high-functioning kindergarten student with autism, had difficulty understanding

Learning About Being Fair

My name is Derrick. I try to be fair and follow the rules. Playing fair is important.

People learn about what is fair as they grow up. Usually by the time people are adults, they know a lot about being fair.

I am still learning about what is fair and what is not fair.

It's important to listen to people who know a lot about being fair. Miss Roberts knows what is fair. My Mom and Dad know what is fair.

I will try to listen to adults when they are talking to me about what is fair.

Fig. 9-1. Excerpts from text of a social story on the topic of fairness for a kindergarten student with HFA. (Original story was printed one concept per page and was accompanied by simple illustrations.)

the concept of *fair*, and was often distressed by situations he perceived as unfair. A social story addressing the issue of fairness explained to Derrick that *others had information* on this topic that may be helpful to him (see Figure 9-1). Social stories are often written in response to situations that are upsetting for a student with HFA/AS. Changes in routine were difficult for Heather, a fourth grader with AS. In particular, she became upset when she had a substitute teacher. A social story describing how a substitute teacher knows what to do immediately eliminated Heather's negative response (see Figure 9-2). In addition to sharing relevant information, most social stories identify desired responses. People who write social stories are encouraged to share information with consideration of a student's perspective, abilities, and interests. As a result, social stories vary in content and ability level, though all are defined by a standard that includes a specific ratio of sentence types (described later). The result is an individualized story that shares accurate information with a reassuring and patient quality.

The effectiveness of each social story varies, and is most likely dependent on many factors. The original article describing social stories theorized that "social stories are most likely to benefit students functioning intellectually in the trainable mentally impaired range or higher who possess basic language skills" (Gray & Garand, 1993, p. 2). Specifically, it was initially suspected that children who are interested in letters and numbers, read from an early age, or demonstrate an interest in books, videos, and visual materials may be most likely to benefit from the use of social stories. Clinical experience reveals that, with modification, social stories may also be effective for more severely challenged children. Swaggart *et al.* (1995) found initial support for the use of social stories "in

Having a Substitute Teacher

My name is Heather. I go to Lincoln Elementary School. I am in the fourth grade. Mrs. Smith is my teacher.

Sometimes Mrs. Smith cannot be at school. We have a substitute teacher. This is okay.

Mrs. Smith writes LESSON PLANS for the substitute teacher. The substitute teacher reads the lesson plans and knows what to do.

The substitute teacher helps Mrs. Smith and the children. If I have questions about what we will be doing, I may ask the substitute teacher. I may ask the substitute teacher other questions. She is there to help me and the other children in my class.

Many things stay the same when we have a substitute teacher.

We will probably have math, reading group, board work, and seat work.

We will probably have recess.

We will probably have spelling or make up work.

We will have lunch.

We will have language and science if there is time. The substitute teacher will tell us if we have time for language and science.

We may do other things. This is okay.

The substitute teacher will tell the children when it is time to go home. The children will leave to go home, like they always do. The substitute teacher will leave to go to her home.

Fig. 9-2. Social story to prepare a student with AS for a substitute teacher.

individual and group settings for individuals with autism who function at a variety of levels" (p. 13).

Developing, writing, and implementing an effective social story requires six elements: (1) determining a topic; (2) gathering individualized information regarding the student and situation; (3) consideration of the guidelines for writing for persons with HFA/AS; (4) adherence to the Social Story Ratio; (5) incorporating student interests into a social story; and (6) introducing, reviewing, and monitoring a social story. These elements are simultaneously considered throughout the process of developing and writing an effective social story. The following sections focus on each of these elements.

The Topic

The first step in developing a social story is to determine the topic. Social stories are often written in response to events that are difficult or distressing for a student; situations that have resulted in confusion or fear. Topics for these stories "identify themselves." For example, a student continually refuses to go outdoors for recess. A social story is developed to explain what children do on a playground. Social stories may also be used to describe a future situation or introduce a new social skill. Anticipating a student's experience, and writing to provide a student with accurate information in advance of when it is needed, may avoid negative responses and improve a student's confidence. In addition, selecting a situation in which a student is already successful makes an excellent topic for a student's "first story."

Gathering Information for a Social Story

Once a topic is identified, detailed information is gathered through observation of the situation and interviews with relevant individuals. This includes information regarding relevant cues, the typical sequence of events, ideas from those involved in the situation, and the perspective of the student with HFA/AS regarding the situation. A social story may not contain all of the information that is gathered. Still, a complete understanding of the situation is needed to determine information that is important to include in a story, as well as that which may be excluded.

Observation of relevant cues will result in a social story outline. These cues create a "backdrop" around which people and events revolve. Cues define a situation. From the perspective of a child with HFA/AS, cues may be focused on as predictable markers of time, consistent and reliable "soldiers" that occur among the relative disorder and chaos of daily life. For others, cues may be undetected, or misinterpreted. Therefore, an observer attempts to simultaneously view the situation from his or her own perspective and the perspective of the student. To develop a story about recess, an observer notes when recess typically begins and ends, the signal that is used, and the criteria for outdoor and indoor recess. Possible "cue variations" are also considered. If the recess bell is out of order, what happens? If an assembly runs past the time for the start of recess, who will know what to do? An accurate assessment of cues and cue variations provides a framework for the development of an effective social story.

In addition to direct observation of the situation, interviewing those who have direct contact with the student often results in valuable information and establishes a team effort. Teachers, custodians, and other professionals often have helpful information regarding the student's responses. Parents are also a valuable resource. They possess insightful, detailed information about their child. Information regarding a child's likes and dislikes, interests, and responses to the given situation *and similar events* can directly influence the content or format of a social story. Authors recognize the expertise of those surrounding a child and listen for information that may be incorporated into a social story.

Students with HFA/AS often have unique ideas and perceptions of a situation, though they may be overlooked as potential experts in the development of their own social story. Taking the time to talk with a student often reveals misperceptions or misinterpretations that are causing difficulty. Structuring the conversation using Comic Strip Conversations (described later in this chapter) helps a student follow the interaction and stay on topic.

Guidelines for Writing for Students with HFA/AS

The guidelines for writing social stories are based on the learning characteristics of students with HFA/AS. These guidelines, together with the Social Story Ratio and efforts to incorporate student interests (described in later sections), help to ensure the patient accepts quality associated with social stories. This improves the likelihood that a social story will be effective for a student.

A Social Story Is Developed According to Several Individual Factors

Consideration of a student's age, reading and comprehension ability, and attention span directly influences the content and format of each social story. For example, a story for a preschool student will contain a few large words per page, and will be accompanied by photographs, simple illustrations, or Picture Communication Symbols (Mayer Johnson, 1992). The social story in Figure 9-3 was written for a preschool student who became upset whenever the washing machine at home was not in use. Prereaders often use social stories with accompanying audio cassette tapes. Stories are recorded with a bell that signals the child to turn the page.

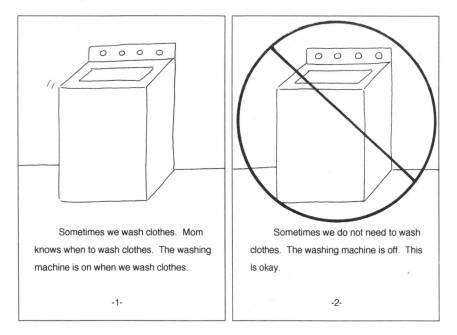

Sometimes we wash clothes. Mom knows when to wash clothes. The washing machine is on when we wash clothes. -1-	Sometimes we do not need to wash clothes. The washing machine is off. This is okay. -2-

Fig. 9-3. Social story for a preschool student with an autistic spectrum disorder.

Recording the story using the voice of a parent, or a person the child most consistently attends to, serves to further personalize a story. In contrast, a social story for an adolescent with AS may be written using advanced vocabulary, fine print, and columns similar to a newspaper article. Writing a social story appropriate for a student's abilities increases the likelihood that the story will be effective.

A Social Story Shares Relevant Information

An author of a social story describes events and cues objectively, as they typically occur, omitting extraneous details. Focusing on the most important information, highlighting events, words, and gestures that carry the greatest meaning, is central to developing a social story. In this way, each social story *excludes* events that are irrelevant, drawing attention to the most important aspects of a situation.

Authors Consider the Possibility of Literal Interpretations

Writing a social story requires the author to share information with "literal accuracy" so that the content of a social story, or individual sentences, may be interpreted literally without any loss or deviation of meaning. One characteristic of language use in students with autism is "literalness…responding to the literal meaning of information, as opposed to the implied meaning" (Twachtman, 1995, p. 137). This is also true of students with AS (Gillberg & Gillberg, 1989, as cited in Attwood, 1996; see discussion in Attwood, 1996), whose extensive use of vocabulary and formal use of language can be misleading and may "detract from the proneness of many of them to concrete misinterpretations" (Gillberg, 1991, p. 142). For example, stating "My birthday party will start at *about* 2:00 on Friday," is preferable to "My birthday party is this Friday at 2:00." The word *about* in this example, and similar words like *usually*, *sometimes*, and *probably*, provide "social story insurance," an accommodation for possible literal interpretation that ensures the accuracy of the story.

Authors Write from a First- or Third-Person Perspective

Most social stories are written from a first-person perspective, usually in the present or future tense. Writing a story in the first person has advantages, as well as potentially negative implications. The major advantage is a social story that is nonthreatening, and assumes individual competence. Instead of a student being told what to do, as in "Brian will try to stand quietly in line," a story using the first-person perspective self-directs: "I will try to stand quietly in line." Recognizing the unique perspective of students with HFA/AS, statements that describe the HFA/AS student's personal feelings, beliefs, or motivations are avoided in a social story. For example, the statement, "I love to go out for recess," may be inaccurate and unrepresentative of a student's actual feelings. Instead, an author may write, "Many children like to go outside at recess," to describe how others respond to the situation. On rare occasions, social stories for adolescents and adults with HFA/AS may be written from the third-person perspective to imitate the style of a newspaper article.

Types of Social Story Sentences and the Social Story Ratio

Social stories are comprised of a combination of up to four different types of sentences: *descriptive*, *perspective*, *directive*, and *control sentences*. Each type of sentence in a social story serves a specific function. A social story may not contain all four different types of sentences, though each social story meets the criteria set by the Social Story Ratio (described later).

Descriptive sentences objectively define where a situation occurs, who is involved, what they are doing, and why. A descriptive sentence may describe a setting or environment, as in this example: "My school has many rooms. One room is called the lunch room. Usually, the children eat lunch in the lunch room."

Descriptive sentences also introduce the most relevant characters in a story and/or their role, as in "Many children stand in the lunch line," "An adult takes the lunch tickets," or "Each child has a turn to buy their lunch." Descriptive sentences may also explain why people behave the way they do: "Standing in a line helps the children get their hot lunches."

Perspective sentences are statements that describe a person's internal states. Perspective sentences may simply describe a physical state or desire: "The children are hungry. They want to eat." They may also describe a person's perceptual perspective: "The children hear the lunch bell." Perspective sentences frequently describe another person's thoughts ("Children know the lunch bell tells them to line up at the door"), feelings ("Some children like to eat and rest at lunch"), or beliefs and motivations ("Some children think the lunch lines are too long, so they bring a lunch from home").

Directive sentences are statements that directly define what is expected as a response to a given cue or situation. These sentences gently direct a student's behavior: "I will try to stand quietly in the lunch line." Considering students with HFA/AS may interpret information literally, this can intensify the influence of directive sentences on a student's behavior. For example, if a directive sentence begins only with "I will..." or "I should...," a student may interpret the statement as a demand requiring absolute compliance instead of as a statement intended to assist in learning and practicing new responses. For this reason, directive sentences always begin with phrases like "I will work on...," "I will try...," or "One thing I might try to say (do) is...." This minimizes the pressure a student may feel to "get it right the first time" or comply exactly to be regarded as successful.

The decision to use directive sentences is based on careful consideration of the individual student. One student may not need directive sentences in a social story, whereas another will not know what to do if directive sentences are excluded. The objective is to keep social stories "least restrictive": to provide accurate information without needlessly limiting a student's choices. Directive sentences may not need to direct, instead they can suggest. One approach is to list a variety of choices. This demonstrates the wide variety of possible responses to a given situation and increases a student's sense of control.

In a social story, a descriptive, perspective, or directive sentence may be written by parents/professionals as a partial statement. In this case, the student completes the sentence. A partial sentence encourages a student to make predictions regarding the next step in a situation, the response of another individual, or his or her own response. In the process of reviewing a social story, the parent/professional helps the student complete the unfinished statement. For example, following a series of sentences describing the process of standing in the lunch line at school, a student is asked to finish this partial directive sentence, "I will try to_____in the lunch line."

Control sentences are statements written by a student to identify strategies the student may use to recall the information in a social story, reassure him- or herself, or define his or her own response. In contrast to directive sentences, these statements provide an opportunity for a student with HFA/AS to control his or her own response by identifying meaningful, personal strategies to handle difficult situations. In writing a control sentence, a student may also incorporate his or her interests or favorite writing style. First, the student reviews the social story, adding control sentences of his or her own. A student interested in reptiles and poetry wrote the following control sentence about delays in the lunch line at school: "Lunch lines and turtles are both very slow. Sometimes they stop, sometimes they go." Another student wrote a different control sentence to help himself remain calm when people change their mind. "When someone says, 'I changed my mind,'" he wrote, "I can think of an idea becoming better. Like a caterpillar changing into a butterfly."

The *Social Story Ratio* defines the proportion of descriptive, perspective, directive, and control sentences in an entire social story. A basic premise of the social story approach is that each story should *describe more than direct*. This premise is reflected in the guidelines for writing social stories, and specifically defined by the Social Story Ratio. One section of a story may contain only descriptive and/or perspective sentences, while another section may contain only directive and/or control sentences. The proportion of these different types of sentences will be consistent with the Social Story Ratio when the story is considered as a whole. This ratio is maintained regardless of the length of a social story:

$$\frac{0\text{-}1 \text{ directive or control sentence(s)}}{2\text{-}5 \text{ descriptive and / or perspective sentences}} = \text{Social Story Ratio}$$

The following excerpt from a social story demonstrates how different types of sentences are combined in a social story:

> The children stand in the lunch line [descriptive]. Many children are hungry [perspective]. Each child will get a lunch [descriptive]. Each child waits for a turn to get their lunch [descriptive]. Lunch lines and turtles are both very slow, sometimes they stop, sometimes they go [control]. I will try to _____ in the lunch line [partial directive].

Combined with the guidelines for writing for students with HFA/AS, the Social Story Ratio completes a standard that defines each social story.

Incorporating Student Preferences and Interests in a Social Story

A student's interests and preferences can directly influence the content, writing style, illustrations, format, or implementation of a social story. Incorpo-

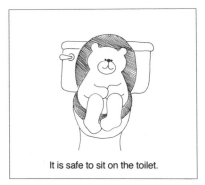

It is safe to sit on the toilet.

Fig. 9-4. Sample page from a social story for a preschool student using a favorite animal as a toileting model.

rating the "inside information" collected from discussions with professionals, parents, and the student, personalizes a social story. In addition, creatively customizing how information is presented may increase a student's motivation to attend to a social story.

A social story may contain references to a student's favorite character, animal, sports figure, or setting. For example, effective toilet training stories for preschool students often incorporate a child's favorite cartoon character or animal as a model (K. A. Quill, personal communication) (see Figure 9-4). To explain to a first-grade student with AS why people sometimes have to wait in line to order food (a practice she found very upsetting), her favorite fast-food restaurant was selected as the setting for the social story.

A social story may also reflect a student's favorite writing style. For example, to assist a second-grade student with HFA who was fascinated with Dr. Suess books (Geisel, 1940), a social story was written in "Dr. Suess style" following a repetitive pattern of rhyming phrases. The story addressed the topic of inappropriate language, describing new words and phrases to express anger and frustration ("Feeling angry is okay. I will try new things to say...").

Illustrations or visual materials that reinforce story content may similarly reflect individual preferences/interests: incorporating photographs, word find puzzles, street signs, or maps. Social stories for a third-grade student interested in the U.S. Postal Service were systematically customized in several ways. The stories were handwritten on elaborate stationery, accompanied by a representative hand drawn "stamp" to illustrate and reinforce story content, and folded and mailed as a personal letter to the student.

Finally, items that hold a student's attention can have a direct impact on how a social story is implemented. For example, a mother casually mentioned she would love it if her child's interest in reading books "would equal the intensity with which he read the back of cereal boxes." Her casual comment resulted in highly customized social stories. Advertisements for social stories were pasted to the backs of cereal boxes, using cereal box vocabulary ("Exclusive Offer! Send no money! Send in box top! Story to arrive in six days or less!"). The child sent cereal box tops to the address listed on the cereal box (the teacher). In return, the teacher sent social stories to her student. The social stories addressed social skills from the educational plan and incorporated cereal box phrases. The student's interest in the process surrounding social stories, as well as the information they contained, dramatically improved

Introducing, Reviewing, and Monitoring a Social Story

The cooperation, understanding, and support of all those working with a student result in a team approach to a social story and a shared responsibility for its implementation. Prior to introducing a story to a student, a rough draft is shared with a student's parents and others directly involved with the student for critical review. This catches inaccuracies and results in important revisions and/or the inclusion of critical details. The final draft of the story is distributed with an implementation plan that outlines review schedules and instructional methods that will accompany the story. In addition, this section describes several other guidelines that apply when introducing and monitoring a social story.

A Social Story Is Introduced to a Student in a Relaxed Manner

A quiet and comfortable environment with limited distractions is best. The parent/professional sits at the student's side and slightly back, talking quietly outside of the student's immediate view. Statements introducing a story range from a simple, "Let's read this story," to a more advanced, "You have been having difficulty in the lunch line. I wrote this story. It may be helpful to you. Let's read it." The story is placed in front of the student, who is encouraged to turn the pages and read the story independently. If an audio cassette tape accompanies the story, the parent/professional first ensures that the student knows how to operate the tape player, and then introduces the story.

Parents and Professionals Carefully Minimize Their Involvement

Support or direction is provided to the student as it is needed. Benjamin, a 4-year-old diagnosed with HFA, attended a preschool for students with developmental disabilities. The classroom was equipped with a large reading loft. To get into the loft, students had to climb a ladder. Each day, Benjamin would climb to the top of the ladder. Despite encouragement, Benjamin would not crawl onto the loft. A social story was written for Benjamin to describe how to climb in and out of the loft. Benjamin could not read, so an audio cassette tape, with a bell to signal when to turn the page, accompanied his story. Benjamin knew how to operate a tape player, and all he needed was a quick introduction to the story. Benjamin's teacher told him, "I have a story for you," demonstrated how to turn the page when the bell sounded, and walked away. After reading the story once, Benjamin turned off the tape player, put down the book, looked over at the loft, walked up to the ladder, and climbed onto the loft for the first time!

A Student May Share the Story with Others

Students often regard the content of a social story as real "news," and want to share the information with others. Hearing a variety of people read the story aloud demonstrates to the student that other people have the same information. Specifically, it is often helpful if those people who will be directly involved in implementing and monitoring the story have the opportunity to read the story with the student. Once a story is in place, parents/professionals may "cue the story": restating key phrases to support a student as he/she learns new responses and social skills.

A Consistent Review Schedule Is Established

Several factors may impact on how often a social story is reviewed by the student with HFA/AS. Often, the review schedule is dependent on the topic of the social story. For example: a social story about different ways to greet people is reviewed each morning; a social story about a holiday celebration is reviewed for a few days before the gathering; and a story describing a daily or weekly activity is initially reviewed just prior to that event. A copy of the review schedule is shared with relevant individuals. Depending on the student and situation, a social story may gradually be reviewed less frequently until it is no longer needed. Mastered stories are kept accessible to a student in a three-ring notebook for future reference.

The Impact of a Social Story Is Carefully Monitored

Occasionally, parents/professionals find it necessary to revise a social story. It may be apparent that a student is interpreting a portion of a story literally, or that part of a story is confusing. Catching these problems early, and rewriting a story accordingly, improves chances for success. Stories can also be revised in response to a student's progress. In this case, eliminating the directive sentences in a story increases student independence.

In summary, a social story is a short story that objectively describes a person, skill, event, concept, or social situation following a specific format and guidelines. Most social stories are developed and written by parents/professionals who begin by determining a topic, observing the situation, and gathering information from those directly involved with a student. This information is considered along with the learning characteristics of students with HFA/AS and a student's individual needs and abilities to determine appropriate vocabulary, story length, and size of print in a social story. In addition, student interests may directly impact on how information is stated or presented. The result is a story customized to maximize a student's motivation and comprehension while presenting social information in a patient and reassuring manner. This team approach is important in developing a social story and later as it is brought to a final draft and implemented. Parents and professionals review the rough draft for final revisions, follow a consistent review schedule, and carefully monitor a student's progress.

COMIC STRIP CONVERSATIONS

A Comic Strip Conversation (CSC) incorporates simple drawings, symbols, and color to illustrate relevant details, ideas, and abstract concepts in selected conversations (Gray, 1994a). A CSC is similar to any conversation, sharing ideas about the past, present, and future; though other characteristics of this approach make it unique. Parents and professionals use CSCs to clarify important information for a student with HFA/AS. Conversations focus on selected topics. Good opportunities for a CSC include situations that are causing difficulty, explaining the responses of others, or preparing for a new situation or unfamiliar event. The content of a conversation is simultaneously illustrated, guided by carefully selected questions that assist a student in sharing information. Each CSC systematically identifies what people do, say, and think. In addition, the use of color identifies the motivation behind actions and statements, and illustrates for a student with HFA/AS the "unseen" aspects of communication. In this way, SCs provide predictability and organization to an interaction.

CSCs originated from the communicative drawings of a 10- year-old girl, Larkin, and were developed with the assistance of an 11- year-old boy, Matthew. Larkin would draw to communicate frustrating situations to her mother, Teri, who would draw in return. In Teri's words:

> My daughter uses a kind of "social stories" process to talk her way through difficult situations. She *draws* or has someone else draw situations that have been confusing or distressing for her. We have learned not only to draw the disturbing situation she requests, but also to draw the sequence of events that leads to an appropriate conclusion to the situation.

Larkin takes great comfort in these drawings and can then use that information to *help herself* in future similar situations. We have taken *her lead* and used this method to help her develop coping skills. My drawings are always in response to Larkin's drawings — unless she is just too agitated about a situation and insists that I draw the situation for her — then I still follow up with my conclusion — sometimes accompanied by a cryptic "social story." (Sasseville, personal communication)

Building from Larkin's example, a systematic approach to sharing information with stick figures, symbols, and color was developed with Matthew, an 8- year-old diagnosed with a disorder on the autistic spectrum. Specifically, Matthew identified colors to represent feelings, which later became the *Conversation Color Chart* (described later) for this method. The approach has been continually revised and expanded through its use with several students (aged 7 through adolescence) with HFA/AS.

CSCs illustrate "the art of conversation." Equipped with a set of markers and a sheet of paper, each person involved in a CSC draws while they talk. Simple stick figures and symbols are used to reenact an event or discuss a future activity. The pictures serve as an ever-present visual reference, supporting students who struggle to comprehend the quick exchange of information in a traditional conversation. In addition, sharing information on a piece of paper requires all of those participating in the conversation to slow down, focusing joint attention on the information that is most critical. Most conversations end with a new drawing or drawings that depict more effective ways to respond to the situation.

CSCs are based on the rationale that pictures and visual supports, found useful in structuring the learning of students with autism (Quill, 1995), may also improve their understanding and comprehension of information shared in a conversation. Temple Grandin has shared her discovery that whereas many people think in words, she thinks in pictures that represent words, ideas, and abstract concepts (Grandin, 1995a). Although no objective research on the CSC approach is available at this writing, experience indicates the approach may be most applicable for students over 4 years of age with HFA/AS. In particular, students who are interested in drawing, books, reading, comic strips, and/or fictional heroes often learn the basics of the approach very quickly. Many students will insist on personalizing the approach, developing their own color chart (described later), and/or adding symbols that they create to represent places, persons, and concepts that are unique to their own experience.

Drawings and Symbols in a CSC

Symbols and drawings in a CSC are kept simple and representative. A CSC uses stick figures to represent people and basic outlines to indicate buildings and objects. Drawings are avoided that contain extraneous details, or that take so much time to draw that the purpose of a conversation is lost in artistic detail. These drawings are never "colored in," as this can cause confusion with the use of color to represent feelings in a CSC (described later).

A student may be encouraged to use identifying features to enhance stick figures and simple drawings. These "personalizations" can add meaning to a conversation as long as they do not require so much time that they delay the flow of a conversation. One student interested in numbers identified each person in his drawings with t-shirts displaying their birth date, and represented places in the community by drawing a simple building with the exact street address over the door. The distinguishing characteristics a student selects are often different from those that would be selected by a parent/professional. This can make a CSC a little difficult for a parent/professional to follow. To minimize confusion, a student and parent/professional may develop a *Personal Symbols Dictionary*, a consistent set of individualized symbols to use as a reference during each CSC. Each student's Personal Symbol Dictionary is continually expanded.

Symbols in a CSC can illustrate abstract concepts and reinforce meaning. The *Conversation Symbols Dictionary* contains a set of eight conversational symbols that are commonly used in a CSC (see Figure 9-5). Abstract conversational concepts, like *listening* and *interrupting*, are represented by symbols that "look like" the concepts they represent. Definitions of these terms are stated in the first person, like a social story, and are defined using visual images. For example, the word *interrupt* is defined as "when my words *bump into* words from other people." Translating abstract social concepts into visual representations provides students with social information they can look at, evaluate, and comprehend.

For students who are more advanced, the talk and thought symbols may be varied to emphasize the meaning of the words they surround. Using sharp edges to indicate anger, irritation, or frustration; or wavy edges to indicate uneasiness, anxiety, or a lack of confidence; helps students "visualize" their own feelings. These slight symbol variations may also be used by a parent/professional to illustrate the emotional states of others. Over the course of several conversations, a student may invent his or her own set of talk symbols to represent various feelings and concepts. These are added to the Personal Symbols Dictionary. Color is also used to identify motivation and emotional states (described in the following section).

The Use of Color in a CSC

The use of color in a CSC identifies the emotional content or motivation behind a statement, thought, or question. For example, the statement "Hi Stephen. Do you want to swim?" varies in its meaning depending on the context in which it is asked and the motivation of the speaker. On a beach the statement indicates a friendly invitation. On the playground, standing near a large puddle,

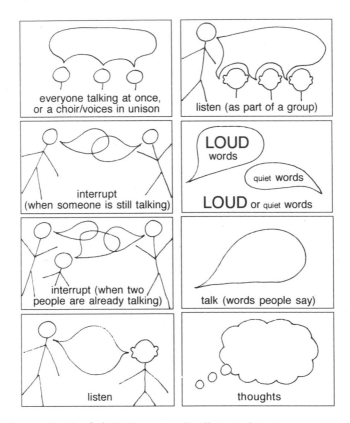

Fig. 9-5. Conversation Symbols Dictionary, used to illustrate abstract conversational concepts.

the identical statement reflects negative intent. The process of deciding "what color" words should be requires a student to review the picture and demonstrates the importance of thoughts, feelings, and motivation in verbal communication.

The use of color in a CSC is carefully structured. The Conversation Color Chart in Figure 9-6 lists eight basic colors and associated meanings. For example, red indicates anger, teasing, an unfriendly statement, or a bad idea. In contrast, green represents a good idea, happiness, or a friendly statement. A student selects a color from the chart prior to writing what people say or think. As soon as a student is introduced to conversation colors, he or she is also taught the limits of their application. Without this distinction, the meanings associated with the colors are potentially confusing if they are applied elsewhere. For example, even though a stop sign is red, that does not *mean* that stopping is a *bad idea*. Establishing rules and limits early for the use of conversation colors avoids unnecessary confusion.

green: good ideas, happy, friendly

red: bad ideas, teasing, unhappy, unfriendly

blue: sad, uncomfortable

brown: comfortable, cozy

purple: proud

yellow: frightened

black: facts, things that we know

orange: questions

combinations of colors: confused

Fig. 9-6. Conversation Color Chart, listing Comic Strip Conversation colors and associated meanings.

Colors are introduced gradually. A student may first gain experience with CSCs using only a black marker, with color introduced later. Colors are introduced over the course of several conversations as feelings become apparent. For example, before a student writes, "I like cookies!" it is suggested that the words be written in green because it is a happy statement. Depending on the ability of the student, the chart may be modified to consist of one or two colors that represent a limited number of basic feelings (green = happy, red = sad). Gradually, new colors and associated meanings are added.

The use of colors in a CSC often becomes as personal as the feelings they represent. Experience with this technique indicates many students with HFA/AS learn this approach very quickly, individualizing the approach with their own color chart and expanding the number of colors and/or associated feelings. Andrea, a secondary student with HFA, worked at a fast-food restaurant. Her manager identified specific behaviors that he viewed as a threat to her continued employment. In the course of a CSC, she was asked to identify what customers might be thinking when she engaged in those behaviors. Andrea responded with a question: "Are they thinking *bad* about *me*?" She quickly turned her attention to the Conversation Color Chart. "I can't find a color for *embarrassed*. Embarrassed would be *pink*." Pink was quickly added to Andrea's color chart. A new picture was drawn to help identify new responses Andrea could use to change what other people were thinking about her. Another student insisted each feeling would have to have its own color; he purchased a set of 24 markers and set up his own color chart.

Many students quickly memorize and internalize color charts and may refer to emotions using colors in casual conversations. Jessica ran up to her teacher in the hall and claimed she had been hearing a lot of "red words" lately. She added that it made her "think yellow." Her teacher asked Jessica to replace the color words with feeling words, and Jessica stated: "When kids yell it scares me." To assist students who are not as adept as "translating" colors into feelings, the parent/professional may respond to a student's color words with a translation. For example, "You're feeling *purple*? Do you mean that something has made you feel *proud*?" Occasionally, a student will refer to colors to express a new level of social understanding. Mark, a second-grade student with AS, arrived at his third CSC session with an important question. "Do you mean if I change the color of my words, I can change the colors of the words that come back to me?"

Parents or professionals may need to correct a student's choice of color. Students often assign colors representing thoughts, feelings, and/or motivations inaccurately. When this occurs, the parent/professional has two options. The first is to wait, providing a few moments of silence for a student to consider the drawing. Stephen, a fourth-grade student diagnosed with a pervasive developmental disorder, was involved in the situation mentioned earlier where another student invited him to swim in a puddle at recess. Stephen had complied. In the CSC reviewing that situation, Stephen was asked to identify the color of the statement, "Do you want to swim?" Stephen immediately picked up the green marker to indicate the invitation was a good idea, began writing, then stopped and looked at the consultant. "Those are red words, aren't they?" he asked. Waiting for a student to finish drawing, even if a "wrong color" has been selected, gives a student the opportunity to self-correct. If waiting isn't effective, the parent/professional acknowledges the student's response, "Yes, that's one idea...," and provides a more accurate answer. "Or maybe those words were red. If they had been red, what would that mean?"

Structuring a CSC

Parents or professionals serve as guides to a CSC, giving it structure and direction without assuming total control. In contrast to a social story that may be written and revised several times, a CSC is a dynamic interaction. Although the approach was initially developed to give visual feedback to students during the course of an important discussion, the drawings often reveal surprising and unexpected information to parents and professionals. Incorporating this new information, along with its implications, is central to a CSC. The art of a CSC lies in knowing when to provide structure and direction versus when to follow a student's lead.

Questions Guide Each CSC

A CSC proceeds similar to an interview, with the parent/professional asking questions in a logical sequence (see Figure 9-7). Each CSC begins by determining where the situation occurs. A *location symbol*, a simple drawing that represents the setting, is placed in the upper left-hand corner of the paper. For

1) **Where are you? What are you doing?**

   (draw location symbol, stick figure, and relevant objects and
   actions)

2) **Who else is here?**

   (draw stick figure)

3) **What happened? What did others do?**

   (draw relevant objects, actions)

4) **What did you say?**

   (use talk symbol)

   What color would those words be?

   (refer to Conversation Color Chart)

5) **What did you think when you said that?**

   (use thought symbol)

   What color would those words be?

   (refer to Conversation Color Chart)

6) **What did others say?**

   (use talk symbol)

   What color would their words be?

   (refer to Conversation Color Chart)

7) **What did others think when they said that/did that?**

   (use thought symbol)

   What color would those words be?

   (refer to Conversation Color Chart)

Fig. 9-7. Questions that guide a Comic Strip Conversation.

example, a parent may open a conversation with, "What will we do at Grandma's house?" while drawing a simple house.

A series of questions continue to guide the conversation, identifying who is present, what they do and say, and what they may be thinking. It may be easier for some students to respond to simple directive statements that guide their drawings, for example, "Draw yourself. Draw other people that were there. Write what you said." The questions provide a framework and identify relevant details early in the conversation. Intended to serve as a guide, it is rarely advisable or possible to follow the series of questions/statements exactly as they are listed in Figure 9-7.

CSCs allow for "time to think." Questions are asked quietly and slowly, providing a student with an opportunity to "look over" the current drawing and formulate a response. Maintaining a relaxed attitude increases the likelihood that the student may initiate and draw spontaneous and unexpected details, or make comments that lead to important topics of discussion. A slower pace also provides time for a parent/professional to carefully consider what to ask next. It is difficult to "go back" in a CSC to ask a missed question. It is also important to recognize opportunities as they occur. It is not uncommon for the interview format to gradually yield to a more natural and casual interaction as the CSC progresses.

A student may have difficulty with organization of ideas and reporting on a situation in sequence. Depending on the student and the topic of conversation, the picture created during a CSC may look more like a conglomerate of random doodles and arrows than a finished picture. In this case, the parent/professional draws a series of numbered boxes, or uses several sheets of numbered papers, identifying what happened first, second, and third. The disadvantage is that many aspects of a situation may need to be drawn repeatedly each time a new box or page is started, a process that requires additional time and may cause a student to lose interest.

The result of a CSC is often surprising. As mentioned earlier, insights a parent/professional gains during the course of a CSC are often important, though unexpected. Jacob, a sixth-grade student with AS, was often drawing pictures in class when he was supposed to be taking notes. Miss Tischler, Jacob's teacher, wanted him to take notes during social studies class. Instead, Jacob drew pictures. In the course of a CSC with the consultant to address this concern, Jacob was directed to write what he thinks about during social studies while Miss Tischler talks to the class. Agitated by the consultant's request, Jacob responded, "I can't *write* what I am *thinking*. I only have *pictures* in my head." The consultant reassured Jacob that it was okay to think in pictures, and asked him to *draw* what he was thinking, instead of writing words. Jacob drew pictures of corn, commenting, "I drew this Tuesday when Miss Tischler was talking about the corn belt and Iowa." The CSC revealed Jacob was "taking notes" by drawing pictures, a format consistent with his style of thinking. To help Jacob more effectively organize his "notes" while utilizing his ability to visualize information, he was introduced to Mindmaps (Wycoff, 1991) in place of traditional note taking.

Concluding a Comic Strip Conversation

Summarizing a conversation and identifying new solutions to the situation concludes a CSC. First, the parent/professional and the student summarize the situation by reviewing the picture of their conversation, beginning with events that happened first and proceeding sequentially. This process is kept brief, identifying the most relevant aspects of the situation and encouraging a student to "see the whole picture." Some students have a tendency to recite the entire conversation verbatim, moving from one drawing to the next as each word of the conversation is "played back." If this occurs, the parent/professional numbers the most relevant cues, and asks the student to review the situation by limiting their comments to numbered parts of the picture only. Summarizing a conversation places visual emphasis on the most relevant facts in a situation and "pulls things together" prior to identifying new solutions to the problem.

With the picture depicting the difficult situation in view, new responses to the situation are "drawn out." Drawing new ways to handle a difficult situation helps a student practice a new skill prior to using it, and provides a lasting picture the student may keep for future reference. Ideas may also be written in the form of a list, crossing off or throwing away solutions that are not feasible, creating a plan to try the next time the situation occurs. If a student cannot identify effective solutions independently, the parent/professional makes suggestions, illustrating how the situation might change if new responses are used. In some cases, the process of listing or drawing new solutions may not be feasible, and it may be more effective for the parent/professional to write a social story for the student based on information from the CSC.

Occasionally, a single solution becomes very apparent, and a review of the conversation, or listing new solutions, is not needed or advisable. For example, the drawing in Figure 9-8 illustrates the content of a conversation with Randy, a bright fifth grader with AS, and his teacher. Randy's teacher was delighted that Randy had a new chess partner, Jesse. She was concerned, though, that Jesse may be rapidly losing interest in playing with Randy. Randy took excessive time to "make his move," and did not seem aware that he was boring Jesse. Randy's teacher assumed the role of Jesse in a CSC. This conversation discussed, and illustrated, Jesse's increasing impatience with Randy. Other factors came to light in the course of this conversation. Playing chess made Randy think about the

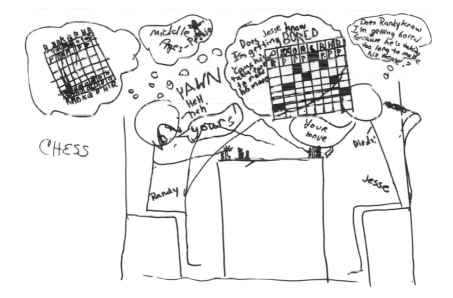

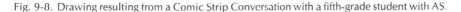

Fig. 9-8. Drawing resulting from a Comic Strip Conversation with a fifth-grade student with AS.

Middle Ages in detail, and visualizing characters and battles associated with that period of history was delaying his moves on the chess board. In addition, Randy felt that Jesse was also guilty of taking too much time to make his moves. A 2-minute sand timer solved the problem, establishing a new rule that each turn had to be completed before the sand ran out.

Conversation pictures, especially those illustrating the use of new, more effective responses to a given situation, are kept accessible to a student and the parent/professional. The picture of a new skill can be reviewed just prior to encountering a situation where it will be applied. One student insisted on having the pictures posted by his desk as a constant reminder to use newly learned skills. Pictures may also be kept in individual notebooks, or as illustrations accompanying social stories, creating a personal encyclopedia of relevant social information.

Group Comic Strip Conversations

Group CSCs are used in a structured group setting, usually involving several students with HFA/AS and a professional serving as a group leader. Students create a visual display of selected interactions that occur in the course of a group discussion. Each group participant, and the group leader, is represented on a chalkboard with a stick figure labeled with their name. Each stick figure also has a blank thought and talk symbol. Students are encouraged to use the stick figures and colored chalk to illustrate how they feel in response to certain statements. For example, Maggie, a teenager with HFA, has difficulty identifying her feelings and expressing them appropriately. During a social skills group meeting, Jason makes a comment that hurts Maggie's feelings. Maggie is encouraged to guess the "color" of Jason's words as she writes what he said in his talk symbol. Maggie selects a representative color to write how Jason's statement makes her feel in her thought symbol. With this information recorded on the chalkboard, Maggie writes a response to Jason in her talk symbol and reads it to him. This process slows an interaction down, makes it less transient, and provides students with an opportunity to "see" how their behavior impacts on the thoughts and feelings of another person. Group conversations require all participants to agree on one color chart for use in the social skills group, with the entire group completing one picture depicting a variety of selected interactions.

In summary, CSCs illustrate the content of a conversation, providing a student with a visual display of information. The process requires parents/professionals to take time to determine the thoughts and feelings of a student in regard to a situation that is presenting difficulty, often resulting in information that helps others understand where a student may be misperceiving or misinterpreting a situation. In addition, a CSC provides an opportunity for parents/professionals to share accurate information with a student, using a format that is understandable. Using colors to represent thoughts, motivations, and feelings; and incorporating symbols that "look like" the social skills they represent; provides students with visual images of abstract concepts. The entire process adapts an interaction to improve student understanding, and enables parents and professionals to share social information that might otherwise be difficult to explain. Illustrating new responses or solutions to a previously difficult situation provides the student with a personal reference to use to review and rehearse newly acquired social skills.

RESEARCH, OUTCOMES, AND FURTHER STUDY

Extensive clinical experience and limited research provide early evidence of the positive potential of both social stories and CSCs. This section summarizes informal observations of these approaches, shares the results of one study, and explores ideas for future research.

In school, clinic, and home settings, students with HFA/AS demonstrate a variety of responses to social stories. Many parents and professionals have shared numerous experiences attributing positive changes in a student's behavior to the use of a social story. At times, students demonstrate new, more effective responses to a skill or situation within a very short period of time, as Benjamin did after reading his loft story, described previously. Changes in behavior for some students are limited to responses defined in the story, whereas other students demonstrate changes in behavior when the story is totally descriptive. Occasionally, a student will identify a situation that is difficult, and independently initiate a request for a social story on that topic. After reading a social story about how to work in a small group, a student with AS exclaimed to his teacher, "You should read this. There is *news* in here!"

Negative responses to social stories are infrequent. Students may not always be receptive to a social story, either stating they don't *like* the information in the story or refusing to read it completely. Negative impact has been attributed to stories that did not adhere to the Social Story Ratio or guidelines. For example, one parent attributed her child's increasing anxiety at school to stories containing too many directive sentences (Gray, 1995). A student's response may also be neutral, with no apparent change in behavior. In most cases, however, social stories that are carefully written and implemented have positive results.

It is not only social stories that may impact the behavior of students, but *anything in writing*. This includes classroom schedules, books, poems, stories, advertisements, or written directions. Written information that is clear and readily understood by most students may, in some cases, be the cause of negative behavior for a student with HFA/AS For example, a posted classroom schedule, if interpreted literally, will quickly be inaccurate as changes in schedule or

delayed starting times occur, and may cause a student with HFA/AS to experience anxiety or confusion. Recognizing and understanding the importance and
influence of written information may expand understanding of student behavior,
especially behaviors that seem to occur "out of the blue" or "without apparent
reason."

Clinicians report CSCs help to clarify a variety of concepts for students
with HFA/AS, and often lead to surprising insights. On occasion, students
display the ability to accurately identify what another person is thinking, feeling,
and/or what is motivating a given response. Usually, these realizations seem to
follow a period of silence, where the parent/professional has provided time for
the student to consider the CSC picture and its implications. Other students
express genuine surprise when presented with the thoughts or motivation of
another individual. Once a more complete "picture" of the situation is illustrated,
they may independently identify the error in their current response to the
situation. For many students, the use of color and symbols seems to serve as a
conversational "screen" that translates abstract or elusive information into a
tangible and usable resource.

To date, objective research is limited to one study of social stories.
Swaggart *et al.* (1995) combined the use of stories with traditional behavioral
social skills training. The study involved three students diagnosed with moderate
to severe autism, two 7- year-old boys, Adam and Darrell, and an 11- year-old
girl, Danielle. Interventions were individually designed to improve Danielle's
greeting behavior and to teach Adam and Darrell to share and play more
effectively with one another. Each morning, a teacher and/or paraprofessional
read an individualized story addressing the target behavior to each student.
Stories contained icons to illustrate and reinforce the meaning of the text. A
second story was read to one of the students to explain the related behavioral
intervention (response-cost). The authors concluded the studies "provide support
for the use of social stories with children with autism... in combination with a
traditional social skills training model" (p. 11) to teach new skills and decrease
undesirable behaviors. Pairing the use of a social story with a behavioral
intervention, however, made it impossible to determine the impact of the social
stories on the positive changes in behavior. In addition, there were differences
in how social stories are defined by Gray (1994b) and Swaggart *et al.* (1995).

Theories as to why, and how, social stories and CSCs "work" are numerous.
The effectiveness of social stories may be tied to how information is presented
and the kind of information that is highlighted. It is suspected that the visual
learning style of students with HFA/AS may explain the relative ease with which
information in a social story or CSC is seemingly understood and applied by
many students. Other visually based approaches, from picture schedules to
checklists based on task analysis, have clarified for students the elements of a
task, and expectations for performance of new skills. It may be that social stories
and CSCs complement traditional approaches by systematically presenting *ad-*

ditional social information. For example, social stories *describe* more than direct, placing important cues and responses in sequence. Similarly, CSCs explore not only environmental factors, but also pragmatics and motivation that add to the context surrounding statements and actions. Describing the context of a given situation, establishing relationships between relevant cues, and defining meaningful responses may place "central coherence" information in writing — or in pictures — for students who are otherwise unable to make those ties independently.

To date, social stories and CSCs have raised as many questions for professionals and parents, as they have answers for students with HFA/AS. Experiences with these instructional techniques often challenge and redefine the possible limits of what students with HFA/AS can be taught, and what they can learn. Considering these approaches developed as the direct result of creative consideration of the perspective of people with HFA/AS, helpful study of social stories and Comic Strip Conversations will most likely reflect attention to first person accounts, as well as innovative thinking and design. Case studies with independent observers, controlled studies of the impact of social stories and CSCs on the behavior of people with HFA/AS, and research into how these instructional techniques are tied to different cognitive and behavioral theories, may provide a starting point.

SUMMARY

This chapter described two instructional techniques, social stories and CSCs, designed to teach social understanding and social skills to students with HFA and AS. A fundamental premise of these instructional techniques is that the "social impairment in autism" *is shared*: experienced by people with HFA/AS and those who live and work alongside them. An individual with HFA/AS may be confused or overwhelmed by specific social situations and interactions. At the same time, parents and professionals may view the responses of the person with HFA/AS as "inappropriate," "stubborn," or occurring "without apparent reason." Consequently, improving social interactions requires strategies designed to address both sides of the social equation, helping others understand the person with HFA/AS, while sharing accurate and specific social information. Parents and professionals are encouraged to abandon all of their assumptions in favor of attitudes of humor, acceptance, and creativity. The perspective of a person with HFA/AS is regarded as equally valid but different, as parents and professionals share the responsibility for social success.

Social stories and CSCs are designed to help parents and professionals respond to students with HFA/AS with understanding for their unique social perspective. These strategies structure how information is exchanged, with recognition of the learning characteristics of these individuals. Visual supports, structured guidelines, individualized accommodations, and efforts to incorporate the interests of students, are essential elements of social stories and CSCs. Extensive informal experience with these approaches, and limited objective study, indicate they are an effective way to share social information and teach new, more effective social understanding and social skills to students with HFA/AS. Experience is resulting in the continual revision of social stories and CSCs. This, coupled with information provided by objective study, will be critical to the improvement and expansion of social stories and CSCs in the coming years.

ACKNOWLEDGMENTS

The author expresses sincere appreciation to Dr. Julie Donnelly, Educational Resource Specialist, Project ACCESS, Springfield, Missouri; Dr. Anthony Attwood, Clinical Psychologist, Queensland, Australia; and Brian Gray, School Psychologist, Jenison Public Schools, Jenison, Michigan, for their critical review of a draft of this chapter. In addition, the author acknowledges the influence of Eric Kortering, Susan McDowell, Terri Sasseville, Larkin Sasseville, and Matthew Graham to the development of the instructional techniques described in this chapter.

REFERENCES

Asperger, H. (1944). Die "Autistischen Psychopathen" im Kindesalter. *Archiv für Psychiatrie und Nervenkrankhieten, 117,* 76–136. 'Autistic psychopathy' in childhood (U. Frith, Trans.). In U. Frith (Ed.), *Autism and Asperger syndrome* (pp. 37–92). Cambridge: Cambridge University Press.
Attwood, T. (1996). Asperger's syndrome: A guide for parents and professionals. Unpublished manuscript.
Baron-Cohen, S. (1995). Autism and mindblindness. In *Mindblindness* (pp. 59–84). Cambridge, MA: MIT Press.
Baron-Cohen, S., Leslie, A. M., & Frith, U. (1985). Does the autistic child have a "theory of mind"? *Cognition, 21,* 37–46.
Cesaroni, L., & Garber, M. (1991). Exploring the experience of autism through firsthand accounts. *Journal of Autism and Developmental Disorders, 21,* 303–313.
Cohen, S. (1990). Autism: A specific cognitive disorder of 'mind-blindness.' *International Review of Psychiatry, 2,* 79–88.
Dalrymple, N. J. (1995). Environmental supports to develop flexibility and independence. In K. Quill (Ed.), *Teaching children with autism: Strategies to enhance communication and socialization* (pp. 243–264). New York: Delmar.
Dawson, G., & Adams, A. (1984). Imitation and social responsiveness in autistic children. *Journal of Abnormal Child Psychology, 12,* 209–226.
Dawson, G., & Galpert, L. (1990). Mother's use of imitative play for facilitating social responsiveness and toy play in young autistic children. *Development and Psychopathology, 2,* 151–162.
Ferrara, C., & Hill, S. (1980). The responsiveness of autistic children to the predictability of social and nonsocial toys. *Journal of Autism and Developmental Disorders, 10,* 51–57.
Frith, U. (1989). *Autism: Explaining the enigma.* Oxford: Blackwell.

Frith, U. (1991). Asperger and his syndrome. In U. Frith (Ed.), *Autism and Asperger syndrome* (pp. 1–36). Cambridge: Cambridge University Press.

Geisel, T. S. (1940, renewed 1968). *Horton hatches the egg*. New York: Random House.

Gillberg, C. (1991). Clinical and neurobiological aspects of Asperger syndrome in six family studies. In U. Frith (Ed.), *Autism and Asperger syndrome* (pp. 122–146). Cambridge: Cambridge University Press.

Gillberg, I. C., & Gillberg, C. (1989). Asperger syndrome — some epidemiological considerations: A research note. *Journal of Child Psychology and Psychiatry, 30*, 631–638.

Grandin, T. (1995a). How people with autism think. In E. Schopler & G. B. Mesibov (Eds.), *Learning and cognition in autism* (pp. 137–156). New York: Plenum Press.

Grandin, T. (1995b). The learning style of people with autism: An autobiography. In K. Quill (Ed.), *Teaching children with autism: Strategies to enhance communication and socialization* (pp. 33–52). New York: Delmar.

Grandin, T., & Scariano, M. (1986). *Emergence: Labeled autistic*. Novato, CA: Arena.

Gray, C. A. (1994a). *Comic strip conversations*. Arlington: Future Horizons.

Gray, C. A. (1994b, October). *Making sense out of the world: Social stories, comic strip conversations, and related instructional techniques*. Paper presented at the Midwest Educational Leadership Conference on Autism, Kansas City, MO.

Gray, C. A. (1995). A close look at directive sentences. *The Morning News, Summer*, 4–7.

Gray, C. A., & Garand, J. (1993). Social stories: Improving responses of individuals with autism with accurate social information. *Focus on Autistic Behavior, 8*, 1–10.

Groden, J., & LeVasseur, P. (1995). Cognitive picture rehearsal: A system to teach self-control. In K. Quill (Ed.), *Teaching children with autism: Strategies to enhance communication and socialization* (pp. 287–305). New York: Delmar.

Happé, F. (1995). *Autism: An introduction to psychological theory*. Cambridge, MA: Harvard University Press.

Happé, F., & Frith, U. (1995). Theory of mind in autism. In E. Schopler & G. B. Mesibov (Eds.), *Learning and cognition in autism* (pp. 177–197). New York: Plenum Press.

Harris, P. (1993). Pretending and planning. In S. Baron-Cohen, H. Tager-Flusberg, & D. J. Cohen (Eds.), *Understanding other minds* (pp. 228–246). London: Oxford University Press.

Hart, C. (1989). *Without reason*. New York: Harper & Row.

Hodgdon, L. (1995). *Visual strategies for improving communication*. Troy, MI: QuirkRoberts.

Kanner, L. (1943). Autistic disturbances of affective contact. *Nervous Child, 2*, 217–250.

Klinger, L. G., & Dawson, G. (1992). Facilitating early social and communicative development in children with autism. In S. F. Warren & J. Reichle (Eds.), *Causes and effects in communication and language intervention* (pp. 157–186). Baltimore: Brookes.

Klinger, L. G., & Dawson, G. (1995). A fresh look at categorization abilities in persons with autism. In E. Schopler & G. B. Mesibov (Eds.), *Learning and cognition in autism* (pp. 119–136). New York: Plenum Press.

Koegel, L. K., & Koegel, R. L. (1995). Motivating communication in children with autism. In E. Schopler & G. B. Mesibov (Eds.), *Learning and cognition in autism* (pp. 73–87). New York: Plenum Press.

Leslie, A. M. (1987). Pretence and representation: the origins of a "theory of mind." *Psychological Review, 94*, 412–426.

Mayer Johnson, R. (1992). *The picture communication symbols books I, II, & III*. Solana Beach, CA: Mayer Johnson.

McDonnell, J. T. (1993). *News from the border*. New York: Tickner & Fields.

Mesibov, G. B., & Stephens, J. (1990). Perceptions of popularity among a group of high-functioning adults with autism. *Journal of Autism and Developmental Disorders, 20*, 33–43.

Moreno, S. (1992). A parent's view of more able people with autism. In E. Schopler & G. B. Mesibov (Eds.), *High-functioning individuals with autism* (pp. 91–103). New York: Plenum Press.

Olley, J. G. (1986). The TEACCH curriculum for teaching social behavior to children with autism. In
      E. Schopler & G. B. Mesibov (Eds.), *Social behavior in autism* (pp. 351–373). New York:
      Plenum Press.
Quill, K. A. (Ed.). (1995). *Teaching children with autism: Strategies to enhance communication and
      socialization*. New York: Delmar.
Schopler, E., Mesibov, G. B., & Hearsey, K. (1995). Structured teaching in the TEACCH system. In
      E. Schopler & G. B. Mesibov (Eds.), *Learning and cognition in autism* (pp. 243–268). New
      York: Plenum Press.
Schuler, A. L. (1995). Thinking in autism: Differences in learning and development. In K. Quill (Ed.),
      Teaching children with autism: Strategies to enhance communication and socialization (pp.
      11–32). New York: Delmar.
Swaggart, B. L., Gagnon, E., Bock, S. J., Earles, E. L., Quinn, C., Myles, B. S., & Simpson, R. L.
      (1995). Using social stories to teach social and behavioral skills to children with autism. *Focus
      on Autistic Behavior, 10*, 1–15.
Twachtman, D. (1995). Methods to enhance communication in verbal children. In K. Quill (Ed.),
      Teaching children with autism: Strategies to enhance communication and socialization (pp.
      133–162). New York: Delmar.
Volkmar, F., & Cohen, D. (1985). The experience of infantile autism: A first-person account by Tony
      W. *Journal of Autism and Developmental Disorders, 15*, 47–54.
Williams, D. (1992). *Nobody nowhere*. New York: Times Books.
Wing, L. (1992). Manifestations of social problems in high-functioning autistic people. In E. Schopler
      & G. B. Mesibov (Eds.), *High-functioning individuals with autism* (pp. 129–142). New York:
      Plenum Press.
Wycoff, J. (1991). *Mindmapping*. New York: Berkley Books.

10

Language and Communication in High-Functioning Autism and Asperger Syndrome

DIANE TWACHTMAN-CULLEN

Communication exists at the intersection of cognition and social behavior.

— Grover J. Whitehurst

INTRODUCTION

For the first time since the *Diagnostic and Statistical Manual* (DSM) was originally published, it lists Asperger's Disorder, more widely known as Asperger syndrome (AS), as a separate category under the general heading of Pervasive Developmental Disorders. Instead of providing definitive answers regarding the relationship between autism and AS, DSM-IV invites an increasing number of questions. This is particularly true regarding its position on language and communication in AS.

According to DSM-IV, "There is no clinically significant general delay in language (e.g., single words used by age 2 years, communicative phrases used by age 3 years)" (p. 62). This statement is misleading for a number of reasons. For one, it treats *language* and *communication* as a single entity, lumping them

DIANE TWACHTMAN-CULLEN • Autism & Developmental Disabilities Consultation Center, Cromwell, Connecticut 06416.

Asperger Syndrome or High-Functioning Autism?, edited by Schopler *et al.* Plenum Press, New York, 1998.

together under the rubric of *delay*. This representation fails to recognize the critical differences between the two concepts. For another, use of the term *clinically significant* is in and of itself unfortunate, for it appears to confer constancy where none exists. In reality, the determination of clinical significance is neither scientific nor precise. Rather, it is both discretionary (i.e., left to the judgment of individual clinicians) and nebulous. As such, it is open to wide interpretation and opinion. Further, given what is known about normal language acquisition with respect to single and multiword combinations, one would be hard-pressed to characterize the ages of acquisition cited in DSM-IV as indicative of a mild, let alone clinically *insignificant*, delay!

It is well accepted among linguists that single words generally emerge somewhere around the child's first birthday (Dale, 1972; James, 1990; Lindner, 1990; McClowry & Guilford, 1982; Owens, 1988). In terms of multiword combinations, Owens (1988) stated that "children begin to combine words into longer utterances at about 18 months of age" (p. 216). According to James (1990), "At 2 years of age, children are using short simple sentences" (p. 74). Even more disquieting, considering the meager characterization of ostensibly "normal" language behavior at age 3 set forth in DSM-IV, is McClowry and Guilford's description of typical 3-year-old language development: "[The 3-year-old] is able to share his knowledge of the world by generating all of the basic sentence patterns and many more complex structures.... *He has the tools to send an unlimited number of messages*" [italics added] (p. 9).

Going strictly by the numbers — that is, the generally accepted norm of first words by 1 year — the DSM-IV example of single words by age 2 would not only constitute a delay, it would constitute a relatively severe one, according to guidelines contained in a report issued by the American Speech–Language–Hearing Association (ASHA). According to ASHA (1989), age delays represent different degrees of deficit at different points in development. The example cited in that report is particularly relevant to DSM-IV's stand on language acquisition. According to ASHA (1989), "A 'one-year delay' in expressive language is more severe in a 2-year-old than it is in a 5-year-old" (p. 117).

Further, DSM-IV's use of the term *delay* is obfuscatory, for it leads one to believe that time factors alone are the only parameters that matter in language acquisition. In addressing the issue of "Criteria For Significant Discrepancy," ASHA specifically argues against the use of discrepancy formulas (i.e., those related to the difference between language ability and chronological age) as the sole criteria for determining the significance of language deficit. According to ASHA (1989):

> The exclusive use of discrepancy formulae as a required procedure for determining eligibility for language intervention should be viewed with extreme caution and avoided whenever possible.... *These formulae should not dictate whether or not a child is identified as having a language disorder*

[italics added] or whether or not speech–language services are warranted. (p. 115)

Finally, use of the term *delay* is also seriously misleading, as it implies that a timely onset of words and phrases is somehow equated with normal language development per se. Nothing could be further from the truth, especially when one considers the issue of *deviance* in language and communication development. ASHA speaks to this issue as well. Holding to an "integrative, broad-based definition of language," ASHA (1989) issued the following:

> Such definitions are inconsistent with the use of a single component or language dimension as the sole criterion for identifying a child as having a language disorder. A language disorder is not simply a disorder of language, but a disorder that reflects potential perceptual, cognitive, and social deficits. (p. 116)

Ironically, while DSM-IV gives overarching significance to the concept of *delayed* language, it remains conspicuously silent on the more cogent issue of *deviant* language use in AS. Toward this end, Wing (1981) found in her study of AS not only delayed speech development, but also deficiencies in the communicative behaviors normally seen in infancy (e.g., joint attention, social referencing, reciprocity). Her views regarding language deviance led her (1991) to criticize the World Health Organization's *International Classification of Diseases* for not including in its description of AS "the abnormalities of verbal and non-verbal communication (as distinct from the formal aspects of language) so graphically described by Asperger" (p. 106). The same criticism obviously applies to DSM-IV.

This notion of language deviance, and the more multidimensional concept of communication, has also been raised by other researchers (Rumsey, 1992; Tager-Flusberg, 1981). Unlike mere language delay, language deviance is not only a central issue in AS, it is, in my opinion, a pathognomonic feature of language use in the disorder. It is also a more comprehensive and telling parameter, in that it takes into account both verbal and nonverbal behavior, as well as the uses of language.

I have taken the time to elaborate on the shortcomings of the DSM-IV position on language acquisition, because the latter has all too often served as a deterrent to diagnosis. Specifically, time and again I have seen textbook patterns of Asperger symptomatology fall short of diagnosis — or worse yet, be assigned other, less appropriate labels — based solely on the presence of any degree of language delay. Likewise, DSM-IV's silence on the more compelling issue of language deviance speaks eloquently to the need for addressing this critically important topic.

Toward this end, the primary focus of this chapter is to address the ways in which the patterns of language use and communication in AS, and in its companionate disorder, high-functioning autism (HFA), deviate from those found in the general population. Recognizing that the development of language does not occur in a vacuum, but rather as part of a social matrix involving significant others, my main premises are as follows: (1) language has an essential communicative base (Bates, 1976; Bruner, 1978; Moerk, 1977; Snow, 1972); (2) it is the communication system, as opposed to the formal aspects of language per se, that bears the major burden of impairment in HFA and AS (Rumsey, 1992; Tager-Flusberg, 1981); and (3) it is in the features of discourse, rather than in those of isolated words and sentences, where the essence of communication impairment may be found in HFA and AS. Pragmatic in focus, and clinical in orientation, this chapter emphasizes the importance of establishing a holistic framework within which to understand and address the language and communication impairment associated with these disorders.

After a brief overview of normal language development, and a description of the components of communication, the focus of attention will be directed to the language and communication characteristics of individuals with HFA and AS. The latter will be addressed within the framework of the social–cognitive underpinnings that scaffold language comprehension and use. Finally, although this chapter is not intended to provide specific information with respect to remediation, it will outline important issues to consider in designing effective intervention programs.

NORMAL LANGUAGE DEVELOPMENT

To more fully appreciate the ways in which language use in autism and AS deviates from the norm, it is first necessary to develop a basic understanding of normal language usage. The phrase *deceptive simplicity* is an apt one to characterize the less-than-auspicious beginnings of the sociocommunicative process in typical children. Specifically, the infant enters the world in a state of unparalleled dependency and helplessness, armed with little, save for the birth cry itself. Yet it is this same helpless being who, with the clamorous announcement of his or her arrival, actually initiates the social exchange that sets up the remarkable "choreography" (Stern, 1977) of which communicative interactions are made. And so it begins — the infant, in partnership with the primary caregiver, sounds the first note toward the extraordinary transformation from dependent creature to competent sociocommunicative being (Kaye, 1982; Stern, 1977).

Under ordinary circumstances this transformation is made so effortlessly that it goes virtually unnoticed. In fact, the ease with which normally developing children acquire speech, language, and communication belies the complexity of the task. Remarkably, according to McClowry and Guilford (1982), "most children in just three or four years develop the basic phonological, semantic, syntactic and pragmatic skills that they need to engage in simple adult-like conversations" (p. 9). It is only when something goes awry — as in the case of autism and Asperger syndrome — that our attention is suddenly directed to the process. And, it is only then, when we analyze the myriad verbal and nonverbal elements, and the subtle ever-changing social nuances that shape the developing language and communication system, that we realize that what is so easily taken for granted, is undoubtedly the most complex skill that human beings are called on to learn.

For most of us, because language use is an effortless, seemingly automatic process, we are unaware of the mechanisms involved in comprehending and processing information, or of those involved in formulating and expressing thoughts and feelings. Given the ease with which the process typically develops, Dale (1972) described language as having an "elusive I-can-do-it-but-I-cannot-tell-you-how property" (p. 3). Notwithstanding that we take it for granted, human language is a powerful vehicle to convey information.

An intact language system is creative, flexible, semantic, and syntactical. Language can transport us into the past or catapult us into the future. We can talk about the here and now, ponder the hypothetical, even consider the nonexistent. In fact, it is not until we *use* language that it attains its highest purpose. And, indeed, language has many purposes. For example, we can use language to make requests, to express dissatisfaction, to ask questions, to give opinions, and to express complex feelings and emotions. We can also use language to speculate and to negotiate, to elaborate, and to direct actions. In addition, we can use language to obtain attention, to deceive, and to implore. It is through language that we both characterize and categorize experience, as well as clarify our positions and correct misconceptions when they occur. Receptively, it is through language that we come to understand the contents of other people's minds — their thoughts, their desires, their fears, their beliefs, their opinions, their feelings, and their perceptives. And, it is in these *uses* of language — the so-called pragmatic elements — that people with autism and AS deviate from typical language users. For these individuals language use is often a high-stress, high-demand activity, particularly when it involves content that is less factually, and more emotionally, based.

THE COMPONENTS OF THE COMMUNICATION SYSTEM

Recognizing that the whole of communication is infinitely greater than the sum of its component parts, it is nonetheless important to consider the latter, not only to avoid misconceptions, but also to develop an appreciation for the interconnectedness and contributions of the separate elements that make up the communication system. In so doing, however, it is acknowledged that this separation is both arbitrary and artificial, and rendered only for the purposes of discussion and clarity.

To the nonprofessional, the terms *speech*, *language*, and *communication* are used interchangeably. Unfortunately, this practice has created a good deal of misinformation and confusion, to wit, DSM-IV's coalescence of the terms *language* and *communication* in its description of AS. Not only are the terms different from each other, they actually represent different aspects of development (Owens, 1988).

Speech

Speech is the main "purveyor" of the vocal delivery system. Defined by Owens (1988) as a complex, neuromuscular, motor behavior, speech is characterized by two types of acoustic features, both of which have implications for message generation and interpretation. The first of these is called the *segmental* feature. It refers to the distinctive sound characteristics of phoneme segments in continuous speech (Crystal, 1975). The second acoustic feature is referred to as *nonsegmental*, and includes such elements as vocal intonation, stress, pitch, timing, and rhythm (Crystal, 1975). Nonsegmental features that serve a grammatical function are referred to as *prosodic* elements (Fay & Schuler, 1980). One example of the latter is the rising intonation at the end of a sentence to signal a question. These nonsegmental features — that is, those elements over and above the words themselves — are also referred to as *paralinguistic codes* (Owens, 1988). Their primary purpose is to add meaning and force to verbal utterances, particularly with respect to attitude and emotion.

It is important to note that it is not the "mechanical transmission" aspects of speech production that are compromised in HFA and AS, but rather the nonsegmental elements that reflect social understanding, and provide information regarding the speaker's attitude and emotional state. Given their power to influence message generation and comprehension, paralinguistic features are more appropriately construed as essential elements of communication.

Language

According to Owens (1988), *language* is defined as a "socially shared code or conventional system for representing concepts through the use of arbitrary symbols and rule-governed combinations of those symbols" (p. 453). The key elements in this definition are the terms *shared* and *conventional*. Unless speaker and listener share the same code (word meanings), true representation of concepts cannot occur. For example, the word *snow* conjures up a visual image of cold, white powdery stuff, because shared understanding of the word *snow* creates a common ground for meaning. Words then constitute the *semantic* (content/meaning) elements of language.

Language must also have form, however, if it is to be of use in communication. Sacks (1989) emphasized the role of language in message generation by characterizing language as the "symbolic currency, to exchange meaning" (p. 39). It should be obvious that information cannot be effectively exchanged unless symbols (words) are combined according to agreed-upon (conventional) rules. Consider, "hungry the is dog." Rendered in this form, the words are meaningless. By simply changing the words around and combining them according to acceptable rules of grammar, a meaningless string of words is transformed into a meaningful sentence (i.e., The dog is hungry). This example illustrates the intrinsic blending of *form* (syntax/grammar) and *content* (semantics) that occurs in message generation.

It is important to note that one of the features common to both HFA and AS is that language form and structure may be superficially intact. In other words, individuals with HFA and AS may produce syntactically correct, complex grammatical structures, while at the same time they evidence difficulty in organizing and using these structures, productively, in ongoing discourse (Tager-Flusberg, 1988). According to Mentis and Thompson (1991), "well developed linguistic knowledge at the sentence level... [does not necessarily translate into] creating a cohesive, coherent text" (p. 199). Thus, despite the emphasis that DSM-IV places on the formal aspects of language behavior, the latter are not necessarily illuminating in the case of HFA and AS. In fact, intact formal language may be quite misleading, especially if it masks the underlying pragmatic deficits that impede one's ability to create cohesive, intelligible discourse.

There is, however, a feature of language that is particularly germane to a discussion of autism and AS. It is one that is not only more encompassing than those of form and content, it is also more dynamic. This feature refers to the function of language; that is, the *use* of language, in context, to communicate one's intent. Known generically as *pragmatics*, this aspect of language behavior has much to do with discourse (i.e., interactional language use), and is most appropriately considered under the rubric of *communication*. Unlike delayed language, disordered pragmatic development is pathognomonic of the type of impairment that is seen in these disorders.

Communication

Owens (1988) defined *communication* as "the process of encoding, transmitting, and decoding signals in order to exchange information and ideas between the participants" (p. 450). Characterized by Muma (1978) as the "primary function of language" (p. 118), communication is a distinctly social phenomenon, requiring both a sender and a receiver (McCormick, 1990; Twachtman, 1995; Willard & Schuler, 1987).

Pragmatics (i.e., the use of language for communication purposes) is best conceptualized as that critical feature of human interaction that represents the intrinsic blending of social, emotional, cognitive, and linguistic factors in the sending and receiving of messages (Baltaxe & Simmons, 1988; Layton & Watson, 1995). Multidimensional in scope, pragmatics encompasses the following three crucial areas of knowledge/skill:

1. The ability to employ speech acts to express intentionality in order to accomplish a given purpose (i.e., function)
2. The ability to make judgments (i.e., presuppositions) about the listener's needs and capabilities, in order to regulate speech style and content vis-à-vis listener and/or situational needs
3. The ability to apply the rules of discourse in order to engage in cooperative conversational exchanges (James, 1990; McCormick, 1990)

Speech acts cover an extremely wide range of pragmatic functions, ranging from those that are relatively simple (e.g., requesting and protesting), to those that are far more complex (e.g., negotiating and conveying humor). Speech acts may be direct (e.g., "Pass the salt") or indirect (e.g., "Can you pass the salt?"). People with autism and AS often have difficulty with indirect requests, in that they fail to understand the speaker's actual intent. For example, the husband of a college professor with AS once informed me that if his wife is given an indirect request such as "Can you pass the salt?" she is likely to respond, "Yes."

Speech acts may also be either literal or nonliteral. In the former case, the speaker means to convey what the words say (e.g., "I need this"). In the latter case, the speaker means to convey something other than what the words say (e.g., "I need this like I need a hole in my head!"). Individuals with HFA and AS have difficulty both in interpreting, and hence in responding to nonliteral (i.e., figurative) language.

To meet the second criterion of pragmatic ability, one needs to be able to make presuppositions (assumptions) about the listener's needs. A certain type of knowledge known as *social cognition* enables people to do this effectively. The latter may be thought of as the "people" sense; that is, the cognitive process by which one comes to understand the world of people — their perspectives, their thoughts, their desires, and their feelings (Geller, 1989). Armed with this type of knowledge, typical individuals are able to make judgments (presuppositions) about their listeners on which to base their own verbal and nonverbal behavior (DeHart & Maratsos, 1984; Geller, 1989). Consequently, typical speakers are not only able to convey information about their own attitudes and feelings, they are also able to use presuppositional knowledge to regulate the verbal and nonverbal subtleties of communication. Geller (1989) stressed the essential role that perspective-taking plays in regulating language to accommodate listener needs. An intrinsic part of communication, adequate presuppositional usage is at the very heart of how speakers and listeners both comprehend and express meaning (Geller, 1989). This aspect of communication constitutes a veritable mine field of difficulty for people with HFA and AS, given the social complexities and perspective-taking requirements that govern its use.

The third main area of pragmatic knowledge is the most comprehensive, taking into account the two that precede it. This aspect of pragmatic ability concerns cooperative conversational exchanges. According to Grice (1975), an early researcher in the field of discourse analysis (i.e., the study of language use over and above the isolated sentence level), conversation is a cooperative event in which participants work together to regulate the ebb and flow of information. Toward this end, Grice (1975) identified four maxims (i.e., discourse rules) that underlie conversational interaction: *quantity, quality, relevance,* and *clarity*. These maxims are particularly germane to the discussion of language use in HFA and AS, as they encompass areas of deficit characteristically demonstrated by these individuals. Despite this, these critical features of discourse are often overlooked — lost in the shuffle, as it were, of syntactically correct, isolated sentence production. Given the discourse needs of people with HFA and AS, Grice's maxims would seem to provide a particularly useful, generic framework for examining the nature of some of the more subtle pragmatic deficits that constrain conversational interaction. In addition, they can also be used to provide a concrete frame of reference for remediation that people with HFA and AS can readily understand and use. Table 10-1 provides examples of how difficulty with each of these maxims may manifest itself in these disorders.

To summarize, the three major domains of pragmatic knowledge encompass specific areas of discourse related to issues of intentionality, topicality (i.e., initiating, maintaining, and changing topics), and code switching (i.e., the ability to adjust one's communicative style to meet listener and/or situational requirements). An example of the latter would be the knowledge that one would speak differently to a child than to an authority figure. Thus, social understanding is foundational to pragmatics, because for communication to be successful both

Table 10-1. The Four Maxims of Conversational Interaction

Maxim 1:	**Quantity** — the rule to be informative without being verbose. Speaking "nonstop" without regard to "social distress" signals is an example of difficulty with *quantity*.
Maxim 2:	**Quality** — the rule to be truthful. Confabulation (i.e., filling in knowledge gaps with false information that the speaker *believes* to be true) is an example of difficulty with *quality*.
Maxim 3:	**Relevance** — the rule to contribute only information that is pertinent to the topic and situation. Tangential comments constitute difficulty with the rule of *relevance*.
Maxim 4:	**Clarity** — the rule that the information conveyed is clear and understandable to the listener. Initiating a conversation in the middle of a thought, without providing background information, is an example of a problem with the rule of *clarity*.

Note. Twachtman (1996) based on the work of Grice (1975).

interactants need to understand not only their own informational needs and perspectives, but also those of their communicative partner (Baltaxe, 1977; Grice, 1975; James, 1990; McCormick, 1990; Owens, 1988). It is this specific type of knowledge that enables typical speakers to fine-tune their messages based on the meanings that they intend to convey. Finally, the term *communicative competence* (Dore, 1986; Gallagher, 1991; Hymes, 1972; Owens, 1988) is used to describe the extent to which speakers in a conversational exchange evidence skill in the three main areas of pragmatics described above.

Paralinguistic Features

No discussion of communication could be complete without taking into account the all-important nonlinguistic (i.e., paralinguistic) information that accompanies verbal discourse. In addition to the acoustic features already noted, these also include gestures, facial expression, eye gaze, and the like. Often, these nonverbal features arc grouped together under the category of *body language*. Eminently "social-sensitive," all of these meaning-carrying elements require social understanding as a prerequisite for use. Employed appropriately, they infuse the message with information regarding the speaker's attitude and emotional state, thus serving a major role in both message generation and sensemaking.

The role of these social–emotional factors in the pragmatics of human communication cannot be overemphasized. As extraordinary as it may seem, Mehrabian (1968), in a set of classic experiments, found that only 7% of the emotional meaning of a message is attributed to the actual words used. He went on to state that, of the other 93%, 55% of the emotional content is expressed through body language (i.e., facial, gestural, and postural), while 38% percent of emotional meaning is attributed to the tone of voice.

Well-known expressions such as "she spoke through clenched teeth" paint an immediate picture of emotional tone, even without the accompanying verbal message. Likewise, the expression "if looks could kill" gives one an appreciation for the powerful effect that facial expression can exert, separate and apart from the words that are uttered. The message-influencing force of vocal intonation and stress is easily seen in the following sequence:

> *I* will not do that.
> I will *not* do that.
> I will not do *that*.

In the first instance, stress on the word *I* sends the message — not *I*, perhaps someone else. In the second, stress on the word *not* communicates — under *no* uncertain terms will I do that. In the third case, stress on the word *that* indicates — not *that*, perhaps something else. Thus, in each instance, most of the meaning is carried not by the words, but by the paralinguistic features related to inflection, intonation, and stress.

The message, then, is far more than the words that comprise it. Unfortunately, the specific components that carry so much of the message — the paralinguistic features of communication — are the very elements that individuals with HFA and AS find the most difficult, both to interpret and to employ. Further, this failure exerts a negative impact on both the message that is received, and that which, in turn, is generated.

Finally, it is important to note that regardless of the specific nature of pragmatic deficit, such deficits are a universal feature of autism and AS, even in the most able individuals. Further, these deficits can and often do exist in the presence of speech that is fluent, and language that is appropriate with respect to grammar, syntax, and lexicality. It is therefore imperative to look beyond the isolated word and sentence level to the richer and infinitely more complex area of discourse if one is to understand the essence of the communicative impairment in these disorders.

Hopefully, the foregoing detailed description of the competencies involved in pragmatic communication will enable the reader to better understand the specific nature of the language and communication deficits that are described in the sections that follow. At the same time, it is hoped that the foregoing discussion has helped the reader to more fully appreciate the plight of those who live in a sociocommunicative world that is largely devoid of the social–emotional context that is so essential to the establishment of meaning and sense-making.

SOCIAL–COGNITIVE DEFICITS IN COMMUNICATION IMPAIRMENT

The fact that pragmatic communication difficulty is common to both autism and AS should come as no surprise to anyone familiar with DSM-IV, given that both disorders share identical descriptions with respect to impairment in social interaction. As social competency is at the heart of pragmatic ability, it is understandable that individuals with impaired social understanding and expression would also be similarly compromised in their comprehension and use of certain aspects of language. Despite the commonality of underlying social deficits, however, there is nonetheless a great deal of variability with respect to the specific ways in which language and communication may be affected in these disorders.

Because pragmatic deficits are a natural outgrowth of impaired social cognition in individuals with HFA and AS, I view such deficits as the final common denominator in the language and communication problems seen in these disorders. Before examining some of the specific characteristics of deviant language use, it is worthwhile to take a general look at the impaired social–cognitive underpinnings that govern the receptive and expressive elements of interactive discourse.

In much the same way that a computer's output is only as good as its programmed input, so too the language use (communicative) deficits in HFA and AS reflect the quality of the input that these individuals receive during communicative interactions. But there the analogy ends, for human beings are far more complex than the most complex computer. As such, human output is based not only on an *understanding* (reception) of input (most of which involves rapidly moving, ever-changing, socially determined information), but also on the ability to *process* this information in an efficient (timely) and effective (meaningful) manner, so that judgments and behavioral adjustments may be made with respect to output (*expression*). This is no small task, given that individuals with HFA and AS are impaired in the social–cognitive underpinnings that govern this type of sociocommunicative decision-making. In order to understand and more fully appreciate the nature of the specific language use deficits in HFA and AS, it is worthwhile to consider three main areas of receptive deficit, and the ways in which they constrain expressive language use.

Theory of Mind

Tager-Flusberg (1993) linked the pragmatic deficits in autism to the deficits that are associated with theory of mind (TOM). The latter refers to the complex, multifaceted ability to infer mental states from behavior (Baron-Cohen, 1995). In so doing, Tager-Flusberg echoed the themes set forth by Baron-Cohen (1988, 1995) and Frith (1989). In expanding on TOM, Baron-Cohen (1995) coined the term *mindblindness* to characterize the inability to "read behavior in terms of mental states" (p. 5) that he feels typifies people with autism. Interestingly, Ozonoff, Rogers, and Pennington (1991) did not find TOM deficits in their AS subjects. The latter finding may represent a true, distinguishing characteristic between HFA and AS, even though higher TOM ability in AS may not have been "naturally occurring." In this regard, even though Frith (1991) acknowledged that individuals with AS may be superior to those with HFA on the belief attribution tasks that underlie one's TOM, she nonetheless hypothesized the following:

> I propose that well-adapted Asperger syndrome individuals may have all the trappings of socially adapted behavior, may have learnt to solve belief attribution problems, but yet may not have a normally functioning theory of mind. The hypothesis allows us to describe behavior as *resembling* the normal pattern but arising from quite abnormally functioning processes. (p. 21)

Finally, it may well be that while individuals with AS are able to solve relatively simple TOM tasks, they may nevertheless evidence TOM deficits at higher levels of complexity (Frith, 1991). In this regard, it has been my clinical experience that the demands of rapidly moving, ongoing discourse do indeed adversely affect the ability of both those with HFA and AS to engage in the mental processes associated with TOM. This is especially true in highly stimulating environments.

Under ordinary circumstances, the ability to "read" social situations and people, and to adjust one's communicative behavior accordingly, is a task that is performed effortlessly, and usually below the level of consciousness. The ability to understand another person's perspective, a key element of TOM, and to infer mental states is governed in large measure by indirect, socially mediated cues. Thus, because individuals with autism and AS have specific difficulty in understanding social information, they are particularly compromised in their ability to engage in the presuppositional behavior — much of which has to do with the attribution of mental states — that is integral to the concept of communicative competence. To complicate matters further, the demands of discourse act to exacerbate the situation.

Nonverbal Elements

Dysprosodies — or disturbances in the intonational elements of speech production — are well-known features of autism (Baltaxe & Simmons, 1992; Fay & Schuler, 1980; Kanner, 1946; Paul, 1987) and AS (Asperger, 1991). Prosodic variation is a particularly powerful communicative device by which even subtle distinctions in word meaning may be conveyed. As in the case of TOM, compromises in using paralinguistic features effectively have their roots in the individual's impaired ability to understand them.

According to Tager-Flusberg (1993), it is the prosodic characteristics of the message that signal whether its meaning is to be taken literally or nonliterally. Further, double entendre, sarcasm, exaggeration, and understatement are all conveyed through prosodic elements (Tager-Flusberg, 1993). Thus, the power of prosody lies in its ability to communicate important information indirectly — not through words, but through the vocal features that carry the real (intended) meaning of the message. Combined with nonvocal elements — eye gaze, posture, facial expression, and gesture — these paralinguistic features may be construed as the receptive and expressive building blocks of successful communication.

People with autism and AS are literal in both their interpretation and use of language (Fay & Schuler, 1980; Rumsey, 1992). The intended meaning of the statement, "No way!" with rising intonation to indicate surprise, will be missed unless specific steps are taken to directly teach the meaning behind the words. Likewise, so too will its semantic counterpart, "You don't say!" Further, a literal interpretation of these messages actually detracts from their communicative intent, creating confusion, and thereby compromising sense-making.

Sometimes the entire meaning of the message is communicated through its paralinguistic features, rather than its words. This creates the type of paradoxical communicative experience that underlies many comedic situations. One is reminded of the rich humor conveyed largely through facial expression and other nonverbal features that characterized the genius of Lucille Ball in *I Love Lucy*, and Jackie Gleason in *The Honeymooners*. It should be apparent that given the lack of facility with paralinguistic information that people with HFA and AS characteristically have, even relatively "obvious" comedic situations would be problematic. Clearly then, it also follows that these individuals would have even more difficulty understanding more subtle humor (Weylman, Brownell, & Gardner, 1988). Consequently, even when people with autism and AS are able to understand the words and the concepts that they represent, they may still be unable to understand the message itself, given the extent to which the latter is dependent on the social-sensitive nonverbal elements that, to a large extent, determine its meaning.

Inference-Making

Inferential reasoning is a cognitive process by which one makes judgments about the physical world based on not only the properties perceived, but more importantly, on information that is not necessarily present at the time. In typical speakers, this "internal information" is selectively applied, according to context, in situations that quite literally call it to mind. For example, seeing a group of children seated around a cake with candles would lead one to infer that someone was having a birthday party. Similarly, seeing someone crying in the waiting room of a hospital would lead one to infer that someone is feeling sad.

Inferential reasoning ability is an area of weakness for even the most able people with autism and AS, given its reliance on indirect cues, many of which are socially determined. In one of his workshops, Dr. Gary Mesibov cited an excellent example of impaired ability to make inferences in a young man with autism who was taking advanced college courses. In seeing this individual carrying a copy of the book *War and Peace*, Dr. Mesibov inquired as to how he liked it. The young man responded, "How did you know I was reading it?" If simple, relatively "concrete" inferences are difficult for even the most intellectually able individuals with HFA and AS, one can *infer* that inferences based on subtle paralinguistic features must be even more difficult. Interestingly, impaired inferential reasoning ability is at the heart of the preference for factual, as opposed to social, information that characterizes people with these disorders.

The specific areas of deviant language use that follow traverse aspects of social cognition and pragmatic communication. The examples used to illustrate specific deficits are often overlapping. This is to be expected, given the intricacies involved in the complex, multidimensional skill of communication.

LANGUAGE AND COMMUNICATION CHARACTERISTICS SEEN IN HIGH-FUNCTIONING AUTISM AND ASPERGER SYNDROME

Literal Language

The propensity for literalness extends beyond difficulty with the paralinguistic features of communication. People with HFA and AS also have problems understanding socially determined shifts in word meaning and/or situational context (Tsai, 1992). This lack of understanding has a profound effect on expressive language. For example, a 7-year-old with AS responded to the question of how to make a friend by listing the component parts of a person: "Atoms, cells, eyes, nose, mouth, arms, legs. P.S. Then say hello" (Twachtman, 1995, p. 136). Notwithstanding the creativity of his answer, his literal interpretation of the words reveals both a unilateral view of the meaning of the word *make* (to construct); a lack of appreciation for the context in which it is rendered; and a lack of understanding of the concept of friendship. An even clearer example of meaning rigidity (i.e., getting stuck on the original perception of the word) is seen in one mother's example of her 4-year-old AS child's insistence that they do not live on Huckleberry Hill Road as their address states, but rather on Huckleberry Hill, because their house is on the *hill*, not on the road.

Literal interpretation and use of language offer one a glimpse into the thought processes of people with HFA and AS. The world of people and things seem to be assigned labels according to the ways in which they are specifically perceived. For example, a mother in Ohio once noted that when her son's soccer coach first yelled, "Time out!" the little boy insisted, "But I didn't do anything." Clearly, that child's interpretation of the term was rooted in his experience with it. Literalness can also give language an odd, pedantic quality. Seip (1995) gave an excellent example of this in relating how one young man with AS referred to a hole in his sock as "a temporary loss of knitting."

Literalness then exemplifies an inflexible cognitive learning style in which meanings are assigned to words as though "set in stone"; that is, based on concrete, factual perceptions, and/or specific experiences, as opposed to a reflection of intangible, abstract, social understanding. Thus, lacking flexibility, individuals with HFA and AS persist in their situation-specific "first impressions" of words regardless of contextually changing situations and/or social usage (Tsai, 1992; Wapner, Hamby, & Gardner, 1981).

Metaphorical Language

The use of metaphorical language — that is, language that holds private, idiosyncratic meaning for its user — is a well-recognized feature of autistic language behavior, particularly at emerging language levels (Fay & Schuler,

1980; Prizant & Schuler, 1987; Rumsey, 1992). In many respects, metaphorical language is prototypic of the syndrome of autism itself. It reflects the individual's use of associative memory to create the private reference (Fay & Schuler, 1980). It also reflects an inflexible, situation-specific, cognitive style that causes individuals with this disability to rigidly "lock on" to a particular association, such that they "miss the forest for the trees" with respect to sense-making. Finally, given that these private references are not shared by interactants, metaphorical language also represents the user's difficulty with perspective-taking and lack of appreciation for the role of shared social understanding in establishing meaning. According to Fay and Schuler (1980), the use of this language strategy "demonstrate[s] communicative intent in the apparent absence of linguistic competence" (p. 57). It should be further apparent that it also reveals a lack of pragmatic competence as well.

Metaphorical language can be used to communicate various types of information. Notwithstanding, its use reflects a lack of linguistic and social competence in coding and expressing information in a manner that is discernible to the listener. For example, several minutes into an activity, Chris, a 9-year-old boy with AS, would often announce to his teacher, "At 12 o'clock we go to Paris." This would soon be followed by behavioral deterioration. When it was learned that this phrase represented Chris's association with an activity that he engaged in at the *end* of his weekly music lesson, it became apparent that the sentence served the purpose of requesting (ordering?) termination of the activity. Without that knowledge the teacher was at a loss to understand Chris's communicative intent. Twachtman (1995) has suggested that this use of metaphoric language may represent a verbal reenactment strategy. Specifically, verbal expressions that produced results in one setting are "recycled" for the purpose of producing the same result in the new setting, in the absence of understanding how to do so in more conventional ways.

Kevin, an 8-year-old boy with AS, hospitalized for a medical condition, told the nursing staff that his name was Wade. His mother was not able to elicit a response from him as to why he gave an erroneous name. Once home, he volunteered the following, "I told them my name was Wade because Wade Duck was afraid of everything, and I was afraid when I was in the hospital." Here, metaphorical language is used to express the emotion, *fear*, at a time when the experience of fear may have made direct verbal expression difficult.

Based on my clinical experience, it would seem that the use of metaphorical language is at its most "poetic," if not its most poignant, in AS. Often it is used to express complex thoughts and feelings (mental states) that the individual is at a loss to express in more standard ways. For example, in the illustration that follows, 14-year-old David communicates a wealth of information (albeit circuitously) about issues of importance to him. He also speaks volumes with respect to the oft-cited problems with common sense that even the highest-functioning people with AS have. In answer to the question regarding what he would do with

$100, David wrote: "I would buy the entire school, McDonald's, and any any any any type of book. I would grow older than my teacher." The idiosyncratic reference to buying the school, and growing older than his teacher suggests a desire for greater control. The idea that the school and McDonald's could be purchased for $100 speaks to the lack of common sense that is often evident in AS (Asperger, 1991).

In the poem "Snowstorm" that follows, David expresses his frustration over not being able to figure out the way things work in his world:

At the window coming at the door,
I saw snow, nothing more.
On the way driving to school,
Mom broke a rule.
She thought it was a snowstorm,
So she turned back home where it was warm.
I was horrified [italics added].
Back in my room I sat and cried.
Then I played with the computer.
I tried to ask mom to send me to school
But couldn't loot her.
Then I watched TV.
I also read books, you see.
That's my vacation behind the front door…
nothing more.

Undoubtedly, the most poignant aspect of this poem is David's *horror* over a "snow day." It is difficult to imagine a 14-year-old boy being unhappy over a day off from school, especially when he is able to engage in some of his favorite activities (e.g., computer, books, TV). Notwithstanding, David communicates *metaphorically* the reason for his disconsolation. The keys to unlocking David's communicative "code" may be found in two sentences. In saying "She thought it was a snowstorm," David reveals his lack of knowledge regarding the nuances that determine whether school will be called off because of weather (e.g., amount of snow; timing of the snowfall; availability of people to plow). In saying "Mom broke a rule," David reveals his attempt to provide his own structure to an ephemeral, inexplicable social world that, in the absence of a well-defined social sense (social understanding), must seem arbitrary and capricious. When asked what the rule was that Mom broke, David replied that people go to school Monday through Friday. A rule-based, discrete understanding of individual events and situations does not easily accommodate extenuating circumstances, like snow. It may well be that — absent a more intrinsic understanding of their social milieus — rules constitute for individuals with HFA and AS their tenaciously held hypotheses about the world in which they live.

It should be obvious that while metaphoric language achieves its highest use with more able individuals, its meaning is nonetheless highly dependent on the listener's ability to "read between the lines" in order to determine the meaning behind the words. Further, the need to "talk around" a subject may well reflect the problems that these individuals commonly have in communicating mentalistic, as opposed to factual, information, especially "when in the heat of the cognitively demanding, or anxious moment."

Topicality

Engaging in conversational discourse requires understanding and use of many interrelated skills. These include being able to initiate, maintain, and terminate topics appropriately, as well as knowing how to appropriately shift topics and repair (clarify) communication when breakdowns occur (James, 1990). Integral to this knowledge is an understanding of how to alternate speaker/listener roles (take turns) in a conversational exchange. In addition, all of these competencies are governed by pragmatic rules that obligate the interactant to adhere to the four maxims of pragmatic communication noted earlier. Thus, contributions to the conversation must be informative without being verbose. They must also be truthful, relevant, and comprehensible to the listener. Application of these competencies is, to a large extent, based on the speaker being able to make appropriate presuppositions regarding the listener's informational needs and perspectives, so that communication may be specifically tailored to the requirements of the particular situation (DeHart & Maratsos, 1984; Geller, 1989). Finally, presuppositions play an important role in signaling the need for repairing conversational breakdown when the latter occurs.

It should be apparent that it is at the juncture of conversational discourse, and the complex judgments that it requires, where "the rubber hits the road" in autism and AS, even at the highest-functioning levels. Communicative competence requires a degree of social understanding, perspective-taking, adaptability, and flexibility that individuals with HFA and AS simply do not possess. Often, they rigidly adhere to topics that center around their special interests (Tager-Flusberg, 1993), regardless of listener reaction. In addition, according to a study by Tager-Flusberg and Quill (as cited in Paul, 1987), they also evidence difficulty with Grice's (1975) maxims governing relevance, quantity, and clarity. Overall, according to Paul (1987), studies of verbal individuals with autism indicate that "the autistic person has little skill in participating in communicative activities involving joint reference or shared topics, and particularly in supplying new information relevant to the listener's purposes" (p. 73). Tager-Flusberg and Anderson (1991) echoed Paul's sentiments regarding the difficulty in supplying new information. Even more telling was their finding that, notwithstanding *linguistic* advances over time, children with autism did not evidence concomitant increases in *conversational competence* (discourse) (Tager-Flusberg & Anderson, 1991).

The following example entitled "Novel of Love" was written by a young man with autism. It provides an excellent illustration of several issues related to topicality. It also demonstrates superficially normal language — appropriate syntax, grammar, and vocabulary — coexisting with distinctly inappropriate pragmatic ability.

"I love you," she said.
"I love you more than I can say."
"I love you, too," he answered.
"My love for you is higher than the highest mountain which is Mount Everest which is over 29,000 feet high."
"My love for you is deeper than the deepest ocean which is the Marianas trench which is over 36,000 feet deep."
! ! ! ! ! !
If you were to drop a rock the size of your head into water 36,000 feet (10,900 meters) deep, it would take the rock about an hour to reach the bottom!
(Courtesy, Gary Mesibov)

The fund of knowledge available to this young man is indisputably remarkable. His manipulation of the tools of language (punctuation marks), and the rules of language (syntax), are quite acceptable, as is his choice of vocabulary. Even so, this "Novel of Love" is distinctly unusual from a pragmatic communication perspective.

A cursory examination of this piece reveals the young man's difficulty with higher-level pragmatic rules of discourse. He evidences specific difficulty with topic relevance and topic maintenance, giving himself over completely to tangentiality as the "novel" ends. Not only does he veer significantly off-topic, he does so precipitously, unmindful of more appropriate ways to segue from one topic to another. Further, there is little evidence that the listener's informational needs and/or perspectives are taken into account. Contrastively, there is abundant evidence of the writer's egocentric focus, that is, his abiding interest in geographical facts. Clearly, in "Novel of Love," the young man demonstrates his excitement, not with the heights and depths of love, but rather with the concrete, straight forward material that anchors that emotion to factual knowledge that he finds interesting and relevant. Witness his effusive and strategic use of exclamation points to punctuate his excitement. "Novel of Love" also provides a suitable vehicle by which to segue into the more predictable world of facts.

Preference for Facts

Informal observation of language use in individuals with autism and AS suggests that they have a predilection for factually based information. Indeed, many of the examples cited in this chapter reveal their tendency either to shy away from social–emotional material or to deal with it in a concrete, factual manner. In the example cited earlier in which David listed how he would spend $100, it is important to note that he does not talk about his *desire* for greater control over his life. Instead, through metaphor, he lists the facts that would enable that to occur: buying the school, and growing older than his teacher. Similarly, literalness in and of itself offers prima facie evidence of the lack of facility with figurative (abstract) language, and the concrete, factualistic thinking that is a stable characteristic of autism and AS, even at the highest-functioning levels.

Notwithstanding a fascinating line of research concerning the alleged inability of people with autism to understand mental states (Baron-Cohen, 1988, 1995; Frith, 1989; Tager-Flusberg, 1993), issues related to mentalistic activities and feeling states nonetheless remain speculative at this time. Harris (1993) observed that children with autism rarely express mental states related to ideas. Tager-Flusberg (1993) compared children with autism and Down syndrome vis-à-vis their use of language related to mental states. She found that although children with autism do talk about desire and emotion, they refer less frequently to cognitive or epistemic states. Undoubtedly, one of the reasons why definitive answers to questions regarding mental states and emotions are not yet available, relates to the high degree of variability and adaptability that is seen in many individuals with autism and AS, particularly at higher-functioning levels (Mayes, Cohen, & Klin, 1993).

Useful information can be obtained clinically, however, through observation and case history. Brian, a fourth-grade boy with AS, was asked to write an essay on what he wanted his future wife to be like, based on his having read a book about a mail-order bride. He deftly listed numerous attributes, all of which related to his own interests. A portion of his lengthy essay follows:

> WANTED: WIFE
> My future wife should be a good bowler. A person who goes to Boston. Likes hot dogs. Doesn't mind that I'm allergic to milk. Is sincere! Likes puzzles. Can read road maps. Likes computers and golfing. [and most poignant of all] *should be enchanted with facts....* [italics added]

Interestingly, Brian's articulate rendering of the characteristics he would like in a wife, stand in stark contrast to his far less articulate expression of emotion in the distressful situation illustrated in the following example:

> The New Jersey ride on the turnpike, going South for "Dying Delaware," the State that's #1.... The days understood me as a rest stop came to me. We stopped near exit 8, maybe 5 miles away, I did not matter unless it came to me. Those things came in my daydream, and Sunoco went further by. Those maps I saw there were in my eye.

These two examples also illustrate the cohesiveness required of discourse in the latter, versus the more isolated sentence production seen in the former example. Brian also evidences difficulty in answering specific questions related to feeling states. For example, when asked, "How did you feel when Kit saved Hannah from the angry mob?" Brian replied, "Dramatic, too dramatic. Trying to kill Hannah, a poor old defenseless woman." Clearly, Brian's use of language demonstrates that he is "ill at ease" in the world of discourse and emotion.

Temple Grandin gives additional insight into possible reasons why factual information may be preferred by people with autism. She notes, *"My mind is like a CD-ROM in a computer — like a quick-access videotape"* (in Sacks, 1995, p. 282). Sacks (1995), based on input from Temple, characterizes the latter's experience as reflecting a lack of "implicit knowledge of social conventions and codes" (p. 270) which form the basis of the presuppositions that govern social interactions. According to Sacks (1995), "Lacking it, she has instead to 'compute' others' intentions and states of mind, to try to make algorithmic, explicit, what for the rest of us is second nature" (p. 270). Even more telling is the explanation that Sacks (1995) offers regarding factual versus social language:

> still quite abnormal in her understanding of ordinary or social language — she still missed allusions, presuppositions, irony, metaphors, jokes — [Temple] found the language of science and technology a huge relief. It was much clearer, much more explicit, with far less depending on unstated assumptions. Technical language was as easy for her as social language was difficult. (pp. 272–273)

Thus, it would seem that the apparent preference for factual information that individuals with HFA and AS evidence, is as much a reflection of their strengths in the more straightforward world of objects and facts, as it is a reflection of their lack of competence in the ephemeral world of ideas, social cues, and feeling states.

"Metability"

It is important to address an additional and somewhat paradoxical aspect of language behavior in AS that I have observed many times in clinical practice. Specifically, notwithstanding the numerous deficiencies in communication that plague these individuals, they nonetheless often evidence surprising facility with discrete aspects of language.

Some people with AS are quite adept at wordplay and puns, ranging from simplistic associations to high-level, witty remarks (Asperger, 1991). For example, one 6-year-old with AS was overheard to say, "I'm not a record player, I'm a record *player*." Interestingly, his interpretation of spoken language was quite literal. In addition, the appropriate use of intonation to highlight the word *player*, contrasted sharply with the unusual cadence, and markedly pedantic quality that characterized his conversational speech.

A 10-year-old boy with AS demonstrated metalinguistic ability when he expressed frustration regarding several aspects of punctuation in the English language. He told his clinician that question marks should not be at the end of a sentence, "because then you can't tell if it's a question until you get there." He even devised his own question symbol to be used at the *beginning* of sentences, commenting, "If they corrected all the problems with the English language, it would be a whole other language!" Such metalinguistic thinking stands in stark contrast to the serious social/pragmatic deficits that characterize these individuals' use of language for communication purposes. It also illustrates an aspect of functioning — seemingly unique to AS — that this writer has termed *metability*.

The Greek prefix *meta* is used here, somewhat generically, to signify the AS individual's penchant for going *beyond* — in this case, beyond simple face-value acceptance of things that the vast majority of people simply accept on face value! The questions that these children ask, and the comments that they make reveal their obsession to know things that either cannot, or cannot easily, be known. Sometimes, as in the case of Kevin, these questions have a decidedly philosophical quality to them. For example, when he was 4, Kevin was obsessed with wanting to know the number *after* infinity. Recently, at age 7, his mother reported the following conversation:

Kevin: "Do we exist forever?"

Mother [Answering according to the tenets of her religion]: "Yes. After we are born, we exist forever."

Kevin: "Do we exist before we are born?"

Mother: "No. We don't exist before we are born. We exist forever after we die."

Kevin: "How do we know we exist after we die, if we don't exist before we are born?"

Kevin's mother refers to her son's quests for such information as *obsessional*. Interestingly, she notes that such questioning abates only when she is able to give an answer that is grounded in more concrete, as opposed to metaphysical, information.

INTERVENTION CONSIDERATIONS

Although this chapter is not intended to serve as a "blueprint" for remediation, it is important to consider the implications of a discourse perspective with respect to intervention. As the essence of the communication impairment in HFA and AS is not found in isolated word and sentence production, traditional assessment procedures may give a false sense of security. Specifically, individuals with these disorders may do well on vocabulary tests, and examinations related to the formal aspects of language. Likewise, they may even do well on aspects of language tested in isolation that would, under the more demanding conditions of interactional discourse, give characteristic difficulty. For example, I have had many clients who exhibited word retrieval difficulty in discourse that was not apparent in confrontation naming tasks performed in isolation. Finally, some aspects of pragmatic behavior do not lend themselves to formal evaluation (e.g., presuppositional knowledge, and judgments with respect to the four maxims of conversational interaction).

With these precautions in mind, it is important to examine the features of discourse as the event is occurring, in order to determine where, and under what circumstances, breakdowns occur. In addition, in addressing the needs of people with these disorders, it is critically important to not be "blinded" by superficially normal language, but rather to look beyond language form and structure to the social–pragmatic dimension of language use. This should include consideration of the complex knowledge base and sociocommunicative decision-making that language use requires. Finally, unless intervention efforts encompass the features of discourse, the essence of the communication impairment in HFA and AS will be sadly neglected.

THE RELATIONSHIP BETWEEN HIGH-FUNCTIONING AUTISM AND ASPERGER SYNDROME

It should be obvious to the reader that both HFA and AS share a common core of social–cognitive deficits that give rise to the impaired pragmatic communication ability that is seen in these disorders. Notwithstanding, variability in the way in which this impaired pragmatic ability is manifested can, and often does, create differences in outward expression in the two disorders. As noted earlier, it has been my clinical experience that people with AS commonly have greater facility with discrete aspects of language than do those with HFA, to wit the examples of metalinguistic behavior noted previously. Similarly, despite the fact that the descriptions of Kanner and Asperger were marked by concordance on all of the main features of autism (Frith, 1991), there is, nonetheless, a distinctiveness about individuals with AS that is emblematical, particularly with respect to the oddities noted in their *style* of communication and social behavior. According to Frith (1991), "Children and adults who are socially inept but often socially interested, who are articulate yet strangely ineloquent, who are gauche and impractical, who are specialists in unusual fields — these will always evoke Hans Asperger's name" (pp. 11–12).

The question that needs to be addressed, however, is whether differences in the outward expression of social–cognitive deficits in AS are sufficiently unique to qualify it as a separate disorder from that of autism. DSM-IV stands on the affirmative side of this issue, stating that in order to qualify for a diagnosis of Asperger's Disorder, "criteria are not met for another specific Pervasive Developmental Disorder or Schizophrenia" (p. 62). Not only does current knowledge (and conventional wisdom) mitigate against so definitive a position, both would seem to lend greater support to the idea that AS and HFA are but different expressions of the same basic disorder. Wing (1991) lent credence to this position in her statement that "the strongest argument for a seamless continuum from Kanner autism to Asperger's syndrome comes from clinical case material where the same individual was typically autistic in his early years but made progress and as a teenager showed all the characteristics of Asperger's syndrome" (p. 103).

All things considered, I view DSM-IV's decision to consider the two disorders as separate entities under the category of Pervasive Developmental Disorders as premature at best, if not overstated, particularly as part of that decision was undoubtedly based on the inaccurate view of language and communication that it sets forth. A less definitive position would have served everyone better, especially because, according to Klin and Volkmar (1995), "the issue of whether Asperger syndrome and Higher Functioning Autism are different conditions is not resolved" (p. 2).

SUMMARY

This chapter has considered the ways in which the patterns of language use in people with HFA and AS deviate from those found in the general population. It has done so within the context of first examining some of the complex, multidimensional features that comprise the communication system, in order to enable the reader to more fully appreciate both the complexities involved in normal communication, and the specific nature of the pragmatic deficits that are seen in these disorders. The information presented is based on the premises that language has an essential communicative base, and that the communication system, as opposed to the formal aspects of language, bears the major burden of impairment in HFA and AS. In addition, I have assumed the position that it is in the features of discourse, rather than in those of isolated word and sentence production, where the essence of communication impairment may be found in these disorders. The latter has significant implications for the type of intervention programming that individuals with HFA and AS need in order to become more competent communicators.

Distinctly clinical in focus, this chapter proceeds from a rejection of the DSM-IV position on language and communication, to a consideration of the common core of social–cognitive deficits that underlie the pragmatic communication impairment that is seen. These deficits are viewed as constituting the primary impairment in the individual's understanding and use of language for the purpose of communication. Further, language deviance, as opposed to language delay, is considered a pathognomonic feature of both disorders. Finally, I have adopted the position that current knowledge would seem to indicate that HFA and AS are different expressions of the same basic disorder, given the nature of the similarities between the two disorders, and in the absence of definitive information to the contrary, this would seem to be a most reasonable position.

REFERENCES

American Speech–Language–Hearing Association. (1989, March). *Issues in determining eligibility for language intervention* (pp. 113–118). Rockville, MD: Research Division at ASHA.

Asperger, H. (1991). 'Autistic psychopathy' in childhood. In U. Frith (Ed.), *Autism and Asperger syndrome* (pp. 37–92). Cambridge: Cambridge University Press.

Baltaxe, C. A. M. (1977). Pragmatic deficits in the language of autistic adolescents. *Journal of Pediatric Psychology, 2*, 176–180.

Baltaxe, C. A. M., & Simmons, J. Q. (1988). Pragmatic deficits in emotionally disturbed children and adolescents. In R. L. Schiefelbusch & L. Lloyd (Eds.), *Language perspectives: Acquisition, retardation and intervention* (2nd ed., pp. 223–253). Austin, TX: Pro-Ed.

Baltaxe, C. A. M., & Simmons, J. Q., III. (1992). A comparison of language issues in high-functioning autism and related disorders with onset in childhood and adolescence. In E. Schopler & G. B. Mesibov (Eds.), *High-functioning individuals with autism* (pp. 201–225). New York: Plenum Press.

Baron-Cohen, S. (1988). Social and pragmatic deficits in autism: Cognitive or affective? *Journal of Autism and Developmental Disorders, 18*, 379–402.

Baron-Cohen, S. (1995). *Mindblindness: An essay on autism and theory of mind.* Cambridge, MA: MIT Press.

Bates, E. (1976). *Language and context: The acquisition of pragmatics.* New York: Academic Press.

Bruner, J. (1978). Learning the mother tongue. *Human Nature*, 42–48.

Crystal, D. (1975). *The English tone of voice.* London: Edward Arnold.

Dale, P. S. (1972). *Language development.* Hinsdale, IL: Dryden Press.

DeHart, G., & Maratsos, M. (1984). Children's acquisition of presuppositional usages. In R. L. Schiefelbusch & J. Pickar (Eds.), *The acquisition of communicative competence* (pp. 237–293). Baltimore: University Park Press.

Dore, J. (1986). The development of conversational competence. In R. L. Schiefelbusch (Ed.), *Language competence: Assessment and intervention* (pp. 3–60). San Diego: College-Hill.

Fay, W. H., & Schuler, A. L. (1980). *Emerging language in autistic children.* Baltimore: University Park Press.

Frith, U. (1989). *Autism: Explaining the enigma.* Oxford: Blackwell.

Frith, U. (1991). Asperger and his syndrome. In U. Frith (Ed.), *Autism and Asperger syndrome* (pp. 1–36). Cambridge: Cambridge University Press.

Gallagher, T. M. (1991). A retrospective look at clinical pragmatics. In T. M. Gallagher (Ed.), *Pragmatics of language: Clinical practice issues* (pp. 1–9). San Diego: Singular.

Geller, E. (1989). The assessment of perspective-taking skills. *Seminars in Speech and Language, 10*, 28–41.

Grice, H. (1975). Logic and conversation. In D. Davidson & G. Harmon (Eds.), *The logic of grammar* (pp. 64–74). Encina, CA: Dickenson.

Harris, P. (1993). Pretending and planning. In S. Baron-Cohen, H. Tager-Flusberg, & D. J. Cohen (Eds.), *Understanding other minds: Perspectives from autism* (pp. 228–246). London: Oxford University Press.

Hymes, D. (1972). Introduction. In C. Cazden, V. John, & D. Hymes (Eds.), *Functions of language in the classrooms*. New York: Teachers College, Columbia University.

James, S. L. (1990). *Normal language acquisition*. Austin, TX: Pro-Ed.

Kanner, L. (1946). Irrelevant and metaphorical language in early infantile autism. *American Journal of Psychiatry, 103*, 242–246.

Kaye, K. (1982). *The mental and social life of babies*. Chicago: University of Chicago Press.

Klin, A., & Volkmar, F. R. (1995). *Guidelines for parents: Assessment, diagnosis, and intervention of Asperger syndrome* (p. 2). Pittsburgh: Learning Disabilities Association of America.

Layton, T. L., & Watson, L. R. (1995). Enhancing communication in nonverbal children with autism. In K. A. Quill (Ed.), *Teaching children with autism: Strategies to enhance communication and socialization* (pp. 73–103). New York: Delmar.

Lindner, T. W. (1990). *Transdisciplinary play-based assessment: A functional approach to working with young children*. Baltimore: Brookes.

Mayes, L., Cohen, D., & Klin, A. (1993). Desire and fantasy: A psychoanalytic perspective on theory of mind and autism. In S. Baron-Cohen, H. Tager-Flusberg, & D. J. Cohen (Eds.), *Understanding other minds: Perspectives from autism* (pp. 450–465). London: Oxford University Press.

McClowry, D. P., & Guilford, A. M. (1982). Normal and assisted communication development. In D. P. McClowry, A. M. Guilford, & S. O. Richardson (Eds.), *Infant communication: Development, assessment, and intervention* (pp. 9–19). New York: Grune & Stratton.

McCormick, L. (1990). Terms, concepts, and perspectives. In L. McCormick & R. L. Schiefelbusch (Eds.), *Early language intervention: An introduction* (pp. 3–36). Columbus, OH: Merrill.

Mehrabian, A. (1968). Communication without words. *Psychology Today, 24*, 52–55.

Mentis, M., & Thompson, S. A. (1991). Discourse: A means for understanding normal and disordered language. In T. M. Gallagher (Ed.), *Pragmatics of language: Clinical practice issues* (pp. 199–227). San Diego: Singular.

Moerk, E. (1977). *Pragmatic and semantic aspects of early language development*. Baltimore: University Park Press.

Muma, J. (1978). *Language handbook*. Englewood Cliffs, NJ: Prentice–Hall.

Owens, R. E., Jr. (1988). *Language development: An introduction*. Columbus, OH: Merrill.

Ozonoff, S., Rogers, S. J., & Pennington, B. F. (1991). Asperger's syndrome: Evidence of an empirical distinction from high-functioning autism. *Journal of Child Psychology and Psychiatry, 32*, 1107–1122.

Paul, R. (1987). Communication. In D. J. Cohen & A. M. Donnellan (Eds.), *Handbook of autism and pervasive developmental disorders* (pp. 61–84). New York: Wiley.

Prizant, B. M., & Schuler, A. L. (1987). Facilitating communication: Language approaches. In D. J. Cohen & A. M. Donnellan (Eds.), *Handbook of autism and pervasive developmental disorders* (pp. 316–332). New York: Wiley.

Quick Reference to the Criteria from DSM-IV. (1994). *Disorders usually diagnosed in infancy, childhood, or adolescence* (pp. 49–79). Washington, DC: American Psychiatric Association.

Rumsey, J. M. (1992). Neuropsychological studies of high-level autism. In E. Schopler & G. B. Mesibov (Eds.), *High-functioning individuals with autism* (pp. 41–64). New York: Plenum Press.

Sacks, O. (1989). *Seeing voices: A journey into the world of the deaf*. Los Angeles: University of California Press.

Sacks, O. (1995). *An anthropologist on Mars*. New York: Knopf.

Seip, J. (Speaker). (1995). *Asperger syndrome: Social skills training for elementary and secondary aged students* (Cassette Recording, ASA). Sylva, NC: Goodkind of Sound.

Snow, C. (1972). Mother's speech to children learning language. *Child Development, 43*, 549–565.

Stern, D. (1977). *The first relationship: Mother and infant*. Cambridge, MA: Harvard University Press.

Tager-Flusberg, H. (1981). On the nature of linguistic functioning in early infantile autism. *Journal of Autism and Developmental Disorders, 11*, 45–56.

Tager-Flusberg, H. (1988). On the nature of language acquisition disorder: The example of autism. In F. Kessel (Ed.), *The development of language researchers: Essays in honour of Roger Brown* (pp. 249–267). Hillsdale, NJ: Erlbaum.

Tager-Flusberg, H. (1993). What language reveals about the understanding of minds in children with autism. In S. Baron-Cohen, H. Tager-Flusberg, & D. J. Cohen (Eds.), *Understanding other minds: Perspectives from autism* (pp. 138–157). London. Oxford University Press.

Tager-Flusberg, H., & Anderson, M. (1991). The development of contingent discourse ability in autistic children. *Journal of Child Psychology and Psychiatry, 32*, 1123–1134.

Tsai, T. Y. (1992). Diagnostic issues in high-functioning autism. In E. Schopler & G. B. Mesibov (Eds.), *High-functioning individuals with autism* (pp. 11–40). New York: Plenum Press.

Twachtman, D. D. (1995). Methods to enhance communication in verbal children. In K. A. Quill (Ed.), *Teaching children with autism. Strategies to enhance communication and socialization* (pp. 133–162). New York: Delmar.

Twachtman, D. D. (1996, Summer). There's a lot more to communication than talking! *The Morning News*, 3–5.

Wapner, W., Hamby, S., & Gardner, H. (1981). The role of the right hemisphere in the apprehension of complex linguistic materials. *Brain and Language, 14*, 15–33.

Weylman, S. T., Brownell, H. H., & Gardner, H. (1988). "It's what you mean, not what you say": Pragmatic language in brain-damaged patients. In F. Plum (Ed.), *Language, communication and the brain.* New York: Raven Press.

Willard, C. T., & Schuler, A. L. (1987). Social transaction: A vehicle for intervention in autism. In T. L. Layton (Ed.), *Language and treatment of autistic and developmentally disordered children* (pp. 265–289). Springfield, IL: Thomas.

Wing, L. (1981). Asperger's syndrome: A clinical account. *Psychological Medicine, 11*, 115–129.

Wing, L. (1991). The relationship between Asperger's syndrome and Kanner's autism. In U. Frith (Ed.), *Autism and Asperger syndrome* (pp. 93–121). Cambridge: Cambridge University Press.

11

Educational Approaches to High-Functioning Autism and Asperger Syndrome

LINDA KUNCE and GARY B. MESIBOV

Research studies on the effectiveness of treatment programs for children with autism have emphasized the link between structured educational intervention and positive child outcomes (Rutter & Bartak, 1973; Rutter, Greenfeld, & Lockyer, 1967; Schopler, Brehm, Kinsbourne, & Reichler, 1971; Schopler, Mesibov, DeVellis, & Short, 1981). Similarly, more recent reviews indicate that optimal treatment programs for children with autism are intensive, structured, educationally-based, and focused on the child's acquisition of basic skills across a broad range of developmental areas (Olley, Robbins, & Morelli-Robbins, 1993; Rogers, 1996; Volkmar & Cohen, 1994). In contrast to the available publications describing highly structured educational programs for more impaired children with autism (see, e.g., Harris & Handleman, 1994; Lovaas, 1981; Schopler, Reichler, & Lansing, 1980), and despite the significant growth of relevant clinical and research literature over the past decade (summarized in this volume; Frith, 1991; Schopler & Mesibov, 1992), professionals have devoted less attention to isolating and empirically evaluating optimal educational interventions for children with high-functioning autism (HFA) or Asperger syndrome (AS).

LINDA KUNCE • Illinois Wesleyan University, Bloomington, Illinois 61702-2900. GARY B. MESIBOV • Division TEACCH, Department of Psychiatry, University of North Carolina at Chapel Hill, Chapel Hill, North Carolina 27599-7180.

Asperger Syndrome or High-Functioning Autism?, edited by Schopler *et al.* Plenum Press, New York, 1998.

Until recently, parents and professionals seeking information on educational interventions for students with HFA or AS have had to rely on three main sources: (1) recommendations embedded in more general publications addressing the full range of students with autism (e.g., Koegel & Koegel, 1995; Quill, 1995), (2) sporadic reports of research, most of which have been conducted from a behavioral perspective using multiple baseline designs (e.g., Kamps, Barbetta, Leonard, & Delquadri, 1994), and (3) relatively informal means of communication such as conference presentations, booklets, newsletters, and the Internet (e.g., Levy, 1988; Moreno, 1991; Pratt, 1995). Although all have served as valuable sources of information, each has its drawbacks for the teacher who has just had a child with HFA or AS included in her or his classroom, has little background in autism, and who is busy juggling the multiple demands of "regular" classroom teaching. For example, general publications on autism can present a breadth of information that is difficult to process and apply, research articles specifically address only a narrowly defined topic (e.g., increasing social initiation), and informal informational sources often fail to identify original sources for intervention ideas or clarify the degree to which recommended strategies have received clinical or empirical support.

In recognition of the need for more accessible and applicable information regarding educational interventions for HFA and AS, there has been a recent rise in professional publications in this area (Fullerton, Stratton, Coyne, & Gray, 1996; Klin & Volkmar, 1995; Myles & Simpson, 1994–1995; Williams, 1995). Although reliably linking suggestions to observed deficits and strengths in the population of interest, this literature inconsistently provides references to original sources for intervention strategies, making it difficult to discern the degree to which intervention ideas have been adapted from other areas and to what degree they have been developed independently by different professionals in response to similar problems (see Chapter 12, this volume, and Siegel, Goldstein, & Minshew, 1996, for important exceptions to this trend). Further, the basis for intervention recommendations more often than not appears to be clinical experience rather than well-designed, controlled studies of intervention effectiveness, indicating a significant need for continued research in this area.

Our goal in the present chapter is to describe how structured teaching approaches can be utilized in the design of educational interventions for students with HFA, AS, and related disorders, especially those who are served in less structured classroom settings. By relating specific intervention ideas to the broader approach of structured teaching, primarily as it has developed in the context of North Carolina's program for the Treatment and Education of Autistic and related Communication handicapped CHildren (TEACCH; Mesibov, Schopler, & Hearsey, 1994; Schopler et al., 1971), we hope to provide a framework from which professionals and parents can most effectively individualize strategies for use with their students and children, and from which researchers can develop and test hypotheses regarding such intervention strategies.

The remainder of this chapter is organized in three major sections. The first section clarifies the target population, addressing whether subsequent recommendations are appropriate for students with HFA, those with AS, or both. The second major section draws on the broader intervention literature as well as the specific experiences of the TEACCH program to explain how structured teaching principles, strategies, and techniques can be applied to promote the educational growth of students with HFA, AS, and related disorders. The third major section illustrates how structured approaches can be used to manage nonacademic yet critical aspects of behavior, such as social behavior, repetitive interests, and emotional swings, that affect students' abilities to learn and cooperate within classroom settings. To clarify the rationale and implementation of intervention strategies, both the second and third sections include case examples highlighting what — in our clinical experience consulting to teachers, school psychologists, and parents — tend to be the most common questions and concerns arising when children with HFA, AS, and related disorders are taught in regular classroom settings.

HFA VERSUS AS AND EDUCATIONAL INTERVENTION

In light of the developing state of the intervention literature specifically targeting nonretarded individuals with pervasive developmental disorders, it is not surprising that we were unable to locate well-controlled research studies investigating whether specific educational interventions were differentially effective for students with AS or HFA. Nevertheless, the question is important and linked inextricably with the larger issue regarding the clinical status of HFA and AS. Most professionals would agree that individuals diagnosed with these disorders share similar patterns of impairments in social interaction, pragmatic communication, and restricted interests and behaviors. However, as the chapters in this volume attest, there is still no consensus in the field regarding whether HFA and AS are best conceptualized as the same disorder, as representing different points along a severity continuum, or as distinct clinical disorders.

Our position is in line with that of Wing (this volume) and Carruthers and Foreman (1989) in suggesting that specific diagnostic labels — HFA, AS, and Pervasive Developmental Disorder Not Otherwise Specified (PDD-NOS) — are less important to the design of educational interventions than a general understanding of the characteristics associated with these categories and a thorough, individualized assessment of the student's strengths, weaknesses, and interests.

Regardless of the specific diagnostic label, HFA or AS, the majority of these students do not meet chronological age expectations for social behavior, communication abilities, and learning styles. The children's characteristics often interfere with their ability to benefit fully, or even at acceptable levels, from traditional teaching techniques and require educational professionals to adapt instructional methods thoughtfully.

The educational and classroom management strategies frequently recommended for students with HFA, AS, and related disorders are manageable. However, implementing these strategies in a regular classroom setting, especially for a teacher lacking experience with these students, can initially appear overwhelming and lead to haphazard trial-and-error attempts to intervene. Therefore, in the following sections we attempt to illustrate how a framework emphasizing structured teaching approaches can be used to help professionals and parents better understand student needs and more effectively design educational interventions.

STRUCTURED TEACHING WITH HFA AND AS

The implementation of structured teaching in classrooms designed specifically for children with autism involves routines, schedules, individual work systems, visual structure, and physical organization of materials. The most intensive use of these techniques has been described elsewhere (Mesibov *et al.*, 1994; Schopler, Mesibov, & Hearsey, 1995), and will be of interest to professionals working with younger or more significantly impaired students. Importantly, the basic aims of structured teaching remain relevant when teaching children with HFA and AS. First, structured teaching seeks to make the world, in this case the classroom environment, as meaningful as possible. When the child genuinely understands what is happening and what is expected, learning is enhanced, and behavior problems decrease. Second, teaching children with autism involves a two-prong approach that focuses on helping the child develop skills and competencies while also recognizing the need for environmental modifications to maximize student strengths and minimize student deficits.

These organizing principles underlie the primary strategies for structuring the classroom environment for students with HFA or AS. The strategies include: (1) understanding autism, (2) understanding the unique child through both formal and informal assessment, (3) making events consistent and predictable, (4) clarifying instructions and expectations, (5) structuring tasks and assignments to promote success, and (6) cultivating and fully utilizing students' compelling interests. Explanation and application of these six strategies begins with a case example.

Strategy #1: Understanding Autism

I've just been told that 11-year-old Alan, a child with high-functioning autism, will be in my fifth-grade class this year. I really don't know much about autism or what to expect. I do know that Alan had a lot of problems last year. I saw him in the principal's office a lot, and I overheard the school librarian describing how he had thrown a fit — yelling at her and hitting his head with his fist — all because the library did not have a certain book he wanted on South American insects. Is this autism? I have had children with special needs in my class before, but I am a bit worried about my ability to teach Alan.

Frequently, regular classroom teachers, similar to the fifth-grade teacher in this example, have limited backgrounds or experiences in autism, even though the foundation for designing effective interventions is a solid understanding of the general characteristics associated with autism spectrum disorders. Children with HFA and AS, like all children with autism, have a developmental disability caused by neurological dysfunction. A failure to understand how the child's atypical behaviors reflect this disability can result in misperceptions such as viewing the child as noncompliant, willfully stubborn, or unmotivated, rather than as confused, involved with repetitive routines, or focusing on less relevant aspects of the situation. Although more capable students are often referred to as mildly impaired in contrast to lower-functioning individuals with autism, it is important to realize that the term *high-functioning* does not imply easy adjustment. Basic impairments in communication and social interaction, as well as associated atypical behaviors and cognitive characteristics, can cause significant difficulties and distress for the person with autism, family members, and teachers.

Difficulties with language and communication can interfere with the student's ability to attend to, process, understand, or remember verbal information. Clinical experience and research evidence (Boucher & Lewis, 1989; Minshew, Goldstein, & Siegel, 1995) suggest that children with HFA have difficulty with receptive language and may fail to benefit fully from verbal instruction. Temple Grandin, a university professor of animal sciences and person with HFA, has written eloquently of her difficulties with language, describing words as "alien" ways of thinking, and saying that she thinks in pictures with no language-based memory (Grandin, 1995).

Even students with apparently well-developed language skills (AS and some HFA) may fail to adapt well in an unmodified classroom environment because of pragmatic social-communication difficulties (Chapter 10, this volume) as well as more general social impairments. For example, as a group, persons with HFA and AS demonstrate relative difficulty in forming and maintaining friendships (Rumsey, Rapoport, & Sceery, 1985), responding empathically to others' distress (Loveland & Tunali, 1991), recognizing emotional expressions (e.g., Bormann-Kischkel, Vilsmeier, & Baude, 1995; Hobson, 1991; Sinclair, 1992), and naturally attending to stimuli on which others are focused (i.e., joint attention, Bowler, 1992). Although most educators are socially skilled, and tend to use social reinforcement, social reasoning, and social cues to help motivate students and keep them on track, students with HFA and AS may miss such cues, misunderstand them, or simply not find them reinforcing or meaningful in the same way as other children.

The unusual repetitive behaviors seen in some persons with HFA or AS, such as finger flicking or pacing, can lead to peer rejection, whereas restricted interests, such as a consuming interest in insects, can interfere with both reciprocal social interaction as well as focus on traditional school subjects (Olley & Stevenson, 1987). In addition, children with HFA and AS, like all children with autism, tend to prefer fixed, often idiosyncratic routines. Changes that are typically welcomed by other children, such as having a substitute or falling snow, may cause distress for the child with HFA or AS and disrupt classroom functioning if not managed effectively.

Finally, students with HFA and AS may fail to pick up on classroom expectations or complete assignments because of associated cognitive difficulties. Although continued research is needed in this area, students with HFA or AS have been shown to have problems understanding abstract concepts (Minshew *et al.*, 1995; Simblett & Wilson, 1993), deficits in sequential processing (Allen, Lincoln, & Kaufman, 1991), difficulty holding items in working memory while considering additional information (Bennetto, Pennington, & Rogers, 1995), problems integrating information from two sensory modalities at once (Olley & Stevenson, 1987; Rosenblatt, Bloom, & Koegel, 1995), and, in general, difficulties organizing time and responses (Chapter 12, this volume). For example, fifth grader Alan, in the case example, might fail to learn from teacher lectures because of a failure to understand abstract terms, problems figuring out which important information is likely to show up on a test, or distraction caused by external (e.g., noise from overhead lights) or internal (e.g., repetitive thoughts about South American insects) stimuli.

In summary, understanding the characteristics of the student's disorder can increase tolerance and lead to more realistic expectations as well as more effective educational interventions (Carruthers & Freeman, 1989; Simblett & Wilson, 1993; Szatmari, 1991; Chapter 7, this volume). In his original description of the children he worked with, Hans Asperger wrote, "the management and guidance of such children essentially requires a proper knowledge of their peculiarities as well as genuine pedagogic talent.... Mere teaching efficiency is not enough" (1944/1991, p. 48). To develop this knowledge, many educators find it helpful to seek out not only the research and professional publications in the field, but also some of the excellent autobiographies and personal essays written by or with persons with HFA (see, e.g., Barron & Barron, 1994; Grandin, 1995; Grandin & Scariano, 1986; Sacks, 1995; Sinclair, 1992).

Strategy #2: Understanding the Unique Child through Assessment

Much of what I have been reading about autism fits with Paul, a child in my second grade classroom, but a lot of it is confusing. It sounds like kids with autism do not talk and are withdrawn, but often Paul just will not stop talking or leave people alone. I feel like I am letting Paul get away with so much — like wandering around the classroom when the other kids have to stay seated. Is he *really* autistic or does he just need some limits set? How do I know what is reasonable to expect?

Along with the characteristics shared by most students with autism, significant variability exists as well, making it inappropriate to apply blanket intervention recommendations without significant individualization. Even students with the *same* diagnosis differ greatly in terms of their cognitive, social, and behavioral characteristics. Students can be gentle or aggressive, rigidly bound by routines or relatively flexible, actively avoidant or in your face whenever possible — all characteristics that can affect the type and degree of structure required in their educational settings. Further, the nonretarded range of functioning is extremely broad, including children who score far above average on intellectual tests as well as those with borderline cognitive ability. This latter group, similar to slow learners among otherwise typically developing children, may require a slower pace, more repetition, and extensive practice to master even basic skills.

Given this diversity, thorough formal and informal assessments are required. Other chapters in this volume (Chapter 12 and 14) review assessment procedures that go beyond traditional psychological assessment batteries to obtain a more complete picture of each child's relative strengths and deficits. In some instances, however, formal tests may reflect what individuals with autism can figure out intellectually, but overestimate their ability to utilize this knowledge in daily interaction (Eisenmajer & Prior, 1991; Happé, 1994; Ozonoff & Miller, 1995; Siegel *et al.*, 1996). Therefore, efficient design of educational strategies requires supplemental informal assessments involving ongoing observations of each child's day-to-day performance in the current classroom as well as close communication and collaboration with parents.

Strategy #3: Structuring for Predictability and Understanding by Using Routines and Schedules

Okay, I understand a lot about autism and a lot about Amy. But what do I *do*? Amy always seems to be out of synch with the rest of the third graders. For example, all the kids will be at their desks ready for math, and Amy will be back in the book corner reading about flags. Sometimes she does not seem to hear me. Sometimes she *knows* what to do, but refuses to get started. And sometimes she tantrums because it is time to *stop* an activity! Amy continually pesters me about going to the library. Last Friday, we had to cancel library and Amy was agitated all day. I am spending more time patrolling Amy than teaching her. How can I help Amy get through the day?

As described earlier, students with HFA and AS may become lost, disorganized, and upset in the regular classroom environment because of communi-

cation difficulties, social confusion, or a greater need for routine and predictability than the other students. A lack of predictability can be very distressing
for students with autism, whether that absence comes from a genuine lack of
consistency in the daily classroom routine or from the child's failure to perceive
that consistency. Two of the most basic intervention strategies to help children
with HFA and AS better understand the workings of their classroom and thus
move through the day with less distress and greater independence involve
establishing consistency and predictability through the use of (1) daily routines
and (2) individualized, pictured or written daily schedules.

Routines

Students with HFA and AS tend to be less anxious, have fewer behavioral
difficulties, and learn better in classrooms where the order of events follows a
regular sequence. In addition, because students with HFA/AS have relative
strengths in rote learning, they can benefit from having practical, productive
routines in place throughout the day. Therefore, educators are encouraged to
develop systematic routines that channel the student's preference for familiarity
into productive behaviors (Dalrymple, 1995; Mesibov et al., 1994; Williams,
1995). For example, routines can be established around daily living skills (e.g.,
wash hands before lunch), work habits (e.g., always putting completed work in
a specific box on the teacher's desk), or social interaction (e.g., play with a peer
for the first 5 minutes during recess each day and then choose a different activity).

Schedules

Routines can enhance predictability for students with HFA and AS and
promote learning; however, classroom life inevitably involves change and requires some flexibility. A broader technique for helping students understand,
accept, and follow the sequence of daily events involves the use of individualized
written schedules. Just as most adults use calendars and appointment books to
stay on track, children with HFA and AS can benefit from having an individualized daily, weekly, or monthly schedule that helps them know what to expect.
Schedules have long been an integral aspect of structured teaching in the
TEACCH program (Mesibov et al., 1994; Van Bourgondien, 1993), and their use
is recommended by others in the field (Dalrymple, 1995; Dewey, 1991; Hodgdon, 1995; Chapters 10 and 12, this volume) as well as by professionals who
work with different populations with similar difficulties in self-organization and
time management (Denckla & Reader, 1993; Mateer & Williams, 1991).

Schedules should be individualized to an appropriate level based on each
child's developmental, cognitive, and behavioral needs. For example, a young

Ms. Waurin's Class Schedule		Amy's Class Schedule
7:44-8:15	Morning Work	____ Morning Work
8:15-9:15	Math	____ Math
9:15-10:00	Activity Time	____ Activity Time
10:00-10:15	Snack	____ Snack
10:15-11:15	Reading	____ Reading
11:15-12:00	Journals/Writing	____ Journals/Writing
12:00-12:45	Lunch & Recess	____ Lunch & Recess
12.45-1:16	Story Time (sometimes Amy	____ Story Time (sometimes Amy
	will go see Mr.Lee)	will go see Mr. Lee)
1:15-2:00	Centers	____ Centers
2:00-2:10	Get ready to go home.	____ Get ready to go home.
2:10	Go home	____ Go home

If I have a problem, I can raise my hand.
Ms. Waurin or Mr. Gold will help me.

Fig. 11-1. Development of a class schedule for a third grader with HFA. Initial attempt at developing schedule is at left. Revised version is at right.

child's daily school schedule might consist of a set of simple line drawings attached to a strip of poster board with Velcro. The pictures indicate the order of activities for the day, such as: picture of morning circle, picture for snack, picture for work time, and so forth.

The first attempt and a subsequent revision of a schedule for Amy, the third grader described in the opening vignette, are shown in Figure 11-1. The revised schedule illustrates ways in which the teacher attempted to make the schedule more meaningful and effective for Amy. First, the teacher's name was removed and replaced with Amy's to personalize the schedule. Second, time periods for activities were removed because Amy did not have independent time telling abilities and asked repetitive questions about the times on her schedule. Further, Amy *could* read times on the hour and became agitated when scheduled activities did not start precisely at these hour marks. Simply removing the time periods from her schedule eliminated both of these problems. Finally, Amy's teacher included lines for Amy to check off as each activity was completed. This helped to clarify the order of events for Amy and to motivate her to complete activities so that she could check them off.

The schedule in Figure 11-2 was developed for a secondary school student, John. John had difficulty transitioning between class lessons without multiple teacher prompts, a genuine concern as he was beginning a job training program that would demand more independent functioning. With the use of the schedule, written reminders (at bottom of schedule), and an individual timer, John learned to move from class to class without repeated adult prompting.

John's Daily Schedule

7:30	-	8:25	English
		8:25	Put away English work. Get out math work.
8:30	-	9:25	Math
		9:20	Put away Math work. Get ready to go to Art class.
		9:25	Go to Art class.
9:30	-	10:25	Art Class.
		10:25	Return to Mr. Hogan's class.
10:30	-	11:25	Computer
11:25	-	12:15	Lunch
12:15	-	1:25	Study Hour (see directions in notebook)
		1:25	Put away study hour work.
1:30	-	2:00	School Job:_____
			(Follow directions in job notebook)
		2:00	Write down unfinished work on Homework sheet.
			Check with Mr. Hogan for extra work.
		2:15	Finished for the day! Have a good afternoon!

Schedule Rules:
1.   If I finish my work before time is up, I can do unfinished
      work from other classes.
2.   When time is up for a class, I put away work.
3.   Cross off each activity when it is finished.

Fig. 11-2. Class schedule for a ninth grader in a self-contained classroom setting for children with learning disabilities and/or mild mental retardation.

Schedules should be as individualized and portable as possible, so that they can supplement the general classroom schedule typically posted for all to see. They can be handwritten, typed and copied, edited and printed daily from a word processor, or even written on a small write-on/wipe-off board that the child keeps at his or her desk. A younger child might use a half-day schedule, whereas an older student might benefit from both a daily schedule as well as weekly and monthly calendars. Whatever the format, the student manipulates the schedule in some way to show when activities are finished (turn over picture, check off, cross off). Further, when changes are anticipated, they should be marked as soon as possible on the student's schedule. Schedules help compensate for the child's difficulties in communication, social interaction, and organization, while taking advantage of the child's preference for predict-ability and routine. As such, the schedule routine helps the child adapt more flexibly and smoothly to the inevitable changes in the daily routine (i.e., It's okay as long as its on my schedule).

Strategy #4: Clarifying Instructions and Expectations: Compensating for Receptive Language Problems

> At 7 years of age, John is usually *where* he is supposed to be *when* he is supposed to be there. He actually seems proud of his schedule and likes to check things off. In fact, I tried to borrow it one day to show the P.E. teacher and John would not let me! *But* he still does not seem to pay attention in class. He fidgets with things as I explain material and seldom contributes to class discussions (except to make comments about airplanes). Finally, he never seems to hear assignments. How can I give instructions more effectively?

A significant proportion of typical education occurs through teacher talk and demonstration, especially directed at large groups of students. Educators give directions, introduce new ideas, and explain concepts through spoken language, and when students do not understand, the first impulse often is to talk more! As described earlier, substantial clinical and research evidence suggests that characteristics associated with HFA or AS can significantly interfere with a student's abilities to learn from traditional teaching methods. Therefore, structured teaching strategies compensate for the difficulties of children with HFA and AS, through a twofold approach: (1) enhancing child competencies and (2) modifying the learning environment.

First, to improve students' understanding of expectations and instructions, educational programs should include components targeting specific communication impairments, whether they involve major expressive language deficits or more subtle social and pragmatic problems. These require traditional and adapted language and communication instruction carried out by the regular classroom teacher. In addition, the expertise of a speech/language therapist well trained in pragmatic intervention is helpful.

Second, enhancement of student communication skills does not replace the need for environmental modifications. That is, a significant proportion of individuals with HFA continue to have difficulties with communication despite years of intervention (e.g., Minshew *et al.*, 1995; Szatmari, Bartolucci, Bremner, Bond, & Rich, 1989). Therefore, exclusively targeting communication skills and waiting to teach academic content until the child can learn in an age-appropriate manner from class lectures and discussions may mean that the child falls further behind in mastering math, science, and other subjects that might otherwise be within his or her grasp. To help students better understand content and instructions, teachers can modify traditional teaching techniques in several ways.

Preferential Seating and Reducing Distractions

Whenever possible, materials and furniture should be arranged in ways that maximize each student's ability to attend to relevant information while simultaneously resisting distractions. Seating the student close to the area in which most teaching occurs is encouraged (e.g., in the front of the classroom near the chalkboard). Not only does this make it easier for the teacher to monitor the student's ability to follow lessons, it also reduces distracting stimuli and makes the relevant classroom activity more apparent (Mesibov *et al.*, 1994; Williams, 1995). In addition, many children with HFA or AS benefit from having an independent work area, perhaps a special desk separated from the general sensory stimulation of the classroom by a partial divider or bookcase. Finally, in classrooms where student desks are frequently rearranged, it can be helpful to keep the desk of the student with HFA and AS in the same familiar, predictable position.

Adjusting the Level of Spoken Language

The advanced vocabularies, excellent reading decoding abilities, and perseverative talking observed in many students with HFA and AS can lead to an overestimation of their receptive language abilities. Research suggests that the ability of these students to understand *complex* language tends to be relatively impaired (e.g., Klin, Volkmar, Sparrow, Cicchetti, & Rourke, 1995; Minshew *et al.*, 1995). Therefore, teachers and others will want to simplify language input to a level the child understands, a strategy that Prizant and Rydell (1993) describe as the "cardinal rule for interacting with individuals with communication impairments" (p. 289). This may entail using shorter sentences, a slower pace, and a less sophisticated vocabulary, as well as accompanying or substituting spoken language with written or pictured information as described below.

Further, children with HFA and AS tend to interpret language literally or concretely. For example, a young child told to grab a chair might actually pick up the chair rather than sit down. When asked "on what grounds" a particular individual was arrested, a very intelligent individual with HFA answered, "Los Angeles." Although this literal understanding can provide moments of humor and insight into our language, teacher use of idioms, metaphors, irony, and sarcasm can contribute to misunderstandings and, at times, be frustrating and upsetting. Such figures of speech should be avoided, carefully explained, and/or explicitly taught as situations allow.

Written Information

Perhaps one of the most effective methods for helping students with HFA and AS is *to write down information.* For example, drawing a student's attention to the written phrase "turn to page 37" is apt to (1) be more efficient than repeating the verbal direction several times and (2) encourage more independent functioning than having a peer find the correct page. Written information has several significant advantages. It reduces reliance on the understanding of oral language while taking advantage of the student's relatively strong reading skills (Minshew, Goldstein, Taylor, & Siegel, 1994; Whitehouse & Harris, 1984). In addition, written information demands less social know-how than verbal interchange and provides the student with a lasting, visual reminder that does not leave the student when the teacher does. For class discussions, written information can be provided in the form of handouts, worksheets, or lists of questions. For independent work, written lists of directions can remind the student how to proceed. Further, whenever possible, students should have an opportunity to learn the same concepts covered in discussion or lectures through reading (e.g., book chapters or directions). Finally, on a related note, visual aids such as maps, pictures, and objects can be more effective for teaching students with HFA/AS than gestures or brief demonstrations.

Strategy #5: Structuring Work Assignments and Tasks

> Karen is doing much better. If I direct her to a specific question on a worksheet during class discussions, she will answer it. Interestingly, the other kids seem surprised at how much she knows! *But* Karen still has a hard time staying on task and finishing assignments. It seems as if she could do better if only she would apply herself. How can I set up assignments to help Karen be more successful?

Despite the most carefully created and predictable classroom environment, regular use of individualized schedules, and modification of traditional teaching techniques to clarify expectations, children with HFA and AS may continue to struggle with assignments (e.g., focusing on the little things while missing the big picture, working too slowly or with no sense of time, and getting confused about how to best prioritize activities so as to complete a task). Difficulties with planning, choosing, integrating, and organizing, generally termed *executive functioning skills*, can interfere with the HFA/AS student's ability to carry out and complete assignments, even when the actual content of the assignment is understood (Chapter 12, this volume). Several compensatory strategies can be used to help students work more systematically and independently to completion.

Organizational Work Systems

It is helpful to have a clear, consistent method for indicating to the students what work needs to be done, how much work there is, when they will be finished, and what will happen after the work is finished. Highly structured work systems using baskets to organize tasks are recommended for younger, less verbal, or

```
                                    Date:_____
 Geometry
 _____  1.  Turn in homework.
 _____  2.  Group lesson, p. 47
 _____  3.  Do problems p. 48, #1 - 21
 _____  4.  Fill out homework sheet & have
            Ms. Garcia sign it.
 _____  5.  9:25 Leave for English
```

Fig. 11-3. A simple work system for a high school student that clarifies expectations regarding: what work to do, how much work is to be done, and what student does when finished.

lower-functioning children with autism (described in Mesibov *et al.*, 1994; Schopler *et al.*, 1995). For higher-functioning or older children, written directions regarding assignments to be completed and external supports for organizing those assignments (e.g., color-coded folders) are most effective.

Effective systems for communicating work expectations to students do not have to be complicated. For example, Figure 11-3 illustrates how the high school teacher in the opening vignette combined the daily geometry class schedule with work directions for Karen, a student with HFA. These directions, written by hand on an index card, explain work expectations. Because Karen knows in advance how much work is expected and when it will be finished, the likelihood of frustration is reduced and the opportunities for independent task completion are enhanced. More sophisticated planners and organizational notebooks can further clarify work expectations by including information that helps the student move more independently through the school day (e.g., school maps, bus schedules, homework/assignment logs, rules for specific classes, pockets for completed work).

Written Task Directions

As explained earlier, written information can help clarify both general instructions and lesson content. Similarly, written directions for *specific tasks* can lead to more successful student performance than oral directions alone (Boucher & Lewis, 1989). *Written* step-by-step directions provide visual, lasting reminders of required steps and the order needed for successful task completion. Written directions enable students to independently complete a variety of tasks and assignments such as: booting up a computer, solving a quadratic equation, cleaning up the class play area, or getting ready for the school day (see Figure 11-4). Their use also has been recommended for individuals with nonverbal learning disabilities (Rourke, 1989, 1995) as well as other populations exhibiting organizational and planning difficulties (Denckla & Reader, 1993; Mateer &

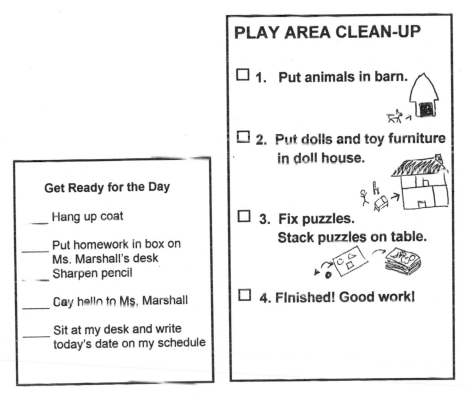

Fig. 11-4. Step-by-step written directions.

Williams, 1991). Similarly, written directions are an example of the parts-to-whole teaching strategy recommended by Klin and Volkmar (1995) for students with AS (i.e., larger tasks are broken down into component parts and presented in the correct sequence).

In preparing written task directions, care should be taken to write directions clearly, spacing them generously so that each step is visually clear to the child. Teaching the child to check off or cross off each step as it is completed helps the child follow steps in the correct sequence. Once the use of written directions becomes routine, they can help motivate and focus students by taking advantage of their desires to do things "just so" and to work to completion when the end point is made clear.

Additional Organizational Supports

In addition to the organizational notebooks and written directions described above, additional explicit supports may be needed for some students. For example, assignments can be clarified for the easily distracted child by reducing the number of items on a page, using larger print, or highlighting areas where the student is to put answers. Similarly, informal assessment may reveal instances in which a child is overlooking important details, such as operands when doing calculations or reading directions on worksheets. Adults can highlight these important pieces of information for the student or, in some instances, teach the student to highlight key information before beginning the task. In addition, visual models — such as a sample page showing where name, date, and margins are to be placed on a page — can make expectations regarding organization clear to the child. Finally, because slow work pace, distractibility, and poor self-management skills can lead to several hours being spent on single assignments, motivation can sometimes be kept higher and the child on task longer, if the number of problems per assignment is reduced.

Other external supports can be used to help students organize belongings and transport materials to and from school. Use of containers and clear labeling can help individuals with organizational problems to function more independently (Dalrymple, 1995; Denckla & Reader, 1993; Mateer & Williams, 1991; Rourke, 1989). Students with HFA and AS can be taught to organize school supplies in backpacks and notebooks, often with the assistance of clear labeling specifying where supplies should go. Similarly, labeling on cupboards, drawers, and cubbies in the classroom can assist the student to independently obtain and return materials. Checklist routines for assignments can be built into the child's day, both at home and at school, to ensure that the student has the needed supplies. Children with more compelling organizational needs may benefit from having two sets of books and school supplies, one kept at home and one at school. Finally, good communication between teacher and parent is critical to maintain organization (Denckla & Reader, 1993; Moreno, 1991). The use of assignment and homework logs or checklists that are filled out daily and used by students, teachers, and parents can be extremely effective not only in increasing student productivity but also in decreasing blaming.

Structuring Assignments in Line with Conceptual Abilities

In some instances, an assignment may be clearly structured, but the abstract or complex nature of the concepts being taught may interfere with the child's ability to complete the task. Studies by Minshew and colleagues (Minshew *et al.*, 1994; Minshew, Goldstein, Muenz, & Payton, 1992; Siegel *et al.*, 1996) suggest that individuals with HFA have relatively intact performance on tasks tapping procedural or mechanical skills such as word identification, naming, and rote or associative memory. In contrast, comprehending and interpretive skills such as abstract thinking, verbal reasoning, and complex memory are relatively impaired. Studies of academic achievement in students with HFA and AS show a similar pattern of relatively strong mechanical (i.e., spelling, reading decoding) and relatively impaired comprehension (i.e., reading comprehension, learning novel material) abilities (Klin *et al.*, 1995; Minshew *et al.*, 1992, 1994, 1995; Venter, Lord, & Schopler, 1992). Math performance has not been clearly identified as either a strength or weakness for students with HFA or AS (e.g., Klin *et al.*, 1995; Minshew *et al.*, 1994).

In classroom life, this means that a child with average to above-average skills in certain areas may struggle with what seem to be straightforward, age-appropriate assignments. For example, given the assignment to write an original sentence for each of his science vocabulary words, one fifth grader wrote the following: "(1) Anatomy is a word on p. 37 in the book. (2) Lung is a word on p. 39 in the book. (3) Vein is a word in the diagram on p. 40...." Rather than being a sign of lazy or impertinent behavior, this work may reflect a tendency to interpret material concretely as well as difficulty with generation of original material on demand. Open-ended questions and assignments, such as this one, tend to be especially challenging because of their demands on flexibility and reasoning, and expectations must be set in light of an individualized assessment of the student's abilities.

When children have difficulty with more complex material, educators can specifically teach comprehension and application skills (Siegel *et al.*, 1996). In addition, teachers can assist students by structuring assignments to make them more concrete. For example, suppose that a fifth grader with HFA has been asked to read a science chapter, abstract relevant information, and write a report. The student may need assistance determining which specific material is important, perhaps by having sentences containing key concepts highlighted or a set of organizing questions. The child may be unable to judge how much is enough when writing his report, becoming agitated or refusing to continue. Therefore, it might be necessary to provide explicit directions regarding the amount of work expected, such as "write 10 sentences" or "write two pages." Explicit directions regarding expected content may be necessary, such as "in your report, answer these four questions." If the student needs even greater structure, sentence stems (e.g., "Volcanoes are found _____ _____") or other organizers can be used (Stratton, 1996; Twachtman, 1995).

In our experience, many children with HFA and AS may do quite well in the primary grades, where the emphasis is on learning and practicing basic mechanical skills such as spelling, reading decoding, and math facts. Increasing difficulty may occur, however, in the upper elementary, middle, and high school years when greater emphasis is placed on application and abstraction of skills and knowledge. Throughout the school years, ongoing informal and periodic formal assessment across content and skill areas is critical to setting appropriate educational objectives and goals.

Providing Help and Creating Help-Asking Routines

Despite careful structuring and attention to the child's readiness to learn specific content, students with HFA and AS will encounter difficulties with assignments. Because of the social impairments associated with these disorders, however, students may not ask for help in a productive manner. Some children become overly dependent, asking for help repeatedly and rarely, if ever, acting independently. Other students work well past the point of frustration and never ask for help. Effective teaching involves observing the student's progress and, when necessary, offering help in a matter-of-fact and concrete manner. It is also important to help the student develop help-asking routines and skills. Rather than simply telling the child to ask for help, this may need to be explicitly taught through role plays or social rules and stories (discussed later). Further, written reminders are often necessary and can be written on the child's daily schedule (see Figure 11-1), written on an index card taped to the child's desk, or even written on a bookmark.

Strategy #6: Motivating Students by Utilizing Special Interests

> You know, Fred is a pretty neat kid. He works so hard to do what comes naturally to the rest of the kids. *But* now that I see what Fred *can* do, it is more clear that he sometimes just is not *motivated* by the lessons I teach. In fact, Fred doesn't seem interested in anything. Well, except for names of trees and flowers and airplanes. I am a pretty creative and fun teacher, but I am at a loss. What am I doing wrong? How can I motivate and interest Fred?

Atypical and restricted patterns of interests and activities were noted in the original writings on autism (Kanner, 1943) and AS (Asperger, 1944/1991). Younger or lower-functioning children may spend long periods of time lining up or spinning objects, whereas older and/or higher-functioning children may exhibit strong interests in topics as typical as dinosaurs, snakes, and volcanoes, or as unusual as gravestones, airline logos, and presidents' terms in office. Kathy Lissner (1992), a young woman with HFA who did not talk until age 4, describes how she daydreamed about numbers as a child, and had focused interests ranging from Indians and rocks to earthquakes and South America. "Everyone else could be talking about...the St. Louis Cardinals," Lissner writes, "and I would say, 'Lima, Peru.' That is all I could think or write about. I was consumed" (p. 304). Temple Grandin (1992), writing about her fixations on sliding glass doors and cattle chutes, has suggested that teachers "need to use fixations to motivate instead of trying to stamp them out" (p. 115). Similarly, several professionals have emphasized the importance of utilizing special interests in developing academic and career skills (Asperger, 1944/1991; Siegel *et al.*, 1996; Szatmari, 1991; Williams, 1995, Chapter 7, this volume).

For example, Fred's special interests in trees and flowers could be used and broadened to help him develop knowledge and skills in several areas, including: history (making a time line coordinating key events in world history with the discovery of various trees), reading and language arts (writing and illustrating a report on a certain group of flowers), science (classification of flora and fauna), math "(Given X roses per square yard in a garden, how many roses in 10 square yards?"), daily living (writing letters to companies asking for information or brochures related to flowers), and peer interaction (making models of favorite forests with a peer). In addition, interests can be used to reinforce less preferred activities as well as to make the school environment more appealing. For example, on finishing math (or some relatively difficult subject), Fred might be allowed to read a book on trees. Further, activities involving his interests could be placed on his daily schedule to remind Fred that he will be able to engage in some preferred activities during the school day.

STRUCTURED APPROACHES TO BEHAVIORS, EMOTIONS, AND OTHER ISSUES OF CONCERN

Implementation of the structured teaching strategies described above enhances student understanding of the classroom environment, ability to complete assignments, and mastery of academic subject matter. Further, when classroom environments are structured, predictable, and as meaningful as possible, students with HFA or AS will experience less frustration and have fewer behavioral outbursts. On the other hand, these techniques do not cure autism, and the social, communication, and behavioral difficulties, although less apparent, still remain. Structured approaches can also be used to address the nonacademic yet critical aspects of behavior that affect students' classroom performance. In this section, the philosophy and techniques of structured teaching — such as the importance of understanding behavior in the context of autism, clarifying expectations, and simultaneously enhancing student skills while modifying the environment — are applied to the following specific areas of concern: (1) social behavior; (2) obsessive talk, repetitive behavior, and sensory responsiveness; (3) emotional swings; and (4) preparation for adulthood.

Addressing Social Behavior, Relationships, and Rules

Mike is doing great academically! We have organized his morning seat work in color-coded folders and I have found it helps to shorten the number of assigned math items. He finishes on time and seems less distressed. *But* Mike still does not have many friends. Sometimes he just does not seem interested and when he does, his odd behaviors put the other kids off. Cari helps him out, but several of the other kids pick on him. How can I help Mike do better socially?

As noted earlier, naive and peculiar social behaviors, in conjunction with a lack of intuitive social understanding, have been well documented in individuals with HFA and AS (Asperger, 1944/1991; Kanner, 1943; Volkmar & Cohen, 1994). As Carol Gray (Chapter 9, this volume) emphasizes, however, "social impairment takes two people." Jim Sinclair (1992), a man with HFA, captures the complexity of social misunderstandings when he explains that problems arise because "people who understand the things I don't understand can't understand how anyone can possibly not understand them" (p. 298). Therefore, in deciding on educational approaches targeting social behaviors, a dual focus is again recommended: It is important not only to enhance the student's social skills, but also to modify the social environment provided for the student.

Teacher–Student Relationships

Educators are typically skilled at establishing rapport with students, reading emotional cues, and motivating others through social and emotional means. However, even highly skilled teachers may doubt their abilities when faced with the atypical social responses of the student with HFA or AS. Remaining empathic with the child and demonstrating respect is critical. Parents, persons with HFA, and professionals in the field have repeatedly emphasized that caring, trustworthy teachers play a key role in each student's educational and occupational success (Grandin, 1990; Moreno, 1991; Ryan, 1992; Williams, 1995).

A neutral, matter-of-fact, yet caring manner has long been recognized as an effective interactional style for adults working with children with autism (e.g., Rutter & Bartak, 1973). Similarly, in describing effective educational approaches for the children he worked with, Hans Asperger emphasized that effective teaching involved giving instruction "in a cool and objective manner without being intrusive" *and* that "genuine care and kindness" as well as "true understanding" were needed as the children "often show a surprising sensitivity to the personality of the teacher" (1944/1991, p. 48). A caring, yet matter-of-fact manner may be especially helpful when working with those individuals with HFA and AS who demonstrate heightened sensitivity to corrections or criticism (Dewey, 1991).

Increasing Student Social Skills

Against the background of a trustworthy educator–student relationship, interventions can specifically target the social skills of the child with HFA and AS. In designing interventions, the reader is referred to the relatively large literature on social (and social-communication) impairments in autism and their treatment, much of which is relevant for persons with HFA and AS (see, e.g., Frea, 1995; Lord, 1993; Mundy & Sigman, 1987; Olley & Stevenson, 1987; Prizant & Wetherby, 1993; Quill, 1995). Recent research suggests that cognitive–behavioral interventions, such as self-management techniques, can be used to teach students with HFA and AS how to increase appropriate social skills and decrease inappropriate social behaviors. For example, Koegel and colleagues found that training children with HFA to use a wrist counter to keep track of appropriate responses in a conversational context resulted in more appropriate behaviors as well as less disruptive behaviors (Koegel, Koegel, Hurley, & Frea, 1992). More detailed descriptions of cognitive–behavioral and self-management techniques for children with autism can be found in Koegel and Koegel (1995) and Quinn, Swaggart, and Myles (1994).

Frequently, teachers and parents ask whether children with HFA or AS benefit from group social skills training. Clinical work indicates that social groups can promote social engagement and enjoyment (Mesibov, 1992; Williams, 1989). On the other hand, prepackaged social skills training programs may be ineffective if they strongly emphasize social and cognitive abilities, such as complex verbal reasoning, that may be impaired in children with HFA or AS. There are few well-designed, controlled studies on the effectiveness of social skills training for children with HFA/AS, and existing data suggest that learning of specific skills may not generalize to improved social competence in daily living (McGee, Krantz, & McClannahan, 1984; Ozonoff & Miller, 1995). If social skills training is to be used, a structured approach is recommended, with group leaders using systematic, explicit instruction (Marriage, Gordon, & Brand, 1995; Ozonoff & Miller, 1995) and taking students' unique and sometimes unusual difficulties into account.

Peer Relationships and Peer-Mediated Intervention

Hans Asperger (1944/1991) wrote that "autistic children are often tormented and rejected by their classmates simply because they are different and stand out from the crowd" (p. 79). Similarly, more recent case studies (Carruthers & Foreman, 1989), parent accounts (Moreno, 1991), and personal accounts (Carpenter, 1992) describe the pain that can accompany peer teasing and rejection, especially for individuals who become aware of their differences and feel inadequate as a result of not "fitting in."

Perhaps the most important step in designing educational interventions addressing social needs is to ensure that the classroom environment is accepting and safe for the student with HFA or AS. Even the best-designed activities for enhancing students' social skills or promoting social interaction will fail if the child is being tripped repeatedly, laughed at when adults are absent, or teased cruelly on the playground. In our experience, the teacher can set a tone for acceptance by modeling this behavior, educating peers about HFA/AS, and enlisting their support. Many teachers have found it helpful to have the student's parent come and speak to the class at a time when the student with HFA or AS is not present. This allows peers to gain an understanding of the student's behaviors, ask questions, and have fears of the unfamiliar decreased.

Research and clinical experiences suggest that simply physically integrating children with autism with nonautistic, typically developing peers is insufficient to promote positive peer interaction (Myles, Simpson, Ormsbee, & Erickson, 1993), and that structuring of activities and provision of instruction or training for peers are necessary (Frea, 1995; Mesibov & Shea, 1996). Interventions that have trained typical peers to initiate, respond to, and maintain interactions with autistic peers have led to increases in social interaction (e.g., Goldstein, Kaczmarek, Pennington, & Shafer, 1992; Odom & Strain, 1986).

While peer-mediated interventions for high-functioning students may not have to be as structured as those for lower-functioning children with autism, classroom teachers can use a number of informal strategies to structure social interactions. For example, peers can be assigned as lunch, free time, and after school companions, with a goal of companionship rather than instruction. Peers can also serve as class time or bus/travel partners, guiding, assisting, and encouraging the student as necessary. Educationally, peers can serve as project partners or tutors. Importantly, Kamps *et al.* (1994) found that a classwide peer-tutoring program for reading fluency led to increases in reading fluency and reading comprehension for *both* the students with HFA and their typically developing peers.

Unstructured or semistructured activities during the school day such as recess, free time, or P.E. can be especially difficult for the child with HFA or AS because of the social demands they impose. Teachers can sometimes help their students be more successful by assigning special roles (e.g., scorekeeper, distributing equipment with a peer) or setting up more structured activities (e.g., playing for a specified amount of time with a familiar activity with only one or two peers). Children with HFA or AS may benefit from semistructured social activities such as scout troops, computer or chess clubs, and, in some cases, sports groups — as long as there is an atmosphere of support and acceptance in the group and adults are ready to provide necessary backup and education for peers.

Social Rules

Children with HFA and AS often find the social world unpredictable and may have difficulty applying their intellectual understanding of appropriate social behavior in "real-life" daily interactions. Not surprisingly, then, our

Dan's Rules

1. Sit at my desk during work times.
2. Raise my hand to talk. Wait until Mrs. Berry calls my name.
3. First I finish my work, then I can work on my projects.
4. No touching other people
5. I can get things from the red basket, rather than from Mrs. Compton's desk.

*If I follow my rules in the morning, I can earn a sticker at 11:30
*If I follow my rules in the afternoon, I can earn a sticker at 2:15.

Fig. 11-5. Sample social rules for a second grader.

experience has been that these students often find clearly stated guidelines regarding others' expectations helpful and reassuring. In an interesting parallel, Asperger explained that one "pedagogic trick is to announce any educational measures not as personal requests, but as objective impersonal law" (1944/1991, p. 48).

Social rules are clearly written statements about appropriate and inappropriate behaviors used to clarify social expectations for the student with HFA or AS (see Figure 11-5). Writing rules down for the child makes them more concrete and provides a lasting visual reminder. Rules can be written on a piece of paper and kept in a special folder, written on an index card and kept in a pocket, or even represented by key words or symbols taped to the child's desk (Twachtman, 1995). When the student engages in inappropriate behavior, the teacher can redirect him or her by pointing to the appropriate rule, thus avoiding repetitive arguments, depersonalizing possible conflicts, and reducing the chance that redirection will be interpreted by the student as criticism.

When developing and implementing social rules, the teachers and students we have worked with have found the following guidelines helpful:

- Individualize rules to the child's unique needs, difficulties, and understanding rather than relying on posted class rules to make expectations clear.
- Consider the child's general level of development as well as awareness of and control over behaviors.
- Write the rule in a neutral yet authoritative manner.
- Write the rules down and provide the child with his or her own copy.
- Review the rules frequently and in a nonpunitive manner with the child, as often as several times a day when they are first implemented.
- Consider writing the positive consequences for following the rules at the bottom of the list to help motivate the student (see Figure 11-5).

In using social rules, professionals should not assume that students will apply rules correctly from one setting to another unless generalization is specifically addressed. Consider making the student's rules portable (e.g., carried in a folder or pocket). Alternatively, separate sets of rules may be necessary for different situations. Educators are encouraged to use social rules judiciously, carefully considering what behaviors are truly important or necessary to change. Like any technique, social rules can be misused and their effectiveness will rely, to a significant degree, on the teacher's ability to be sensitive and creative, rather than critical and punitive, in finding a fit between the child and the classroom environment.

Although social rules help clarify expectations for appropriate behavior, their use alone does not teach the child why certain behaviors are appropriate and others inappropriate. Therefore, this technique is complimented nicely by the Social Story and Comic Strip Conversation techniques (see Gray, 1995, and this volume) that enable teachers and parents to teach social reasoning through visual rather than verbal means.

Understanding Social Preferences

Educators and mental health professionals tend to value highly social relationships, a preference that may not be shared by all students with HFA and AS. Teachers are encouraged to remember that some alone time is not only okay, but may actually provide some students with much needed respite during the school day. In our experience, shared by others (e.g., Moreno, 1991; Pratt, 1995), students with HFA and AS benefit from having a quiet place where they can go either to cool down in times of stress or simply to get away for a while during the school day. This could be a corner in the classroom, a bench in the hallway, or a table in the library. One teacher of a second grader with AS set up a desk in the back of the room, using a cardboard divider to minimize stimulation and provide a sense of privacy. This was labeled as the child's "office," and the second grader used it eagerly at approved and needed times during the school day.

Setting Realistic Expectations and Priorities

Although the various approaches described above can and should be an important part of the educational curriculum for students with HFA and AS, a note of caution regarding their use is important. These interventions, which yield important and positive changes in behavior, do not "cure" children with HFA and AS. Even after intervention efforts, students may fail to generalize skills appropriately (e.g., Goldstein & Cisar, 1992; Marriage et al., 1995;

Ozonoff & Miller, 1995) and/or continue to exhibit peculiar or disruptive social behaviors (e.g., Roeyers, 1996). Therefore, most students with HFA and AS continue to require significant support from teachers over time. Setting realistic expectations is essential and failure to do so can cause increased frustration to the degree that the ultimate goal of helping the child enjoy social interactions may be sacrificed. For example, Simblett and Wilson (1993), in a case study of three adults with AS, suggested that long periods of behavior modification targeting the individual's social deficits may actually have exacerbated social problems by prompting unrealistically high expectations, creating excessive demands, and, in turn, leading to high amounts of conflict. Similarly, Wolff (Chapter 7, this volume) in writing about her work with schizoid disorder of childhood stresses the need to accept the individual over insistence on social conformity.

In summary, then, it is important for educators to remember that the students' unusual social behavior is part of the disorder. Although intervention efforts are important, not every behavior needs to be addressed by every individual who comes in contact with the student. The teacher who insists on natural eye contact before teaching long division, for example, may find that the student with HFA/AS makes little academic progress over the year. A combination of accepting odd but unobtrusive behaviors while trying to change those that are offensive to others usually works best.

Managing Obsessive Talk, Repetitive Behaviors, and Sensory Responsiveness

> Alright, what about Jeanette's "unusual" behaviors? I am embarrassed to say it, but they sort of bother me. There is her pencil flipping. She will do that for long periods of time, and sometimes at recess, she will stand and flap her hands. Also, Jeanette is so alert to noises and so picky about her food. And, well, there is her interest in door frames. I try to ignore the time she spends observing and talking about door frames, but sometimes her comments are *way* off topic and, well, sometimes, I just get fed up with the 100th question of the day about which door I like best. What should I do, if anything, about these behaviors?

Repetitive behaviors, restricted interests, and sensory over- and underresponsiveness are characteristics over which the child may have little awareness and even less control, although awareness and control may increase with age and level of functioning (Cesaroni & Garber, 1991; Sinclair, 1992). At times, these behaviors may signal agitation, excitement, or a lack of understanding. At other times, the behavior may actually represent the child's best attempt to respond as expected. Therefore, designing intervention and management methods for these concerns needs to begin with a careful assessment.

Responding to Obsessive or Repetitive Talk

When confronted with obsessive talk in the classroom, it is helpful to begin with an assessment of: (1) who the talk is really bothering (child? teacher? peers? nobody?), (2) the degree to which the talk is interfering with the student's ability to learn, (3) whether the interest can be utilized in a more constructive manner, (4) whether the student has sufficient opportunities to discuss this interest, and (5) whether the child needs to learn more effective social or communication routines. If the obsessive talk intrudes and interferes with more important activities, it can be effective to use clear limits to contain the behavior. For example, talking about a special topic might be confined to specific times and places that are written on the student's daily schedule. Some students can learn to control the behavior with the help of a written rule or social story that both explains how others perceive repetitive talk and teaches more appropriate turn-taking conversational skills (see Chapter 9, this volume). Another option is to provide a clear ending point by giving the child a certain number of question or comment cards that are handed to others each time the topic is brought up. When the cards are used up, the topic is finished for the day.

Managing Repetitive Behaviors and Stereotypies

Teachers often ask whether or not they should try to limit or eliminate repetitive motor behaviors such as hand flapping, ear bending, rocking, or pacing. These behaviors often increase during stressful or unstructured times and can be seen as barometers indicating the child's stress levels and confusion. Therefore, the teacher might want to begin the assessment process for these behaviors by reexamining the child's environment: Is the child understanding what is going on? Next, the teacher should assess to what degree the behavior intrudes on others and interferes with learning. Some children with HFA and AS can engage in repetitive behaviors without offending others and while following what is going on around them; others cannot.

Depending on the results of the informal assessment and discussions with the student's parents, the following techniques can help manage stereotypic behavior. First, the student can be redirected to a more meaningful, structured activity. Second, a more appropriate or socially acceptable behavior might be substituted. For example, one young woman who repeatedly flipped a pencil with a long string attached (thus earning many questioning looks) was given a small pom-pom in the colors of a favorite sports team (thus earning many supporting smiles from fellow fans). Finally, for the older or more socially aware child, social stories and social rules can be used to explain others' perceptions of these behaviors and to identify appropriate times and places in which the student can engage in the behavior (e.g., during a free period in class or during downtime after school at home).

Sensory Responsiveness

Although not part of the diagnostic criteria for either autism or AS, significant percentages of these children demonstrate intense (hypersensitive) or very limited (hyposensitivity) responsiveness to sensory stimuli. For students with HFA or AS, certain sounds (e.g., tone of a peer's voice, fire drill buzzer), tastes (specific foods), and tactile sensations (being touched, being hugged, wearing certain clothes) may be experienced as aversive and underlie behavioral outbursts. Similarly, sensory responsiveness may also cause problems in the classroom because of a student's fascination with certain stimuli (e.g., electronic sounds, staring at lights or fan blades) or difficulties adjusting to changes in stimulation.

Open discussion with the student, parents, and others who know the student can help identify sensitivities and suggest intervention strategies. Although personal accounts suggest that some children may be helped through sensory integration/occupational therapy, classroom management usually takes the form of organizing the environment to minimize these difficulties. For example, headphones can be used to reduce noise, students are not forced to eat disliked foods, and adults do not touch students in ways they find aversive. Structuring around sensory issues might involve such strategies as incorporating touch into a daily routine (e.g., high five after taking a turn in P.E.), permitting a high school student to leave class a few minutes early to avoid the crush in the halls, or seating a student near the front of the classroom to decrease visual stimulation. Clever and original methods often work as with the teacher who, after unsuccessfully trying for weeks to stop a child with HFA from flipping and staring at book pages during lessons, simply copied the page for the day's lesson and gave this to the child rather than the book. The student was content and focus on the lesson increased.

Managing Emotional Swings and Crises

Bret, in my ninth grade homeroom, has not had a real "tantrum" for several weeks now. But I wonder how I will handle the situation if he gets really upset again. Frankly, it makes me a bit nervous. What if he starts hitting himself in the head again? How can I best manage Bret's emotional swings and tantrums?

The best behavior management is proactive management. All of the strategies discussed so far — using routines and schedules to build predictability into the child's day, utilizing written directions, clarifying social rules, and so forth — are proactive in that the primary goal is to help the child find the classroom environment more meaningful, thereby reducing frustration and outbursts, which are most frequently related to confusion and change. On the other hand, unexpectedly strong emotional swings or inappropriate emotional responses (e.g., uncontrollable laughter with no apparent trigger) do occur in individuals with autism. Research indicates that a percentage of persons with HFA and AS exhibit a variety of mood and behavioral symptoms such as hyperactivity, obsessiveness, high levels of anxiety, compulsive behaviors, and tics (Szatmari *et al.*, 1989; Tsai, 1996). When psychiatric symptoms are intense and chronic, pharmacological treatment can provide some relief (McDougle, Price, & Volkmar, 1994; Szatmari, 1991). Further, although traditional, insight-oriented psychodynamic psychotherapy is not recommended, adolescents and adults may benefit from the structure and guidance provided by supportive counseling directed toward solving real-life problems (Mesibov, 1992).

On a more routine basis in the classroom, emotional swings or outbursts can be used as signals for the teacher to reevaluate the environment to make sure that the child is understanding information, that events are predictable, and that sensory problems are taken into account. If the evaluation indicates problems in any of these areas, the child may be experiencing high levels of tension and frustration. Therefore, restructuring along the lines of the recommendations made throughout this chapter may be needed. On the other hand, even with the best-laid plans crises do occur and some guidelines are useful. First, teachers should maintain a calm, matter-of-fact tone. Second, even students with relatively good language skills and high social interest may find it difficult to mobilize their verbal understanding and social reasoning abilities during times of conflict and distress. Therefore, using short verbal phrases, simplifying interactions, and keeping contact brief and to the point can be helpful. Third, many students respond more appropriately during a crisis when directions are given in writing (e.g., being handed a slip of paper with directions to "Go to the quiet area"). Appropriate social behavior can be taught most effectively during calm periods and in neutral settings, not in the midst of a behavioral conflict. It can be helpful to teach students coping strategies such as putting their distress in writing, using relaxation techniques, or taking a walk. In addition, explicit plans for handling stressful situations can be formulated, written out, and kept by both the student and teacher for future use. (For additional recommendations regarding coping plans see Hodgdon, 1995, and Groden & LeVasseur, 1995.)

Educating for Adulthood

> Compared to how I felt at the beginning of the school year, I am surprised at how much I have come to really care about Barry. He has certainly helped develop my talents as a teacher! Besides, he is just such a *neat* kid. I worry

some about what will happen to Barry in the future? What will he be like as an adult? Do I need to be doing anything special now to help him in the future?

Long-term outcome studies suggest a wide range of ability and functioning levels in adulthood (Burt, Fuller, & Lewis, 1991; Rumsey *et al.*, 1985; Szatmari *et al.*, 1989; Venter *et al.*, 1992). Some individuals have excellent outcomes. The overwhelming majority will continue to show some level of social and behavioral impairments, however, and these difficulties are likely to affect the person's ability to be integrated fully into the community, hold jobs, and live independently.

Starting in the earliest grades, teachers can work toward successful long-term functioning by explicitly teaching basic skills and work habits (e.g., waiting for one's turn, holding a conversation, asking for help when needed, following a work schedule) as well as daily living skills (e.g., eating neatly, ordering from a menu, grocery shopping) and leisure skills (e.g., going to a movie, playing games). By teaching students how to make use of explicit external supports such as daily schedules and written directions within the structured school environment, teachers are providing students with valuable skills that can be made portable and be moved with them into less structured and less supportive work environments (Van Bourgondien, 1993). Because a significant proportion of students with HFA and AS end up underemployed given their basic cognitive abilities, it is important to begin vocational planning and training early. For younger students, this may entail functional academics as well as real-life work practice through school jobs (e.g., delivering messages, sorting mail, collating papers, cleaning in the cafeteria, shelving books in the library, entering student grades on a computer). Szatmari (1991) has warned that formal job training often occurs "too late in the child's education history for maximal benefit" (p. 90). Similarly, in our experience, it is important to begin exploring job training options and services sooner rather than later, certainly by the time the student enters high school.

Teachers play a key role in mentoring and motivating students with HFA and AS. However, it is also helpful to remember that most teachers or professionals typically are involved in the child's life for a relatively brief span — from a few months to a year or two. In contrast, the student's parents will remain their child's primary advocate far into the individual's adulthood. Therefore, collaboration between teacher and parent carries a special significance. The more the parents understand about their child's strengths and difficulties, the more effectively they can assist future professionals in designing not only educational programs, but also appropriate job training, employment opportunities, and living arrangements.

SUMMARY AND CONCLUSION

One of the primary goals of this chapter has been to present educational strategies for students with HFA and AS from within the framework of structured teaching as used in the TEACCH program (Mesibov *et al.*, 1994). This approach emphasizes that the design of effective educational interventions depends on an understanding of autism as well as of each student's unique pattern of strengths, weaknesses, and interests. Although the importance of targeting specific child skills to enhance competencies is acknowledged, structured teaching for students with HFA and AS underscores the importance of modifying the classroom environment to make it predictable (through the use of routines and schedules) and implementing teaching techniques that genuinely clarify instructions, expectations, and assignments for students with HFA and AS.

This review did not attempt to distinguish between HFA and AS with regard to recommended educational approaches, in part because of the lack of consensus regarding the separate clinical status of these diagnoses, and mostly because of the lack of empirical evidence demonstrating differential responses to intervention strategies.

In light of the developing research literature on cognitive, neuropsychological, and academic profiles in HFA and AS, as well as the developing clinical consensus regarding effective educational interventions, there is a clear need for controlled research on the general effectiveness of educational strategies for persons with HFA or AS. More specifically, evidence of differential effectiveness of techniques for students meeting criteria for AS as opposed to those for HFA not only would assist educators and parents in designing more effective educational programs, but also could provide evidence regarding the diagnostic status of these disorders.

ACKNOWLEDGMENTS

Many of the ideas and techniques included in this chapter grew out of three decades of collaboration by professionals, families, teachers, and students with HFA or AS affiliated with the TEACCH program. Further, although we discuss intervention suggestions from the perspective of structured teaching as used in the TEACCH program, many of the specific recommendations have been made by others in the field.

REFERENCES

Allen, M. H., Lincoln, A. J., & Kaufman, A. S. (1991). Sequential and simultaneous processing abilities of high-functioning autistic and language-impaired children. *Journal of Autism and Developmental Disorders, 21*, 483–502.

Asperger, H. (1944/1991). Autistic psychopathy in childhood. In U. Frith (Ed. and Trans.), *Autism and Asperger syndrome* (pp. 37–92). Cambridge: Cambridge University Press. (Original work published 1944)

Barron, J., & Barron, S. (1994). *There's a boy in here*. New York: Avon Books.

Bennetto, L., Pennington, B. F., & Rogers, S. J. (1995). Intact and impaired memory functions in autism. *Child Development, 67*, 1816–1835.

Bormann-Kischkel, C., Vilsmeier, M., & Baude, B. (1995). The development of emotional concepts in autism. *Journal of Child Psychology and Psychiatry, 36*, 1243–1259.

Boucher, J., & Lewis, V. (1989). Memory impairments and communication in relatively able autistic children. *Journal of Child Psychology and Psychiatry, 30*, 99–122.

Bowler, D. M. (1992). "Theory of mind" in Asperger's syndrome. *Journal of Child Psychology and Psychiatry, 4*, 877–893.

Burt, D. B., Fuller, P. S., & Lewis, D. L., (1991). Brief report: Competitive employment of adults with autism. *Journal of Autism and Developmental Disorders, 21*, 237–242.

Carpenter, A. (1992). Autistic adulthood: A challenging journey. In E. Schopler & G. B. Mesibov (Eds.), *High-functioning individuals with autism* (pp. 289–306) New York: Plenum Press.

Carruthers, A., & Foreman, J. (1989). Asperger syndrome: An educational case study of a preschool boy. *Australian and New Zealand Journal of Developmental Disabilities, 15*, 57–65.

Cesaroni, L., & Garber, M. (1991). Exploring the experience of autism through first hand accounts. *Journal of Autism and Developmental Disorders, 21*, 303–313.

Coyne, P. (1996) Organization and time management strategies. In A. Fullerton, J. Stratton, P. Coyne, & C. Gray (Eds.), *Higher functioning adolescents and young adults with autism* (pp. 53–70). Austin, TX: Pro-Ed.

Dalrymple, N. J. (1995). Environmental supports to develop flexibility and independence. In K. A. Quill (Ed.), *Teaching children with autism* (pp. 243–264). New York: Delmar.

Denckla, M. B., & Reader, M. J. (1993). Education and psychosocial interventions: Executive dysfunction and its consequences. In R. Kurlan (Ed.) *Handbook of Tourettes syndrome and related tic and behavioral disorders* (pp. 431–451). New York: Dekker.

Dewey, M. (1991). Living with Asperger's syndrome. In U. Frith (Ed.), *Autism and Asperger syndrome* (pp. 184–206) Cambridge: Cambridge University Press.

Donnelly, J., & Levy, S. (1995). Strategies for assisting individuals with high-functioning autism and/or Asperger syndrome. In *Proceedings of the 1995 National Conference on Autism* (pp. 85–95). Silver Springs, MD: Autism Society of America.

Ehlers, S., & Gillberg, C. (1993). The epidemiology of Asperger syndrome: A total population study. *Journal of Child Psychology and Psychiatry, 34*, 1327–1350.

Eisenmajer, R., & Prior, M. (1991). Cognitive linguistic correlates of theory of mind ability in autistic children. *British Journal of Developmental Psychology, 9*, 351–364

Frea, W. D. (1995). Social-communicative skills in higher-functioning children with autism. In R. L. Koegel & L. K. Koegel (Eds.), *Teaching children with autism: Strategies for initiating positive interactions and improving learning opportunities* (pp. 53–66). Baltimore: Brookes.

Frith, U. (Ed.). (1991). *Autism and Asperger syndrome.* Cambridge: Cambridge University Press.

Fullerton, A., Stratton, J., Coyne, P., & Gray, C. (Eds.). (1996). *Higher functioning adolescents and young adults with autism.* Austin, TX: Pro-Ed.

Ghaziuddin, M., Butler, E., Tsai, L., & Ghaziuddin, N. (1994). Is clumsiness a marker for Asperger syndrome? *Journal of Intellectual Disability Research, 38*, 519–527.

Goldstein, H., & Cisar, C. L. (1992). Promoting interaction during sociodramatic play: Teaching scripts to typical preschoolers and classmates with disabilities. *Journal of Applied Behavior Analysis, 25*, 265–280.

Goldstein, H., Kaczmarek, L., Pennington, R., & Shafer, K. (1992). Peer-mediated intervention: Attending to, commenting on, and acknowledging the behavior of preschoolers with autism. *Journal of Applied Behavior Analysis, 25*, 289–305.

Grandin, T. (1990). Needs of high-functioning teenagers and adults with autism: Tips from a recovered autistic. *Focus on Autistic Behavior, 5*, 1–16.

Grandin, T. (1992). An inside view of autism. In E. Schopler & G. B. Mesibov (Eds.), *High-functioning individuals with autism* (pp. 105–126). New York: Plenum Press.

Grandin, T. (1995). *Thinking in pictures and other reports from my life with autism.* New York: Doubleday.

Grandin, T., & Scariano, M. (1986). *Emergence: Labeled autistic*. Novato, CA: Arena.

Gray, C. A. (1995). Teaching children with autism to "read" social situations. In K. A. Quill (Ed.), *Teaching children with autism* (pp. 219–241). New York: Delmar.

Groden, J., & LeVasseur, P. (1995). Cognitive picture rehearsal: A system to teach self-control. In K. A. Quill (Ed.), *Teaching children with autism* (pp. 287–305). New York: Delmar.

Happé, F. G. E. (1994). An advanced test of theory of mind: Understanding of story characters' thoughts and feelings by able autistic, mentally handicapped, and normal children and adults. *Journal of Autism and Developmental Disorders, 24*, 129–154.

Harris, S. L., & Handleman, J. S. (Eds.). (1994). *Preschool education programs for children with autism*. Austin, TX: Pro-Ed.

Hobson, R. P. (1991). Methodological issues for experiments on autistic individuals' perception and understanding of emotion. *Journal of Child Psychology and Psychiatry, 32*, 1135–1158.

Hodgdon, L. Q. (1995). Solving social-behavioral problems through the use of visually supported communication. In K. A. Quill (Ed.), *Teaching children with autism* (pp. 265–286). New York: Delmar.

Jordan, R., & Powell, S. (1995). *Understanding and teaching children with autism*. New York: Wiley.

Kamps, D. M., Barbetta, P. M., Leonard, B. R., & Delquadri, J. (1994). Classwide peer tutoring: An integration strategy to improve reading skills and promote peer interactions among students with autism and general education peers. *Journal of Applied Behavior Analysis, 27*, 49–61.

Kanner, L. (1943). Autistic disturbances of affective contact. *Nervous Child, 2*, 217–250.

Klin, A., & Volkmar, F. R. (1995). *Asperger syndrome: Some guidelines for assessment, diagnosis, and intervention*. Pittsburgh: Learning Disabilities Association of America.

Klin, A., Volkmar, F. R., Sparrow, S. S., Cicchetti, D. V., & Rourke, B. P. (1995). Validity and neuropsychological characterization of Asperger syndrome: Convergence with nonverbal learning disabilities syndrome. *Journal of Child Psychology and Psychiatry, 38*, 1127–1140.

Koegel, L. K., Koegel, R. L., Hurley, C., & Frea, W. D. (1992). Improving social skills and disruptive behavior in children with autism through self-management. *Journal of Applied Behavior Analysis, 25*, 341–352.

Koegel, R. L., & Frea, W. D. (1993). Treatment of social behavior in autism through the modification of pivotal social skills. *Journal of Applied Behavior Analysis, 26*, 369–377.

Koegel, R. L., & Koegel, L. K. (1995). *Teaching children with autism: Strategies for initiating positive interactions and improving learning opportunities*. Baltimore: Brookes.

Levy, S. (c. 1988). *Identifying high functioning children with autism*. Bloomington: Indiana Resource Center for Autism, Indiana University.

Lissner, K. (1992). Insiders point of view. In E. Schopler & G. B. Mesibov (Eds.), *High-functioning individuals with autism* (pp. 303–306). New York: Plenum Press.

Lord, C. (1993). Early social development in autism. In E. Schopler, M. E. Van Bourgondien, & M. M. Bristol (Eds.), *Preschool issues in autism* (pp. 61–94). New York: Plenum Press.

Lovaas, O. I. (1981). *Teaching developmentally disabled children: The me book*. Austin, TX: Pro-Ed.

Loveland, K. A., & Tunali, B. (1991). Social scripts for conversational interactions in autism and Down syndrome. *Journal of Autism and Developmental Disorders, 21*, 177–186.

Marriage, K. J., Gordon, V., & Brand, L. (1995). A social skills group for boys with Aspergers syndrome. *Australian and New Zealand Journal of Psychiatry, 29*, 58–62.

Mateer, C. A., & Williams, D. (1991). Effects of frontal lobe injury in childhood. *Developmental Neuropsychology, 7*, 359–376.

McDougle, C. J., Price, L. H., & Volkmar, F. R. (1994). Recent advances in the pharmacotherapy of autism and related conditions. *Child and Adolescent Psychiatric Clinics of North America, 3*, 71–89.

McGee, G. G., Krantz, P. J., & McClannahan, L. E. (1984). Conversational skills for autistic adolescents: Teaching assertiveness in naturalistic game settings. *Journal of Autism and Developmental Disorders, 14*, 319–330.

Mesibov, G. B. (1992). Treatment issues with high-functioning adolescents and adults with autism. In E. Schopler & G. B. Mesibov (Eds.) *High-functioning individuals with autism* (pp. 143–155). New York: Plenum Press.

Mesibov, G. B., Schopler, E., & Hearsey, K. A. (1994). Structured teaching. In E. Schopler & G. B. Mesibov (Eds.), *Behavioral issues in autism* (pp. 195–207) New York: Plenum Press.

Mesibov, G. B., & Shea, V. (1996). Full inclusion and students with autism. *Journal of Autism and Developmental Disorders, 26,* 337–346.

Minshew, N. J., Goldstein, G., Muenz, L. R., & Payton, J. B. (1992). Neuropsychological functioning in nonmentally retarded autistic individuals. *Journal of Clinical and Experimental Neuropsychology, 14,* 749–761.

Minshew, N. J., Goldstein, G., Taylor, H. G., & Siegel, D. J. (1994). Academic achievement in high functioning autistic individuals. *Journal of Clinical and Experimental Neuropsychology, 16,* 261–270.

Minshew, N. J., Goldstein, G., & Siegel, D. J. (1995). Speech and language in high-functioning autistic individuals. *Neuropsychology, 9,* 255–261.

Moreno, S. J. (1991) *High-functioning individuals with autism.* Crown Point, IN: MAPP Services.

Mundy, P., & Sigman, M. (1987). Specifying the nature of the social impairment in autism. In G. Dawson (Ed.), *Autism: Nature, diagnosis, and treatment* (pp. 3–21). New York: Guilford Press.

Myles, B. S., & Simpson, R. L. (1994–1995). Reflections on "an analysis of characteristics of students diagnosed with higher-functioning autistic disorder." *Exceptionality, 5,* 49–53.

Myles, B. S., Simpson, R. L., Ormsbee, C. K., & Erickson, C. (1993). Integrating preschool children with autism with their normally developing peers: Research findings and best practices recommendations. *Focus on Autism Behavior, 8,* 1–18.

Odom, S. L., & Strain, P. S. (1986). A comparison of peer-initiation and teacher-antecedent interventions for promoting reciprocal social interaction of autistic preschoolers. *Journal of Applied Behavior Analysis, 19,* 59–71.

Oke, N. J., & Schreibman, L. (1990). Training social initiations to a high-functioning autistic child: Assessment of collateral behavior change and generalization in a case study. *Journal of Autism and Developmental Disorders, 20,* 479–497.

Olley, J. G., Robbins, F. R., & Morelli-Robbins, M. (1993). Current practices in early intervention for children with autism. In E. Schopler, M. E. Van Bourgondien, & M. M. Bristol (Eds.), *Preschool issues in autism* (pp. 223–245). New York: Plenum Press.

Olley, J. G., & Stevenson, S. E. (1987). Preschool curriculum for children with autism: Addressing early social skills. In G. Dawson (Ed.), *Autism: Nature, diagnosis, and treatment* (pp. 346–366). New York: Guilford Press.

Ozonoff, S., & Miller, J. N. (1995). Teaching theory of mind: A new approach to social skills training for individuals with autism. *Journal of Autism and Developmental Disorders, 25,* 415–433.

Pratt, C. (1995, September). *Involving high-functioning students with autism in the general education community.* Paper presented at MAAPing the Future Conference sponsored by MAAP Services and the Indiana Resource Center for Autism, Indianapolis.

Prizant, B. M., & Rydell, P. J. (1993). Assessment and intervention considerations for unconventional verbal behavior. In J. Reichle & D. P. Wacker (Eds.), *Communicative alternatives to challenging behavior: Integrating functional assessment and intervention strategies* (pp. 263–297). Baltimore: Brookes.

Prizant, B. M., & Wetherby, A. M. (1993). Communication in preschool autistic children. In E. Schopler, M. E. Van Bourgondien, & M. M. Bristol (Eds.), *Preschool issues in autism* (pp. 95–128). New York: Plenum Press.

Quill, K. A. (Ed.). (1995). *Teaching children with autism.* New York: Delmar.

Quinn, C., Swaggart, B. L., & Myles, B. S. (1994). Implementing cognitive behavior management programs for persons with autism: Guidelines for practitioners. *Focus on Autistic Behavior, 9,* 1–13.

Roeyers, H. (1996).The influence of nonhandicapped peers on the social interactions of children with a pervasive developmental disorder. *Journal of Autism and Developmental Disorders, 26,* 303–320.

Rogers, S. J. (1996). Brief report: Early intervention in autism. *Journal of Autism and Developmental Disorders, 26,* 243–246.

Rosenblatt, J., Bloom, P., & Koegel, R. L. (1995). Overselective responding: Description, implications, and intervention. In R. L. Koegel & L. K. Koegel (Eds.), *Teaching children with autism: Strategies for initiating positive interactions and improving learning opportunities* (pp. 33–42). Baltimore: Brookes.

Rourke, B. P. (1989). *Nonverbal learning disabilities: The syndrome and the model.* New York: Guilford Press.

Rourke, B. P. (1995). *Syndrome of nonverbal learning disabilities: Neurodevelopmental manifestations.* New York: Guilford Press.

Rumsey, J., Rapoport, J., & Sceery, W. (1985). Autistic children as adults: Psychiatric, social, and behavioral outcomes. *Journal of the American Academy of Child Psychiatry, 24,* 465–473.

Rutter, M., & Bartak, L. (1973). Special educational treatment of autistic children: A comparative study — II. Follow-up findings and implications for services. *Journal of Child Psychology and Psychiatry, 14,* 241–270.

Rutter, M., Greenfeld, D., & Lockyer, L. (1967). A five to fifteen year follow-up study of infantile psychosis. *British Journal of Psychiatry, 113,* 1183–1199.

Ryan, R. M. (1992). Treatment-resistant chronic mental illness: Is it Asperger's syndrome? *Hospital and Community Psychiatry, 43,* 807–811.

Sacks, O. (1995). *An anthropologist on Mars.* New York: Knopf.

Schopler, E., Brehm, S., Kinsbourne, M., & Reichler, R. J. (1971). The effect of treatment structure on development in autistic children. *Archives of General Psychiatry, 24,* 415–421.

Schopler, E., & Mesibov, G. B.(Eds.). (1992). *High-functioning individuals with autism.* New York: Plenum Press.

Schopler, E., Mesibov, G. B., DeVellis, R. F., & Short, A. (1981). Treatment outcome for autistic children and their families. In P. Mittler (Ed.), *Frontiers of knowledge in mental retardation: Social, educational, and behavioral aspects* (pp. 293–301). Baltimore: University Park Press.

Schopler, E., Mesibov, G. B., & Hearsey, K. (1995). Structured teaching in the TEACCH system. In E. Schopler & G. B. Mesibov (Eds.), *Learning and cognition in autism* (pp. 243–268). New York: Plenum Press.

Schopler, E., Reichler, R. J., & Lansing, M. (1980). *Individualized assessment and treatment for autistic and developmentally disabled children.* Austin, TX: Pro-Ed.

Siegel, D. J., Goldstein, G., & Minshew, N. J. (1996). Designing instruction for the high-functioning autistic individual. *Journal of Developmental and Physical Disabilities, 8,* 1–19.

Simblett, G. J., & Wilson, D. N. (1993). Asperger's syndrome: Three cases and a discussion. *Journal of Intellectual Disability Research, 37,* 85–94.

Sinclair, J. (1992). Bridging the gaps: An inside-out view of autism (or, do you know what I don't know?). In E. Schopler & G. B. Mesibov (Eds.), *High-functioning individuals with autism* (pp. 294–302). New York: Plenum Press.

Stratton, J. (1996). Adapting instructional materials and strategies. In A. Fullerton, J. Stratton, P. Coyne, & C. Gray (Eds.), *Higher functioning adolescents and young adults with autism* (pp. 53–70). Austin, TX: Pro-Ed.

Szatmari, P. (1991). Asperger's syndrome: Diagnosis, treatment, and outcome. *Psychiatric Clinics of North America, 14,* 81–92.

Szatmari, P., Bartolucci, G., Bremner, R., Bond, S., & Rich, S. (1989). A follow-up study of high-functioning autistic children. *Journal of Autism and Developmental Disorders, 19,* 213–225.

Tsai, L. (1996). Brief report: Comorbid psychiatric disorders of autistic disorder. *Journal of Autism and Developmental Disorders, 26,* 159–163.

Twachtman, D. D. (1995). Methods to enhance communication in verbal children. In K. A. Quill (Ed.), *Teaching children with autism* (pp. 133–162). New York: Delmar.

Van Bourgondien, M. E. (1993). Behavior management in the preschool years. In E. Schopler, M. E. Van Bourgondien, & M. M. Bristol (Eds.), *Preschool issues in autism* (pp. 223–245). New York: Plenum Press.

Venter, A., Lord, C., & Schopler, E. (1992). A follow-up study of high-functioning autistic children. *Journal of Child Psychology and Psychiatry, 33,* 489–507.

Volkmar, F. R., & Cohen, D. J. (1994). Autism: Current concepts. *Child and Adolescent Psychiatric Clinics of North America, 3,* 43–52.

Whitehouse, D., & Harris, J. C. (1984). Hyperlexia in infantile autism. *Journal of Autism and Developmental Disorders, 14,* 281–289.

Williams, K. (1995). Understanding the student with Asperger syndrome: Guidelines for teachers. *Focus on Autistic Behavior, 10,* 9–16.

Williams, T. I. (1989). A social skills group for autistic children. *Journal of Autism and Developmental Disorders, 19,* 143–155.

12

Assessment and Remediation of Executive Dysfunction in Autism and Asperger Syndrome

SALLY OZONOFF

Impaired executive functions have been documented in individuals with autism and Asperger syndrome (AS) across all ages and functioning levels, using a wide variety of different tasks (McEvoy, Rogers, & Pennington, 1993; Ozonoff, Pennington, & Rogers, 1991; Prior & Hoffmann, 1990; Rumsey, 1985; Rumsey & Hamburger, 1988). Although impairments in abilities such as planning, organization, flexibility, and self-regulation are critical to everyday functioning and school success, little attention has been paid to their remediation. There is a large and growing body of literature devoted to treatment of the communication and social disabilities associated with autism and AS (e.g., Lord, 1988; Marriage, Gordon, & Brand, 1995; Mesibov, 1984; Ozonoff & Miller, 1995; Chapters 9 and 10, this volume), but virtually nothing has been written about managing the executive deficits these individuals demonstrate. This chapter begins by providing a definition of executive function and current hypotheses about the neural substrate of these cognitive processes. This is followed by a review of the research literature on executive dysfunction in autism and AS. The second half of the chapter discusses strategies for assessment and remediation of such problems.

SALLY OZONOFF • Department of Psychology, University of Utah, Salt Lake City, Utah 84112.

Asperger Syndrome or High-Functioning Autism?, edited by Schopler et al. Plenum Press, New York, 1998.

EXECUTIVE FUNCTIONS AND THE FRONTAL LOBES

The term *executive function* encompasses a wide range of abilities, including planning, organization, goal-selection, flexibility, self-regulation, inhibition, and set maintenance (Lezak, 1995; Stuss & Benson, 1986). They are so-called "executive" functions because they are similar to the responsibilities of a business or company executive: they involve setting goals, monitoring progress toward goals, and recognizing when goals have been achieved (Denckla & Reader, 1993). What all executive processes appear to have in common is that they are goal-directed and future-oriented (Welsh & Pennington, 1988).

These cognitive processes are thought to be mediated by the frontal lobes of the brain (Duncan, 1986; Stuss & Benson, 1986). Damage to this region results in a classic pattern of behavioral and cognitive abnormalities, including executive function deficits. For example, individuals who have sustained frontal damage often exhibit repetitive, aimless movements and speech, lack of insight, social isolation, shallow or flat affect, and lack of appreciation for social rules (Damasio & Van Hoesen, 1983; Stuss & Benson, 1986). Impairment in communication and social discourse is evident as either a failure to initiate conversation or a tendency to engage in lengthy, tangential monologues (Duncan, 1986). In the cognitive domain, frontal patients demonstrate classic executive dysfunction: They have difficulty inhibiting familiar or prepotent responses, tend to perseverate on ideas or topics, have a diminished capacity for planning, tend to focus on one aspect of information, neglecting other relevant dimensions, and have difficulty integrating details and managing multiple sources of information (Duncan, 1986; Luria, 1966; Mateer & Williams, 1991; Stuss & Benson, 1986).

Both the social and cognitive impairments that follow frontal damage are reminiscent of the symptoms of autism. Clearly, a hallmark deficit of autism is in the domain of social relating: Individuals with autism, like those with frontal lobe damage, have difficulty taking the mental perspective of others (Baron-Cohen, 1989; Baron-Cohen, Leslie, & Frith, 1985), understanding social rules and conventions, and interpreting interpersonal interactions. The behavior of people with autism often appears rigid and inflexible; children with autism can become distressed over minor changes in their environment or routines. They may repetitively engage in one stereotyped behavior for long periods of time or focus on one narrow, idiosyncratic interest to the exclusion of other age-appropriate activities. In the cognitive domain, many individuals with autism have excellent rote memory capacities, storing seemingly endless bits of information on topics of interest, but have difficulty applying this knowledge in a meaningful or commonsense manner (Hermelin & O'Connor, 1970). They often get stuck on one way of solving a problem and have difficulty shifting cognitive set from one strategy to another. The term *stimulus overse-*

lectivity has been used to describe the tendency of autistic individuals to respond to only a subset of environmental cues, often irrelevant ones, during learning situations (Lovaas, Koegel, & Schreibman, 1979). Finally, autistic individuals often seem narrowly focused on details and have difficulty "seeing the forest for the trees" (Frith, 1989).

The cognitive and behavioral similarities between individuals with autism and patients with frontal lobe disease led Damasio and Maurer (1978) to hypothesize that autism might be the result of damage to frontal cortex and related structures. Neurological evidence for this hypothesis is mixed, however. Whereas many studies have found abnormalities in the limbic system (Bauman & Kemper, 1985, 1988) and cerebellum (Bauman & Kemper, 1988; Courchesne, Yeung-Courchesne, Press, Hesselink, & Jernigan, 1988; Ritvo *et al.*, 1986), no structural abnormalities in the frontal region have been documented. Studies of cortical function, however, are somewhat more suggestive of frontal involvement. An early investigation found depressed cerebral blood flow in right frontal cortex during resting in mentally retarded adults with autism (Sherman, Nass, & Shapiro, 1984). Similarly, a more recent single photon emission computed tomographic (SPECT) study of four young adults with autism found reduced blood flow to the right, left, and midfrontal lobes (George, Costa, Kouris, Ring, & Ell, 1992). Reduced frontal metabolism has also been reported in children and adolescents with high-functioning autism and AS (Gillberg, 1994) and preschool children with autism (Zilbovicius *et al.*, 1995). Finally, autistic children were found to differ from chronological and mental age controls in frontal EEG power (Dawson, Klinger, Panagiotides, Lewy, & Castelloe, 1995).

Thus, although the behavior and cognition of autistic and frontal lobe patients are similar in many ways, it is not yet clear whether they share the same underlying neurological insult. Furthermore, although executive functions are sometimes considered synonymous with "frontal lobe functions," it has become increasingly clear that many areas of the brain contribute to the successful execution of processes like planning, organization, and flexibility (Anderson, Bigler, & Blatter, in press; Denckla & Reader, 1993; Deutsch, 1992; Mountain & Snow, 1993). Because the frontal lobes are richly connected with many other parts of the brain, it is difficult to determine the precise contribution of any one region to performance on a complex cognitive task. This caveat is especially critical to remember when communicating assessment results to parents. When their child is diagnosed with executive function deficits, the inference that he or she has sustained brain damage may alarm parents. It is important to reassure them that poor performance on executive function tests may have a variety of determinants, that the neural underpinnings of such deficits are as yet poorly understood, and that their child's test results do not necessarily indicate that he or she has sustained frontal damage.

EMPIRICAL INVESTIGATIONS OF EXECUTIVE FUNCTION

Research on Autism

In the last decade, the behavioral correspondence between autism and frontal lobe damage has stimulated a large amount of research on the executive function abilities of individuals with autism and AS. Table 12-1 summarizes all studies of executive function conducted with these groups to date. Over 80% of these investigations have documented deficient performance in individuals with autism spectrum disorders on executive function tests.

As can be seen in Table 12-1, by far the most frequently used executive function measure with autistic samples has been the Wisconsin Card Sorting Test (WCST), a task generally considered to tap cognitive shifting ability. This task

Table 12-1. Studies of Executive Function in Autism and
Asperger Syndrome

Study	Task(s) used	Autism < control differences?
Waterhouse & Fein (1982)	MFFT	Yes
Bryson (1983)	Stroop	No
Rumsey (1985)	WCST	Yes
Schneider & Asarnow (1987)	WCST	No
Rumsey & Hamburger (1988)	WCST	Yes
	Trail Making Test	Yes
Prior & Hoffmann (1990)	WCST	Yes
	Milner mazes	Yes
Rumsey & Hamburger (1990)	WCST	Yes
Szatmari et al. (1990)	WCST	Yes
Eskes et al. (1990)	Stroop	No
Ozonoff et al. (1991a)	WCST	Yes
	Tower of Hanoi	Yes
Minshew et al. (1992)	WCST	No
	Trail Making Test	No
	Object Sorting Test	Yes
Hughes & Russell (1993)	Windows	Yes
McEvoy et al. (1993)	Spatial reversal	Yes
Hughes et al. (1994)	Tower of London	Yes
Ozonoff et al. (1994)	Go–NoGo	Yes
Ozonoff & McEvoy (1994)	WCST	Yes
	Tower of Hanoi	Yes
Berthier (1995)	WCST	Yes
	Tower of Hanoi	Yes
Bennetto et al. (1996)	WCST	Yes
	Tower of Hanoi	Yes

Note: MFFT = Matching Familiar Figures Test, WCST = Wisconsin Card Sorting Test.

is administered by placing four cards, varying along the dimensions of color, shape, and number, in front of the subject. A deck of cards varying along these same dimensions is presented and the subject is asked to match them with one of the four "key" cards. The examiner provides feedback about the accuracy of responses, but the sorting strategy is not revealed to the subject. Once 10 consecutive cards have been correctly placed, the underlying sorting principle changes, without notice or comment from the examiner, and responses according to the previous category now receive negative feedback. The primary variable of interest is the number of perseverative responses, defined as the number of trials in which the subject continues sorting by a previously correct category despite negative feedback (Heaton, 1981).

Rumsey (1985) used this measure to study verbal, high-functioning adult men with residual-state autism, finding that the number of perseverations was significantly higher in the autistic individuals than in a normal control sample matched on age. In subsequent investigations, Rumsey and Hamburger (1988, 1990) found that autistic individuals sorted significantly fewer WCST categories than controls with severe dyslexia. Thus, the impairment of those with autism was not just a general consequence of having a developmental disorder, but appeared specific to autism.

Prior and Hoffmann (1990) administered a modified version of the WCST to children with autism and matched controls. All ambiguous cards were removed from the deck and subjects were explicitly told when to shift set. Despite such simplifications, the autistic group made significantly more errors and perseverative responses than controls. The children with autism also performed significantly less well than controls on the Milner Maze Test, demonstrating deficits in planning and difficulty learning from mistakes. The autistic group "perseverated with maladaptive strategies, made the same mistakes repeatedly, and seemed unable to conceive of a strategy to overcome their difficulties" (p. 588).

The WCST was administered to individuals with high-functioning autism by Szatmari and colleagues (Szatmari, Tuff, Finlayson, & Bartolucci, 1990). This study was particularly interesting because 80% of the control group met criteria for attention deficit/hyperactivity disorder (ADHD) or conduct disorder, two childhood conditions also hypothesized to involve executive dysfunction (Chelune, Ferguson, Koon, & Dickey, 1986; Lueger & Gill, 1990). Despite this conservative choice of control group, autistic subjects still made significantly more perseverative errors on the WCST than the comparison sample.

Similarly, Ozonoff, Pennington, and Rogers (1991a) reported elevated rates of perseveration on the WCST in high-functioning children with autism. In addition, they administered the Tower of Hanoi, another executive function measure widely used with autistic samples. This disk-transfer task requires subjects to plan and carry out a sequence of moves that transforms a random arrangement of disks into a pyramidal goal configuration (Borys, Spitz, &

Dorans, 1982). In this study, performance on the Tower of Hanoi was best able to discriminate between autistic children and learning-disabled controls, classifying 80% of subjects correctly. These results were somewhat surprising, as one-quarter of the learning-disabled control sample met criteria for ADHD. This study replicates the findings of Szatmari *et al.* (1990) that nonretarded children with autism are impaired on measures of executive function, even relative to children with other executive function disorders. Ozonoff and McEvoy (1994) demonstrated that deficits on both the Tower of Hanoi and WCST were stable over a 2½-year follow-up period, with a tendency for executive function abilities to decline relative to controls over time.

Only two investigations have failed to find deficits on the WCST in autistic individuals (Minshew, Goldstein, Muenz, & Payton, 1992; Schneider & Asarnow, 1987), although experimental design factors may account for these findings. Whereas Minshew *et al.* (1992) found no group differences on the WCST, they did, however, document deficits on a different executive function measure, the Goldstein–Scheerer Object Sorting Test (described below), in which autistic subjects were less able to shift set than controls.

The only investigation to examine executive functions in preschool-age autistic children was conducted by McEvoy *et al.* (1993). They used several developmentally simple measures of prefrontal function first developed for use with nonhuman primates and human infants (Diamond & Goldman-Rakic, 1986). In the spatial reversal task, an object is hidden in one of two identical wells outside of the subject's vision. The side of hiding remains the same until the subject successfully locates the object on four consecutive trials, after which the side of hiding is changed to the other well. Thus, successful search behavior requires flexibility and set shifting. Significant group differences were found, with the autistic sample making more perseverative errors than children in either the mental- or chronological-age-matched groups.

An early investigation used the Matching Familiar Figures Test (MFFT) to study executive functions in autistic children (Waterhouse & Fein, 1982). The MFFT is a match-to-standard task developed to examine impulsivity (Kagan, 1965). Subjects are shown a picture and four comparison figures, from among which they must choose the one that is identical. The comparison stimuli differ from each other and the standard in minor detail only. Both accuracy and time to respond are recorded. A pattern of short decision time, coupled with high error rate, is taken to indicate impulsivity. This study found a significantly higher error rate and more impulsive patterns of responding in children with autism, relative to controls (Waterhouse & Fein, 1982).

Finally, two studies administered the Stroop Color-Word Test (Stroop, 1935) to children with autism. This task measures the ability to selectively respond to one dimension of a multidimensional stimulus. In the critical color-word interference condition of this task, subjects are given color words printed in mismatching ink (e.g., RED printed in green ink) and instructed to name the color of the ink. This requires selective attention to a relatively less salient dimension of the stimulus, while inhibiting a more automatic response (Dempster, 1991; MacLeod, 1991). The interference created, evident as lower accuracy and longer response time, is known as the "Stroop effect." Both studies, however, failed to find deficits on the Stroop test in autistic children (Bryson, 1983; Eskes, Bryson, & McCormick, 1990). Although the tasks reviewed above rely primarily on the executive functions of flexibility and planning, the Stroop is thought to measure inhibition. One interpretation of these results is that inhibition is a relatively spared component of executive function in individuals with autism, in contrast to the deficits apparent on most tests of flexibility and planning.

This hypothesis stimulated a recent research trend, in which computerized experimental paradigms have been used to examine specific aspects of executive function (i.e., to isolate flexibility from planning, inhibition from flexibility, and so on). Hughes, Russell, and Robbins (1994) used a computerized task that examined the ability to shift set while controlling for a number of other executive processes (e.g., inhibition, rule reversal, transfer of learning). Significant differences between autistic and control samples were found, with autistic individuals engaging in highly perseverative and inflexible strategies. Several researchers using computerized attentional tasks have found that individuals with autism have great difficulty moving their attention from one spatial location to another relative to controls (Casey, Gordon, Mannheim, & Rumsey, 1993; Courchesne, Akshoomoff, & Ciesielski, 1990; Wainwright-Sharp & Bryson, 1993). Ozonoff, Strayer, McMahon, and Filloux (1994) found severe deficits in the ability to shift set on a computerized Go–NoGo task. The performance of children with autism was deficient relative not only to age- and IQ-matched nondisabled controls, but also to individuals diagnosed with Tourette's syndrome, another neurodevelopmental disorder that may involve executive dysfunction (Pennington & Ozonoff, 1996). In contrast, performance on two tests of inhibition was no different in individuals with autism and controls (Ozonoff & Strayer, 1997).

Research on Asperger Syndrome

Given the interest in executive function as a potential core neuropsychological deficit of autism spectrum conditions, there have been surprisingly few studies of the executive function skills of individuals with AS. The Szatmari et al. (1990) study reported above was the first of only three investigations to examine the executive functions of AS individuals. In this study, AS was diagnosed using a modified version of Wing's (1981) criteria, including isolated behavior, impaired social interaction, and either odd speech, impaired nonverbal communication, or bizarre preoccupations. All AS subjects had onset of disorder prior to age 6 years, but none had ever been diagnosed as autistic. These researchers found that the AS group performed more poorly than the control group on the WCST (an average of one standard deviation worse), but the group difference was not statistically significant.

Ozonoff, Rogers, and Pennington (1991b) also examined executive function abilities in subjects with AS. These researchers diagnosed AS using modified draft ICD-10 criteria (World Health Organization, 1989). Specifically, all AS subjects demonstrated impaired social interactions and restricted behaviors and interests. None displayed general language retardation at the time of testing; however, some of the AS subjects had demonstrated communication abnormalities earlier in their development. On an executive function composite that reflected performance on both the WCST and the Tower of Hanoi, AS subjects performed significantly less well than age- and IQ-matched controls, with 90% performing below the mean of the control group. There was no significant difference between the performance of the AS and high-functioning autistic groups, suggesting that executive function was a common impairment shared by all autism spectrum disorders.

Finally, a recent study by Berthier (1995) found that subjects with AS performed less well than normal controls on both the WCST and the Tower of Hanoi. In this investigation, the criteria for diagnosing AS were not explicitly stated. These studies suggest that executive functions are as impaired in individuals with AS as those with autism. However, because standardized diagnostic criteria were not used in these studies, it is difficult to determine whether the three samples identified the same kinds of individuals. Also, it was not made clear in most of these studies how autism was ruled out in cases of AS. Therefore, it is important that research on the executive skills of individuals with AS continue now that standardized criteria (e.g., DSM-IV; American Psychiatric Association, 1994) are available.

To summarize this review of the literature, it is clear that individuals with autism spectrum disorders demonstrate evidence of executive-type deficits not only in their behavior, as richly described in clinical accounts of the syndrome (Frith, 1989; Kanner, 1943; Wing, 1981), but also on empirical, research-validated instruments of executive function. There is some suggestion from this research that the executive functions most affected in individuals with autism are those of flexibility and planning/organization. This helps more precisely identify the nature of the cognitive impairments underlying autism and suggests where we should focus our intervention efforts. In the next section, techniques for assessing executive functions are presented, as this is the first step toward remediating these impairments.

ASSESSMENT OF EXECUTIVE FUNCTIONS

A number of components are necessary in a complete evaluation of executive function, including neuropsychological testing, behavioral observations, and parent and teacher interviews.

Neuropsychological Testing: Specific Tests of Executive Function

A number of tests thought to tap the executive system exist. Many of these were described above in the critique of the research literature. They will be briefly reviewed here, but the reader is referred to earlier sections for more detail on administration and interpretation. To some extent, these tests can be categorized according to the executive functions on which they rely most heavily (e.g., inhibition, organization, flexibility). Although some consensus has been reached on the primary executive processes required by the measures described below, it is important to note that controversy still exists (Pennington & Ozonoff, 1996) and multiple executive and nonexecutive processes appear important to successful performance on such tests (Ozonoff, 1997a,b).

Tests of Flexibility

Tests of flexibility require subjects to shift their thought processes or behavior to conform to changing demands of a situation (Lezak, 1995). Impairments in flexibility may be evident as: (1) perseveration, the inappropriate repetition of previously correct behavior, (2) stimulus-bound behavior, the inability to dissociate from the external features or demands of a situation and drive behavior instead by internal rules or strategies (Lhermitte, 1986), or (3) concrete, rigid approaches to problem-solving.

The *WCST*, described above, is the most frequently used neuropsychological test of executive processes. It measures flexibility by requiring subjects to shift from a prepotent, previously reinforced cognitive set to a new strategy that the individual must generate (Grant & Berg, 1948; Heaton, 1981). Numerous studies have demonstrated that individuals with frontal damage perform poorly on this test (e.g., Grafman, Jonas, & Salazar, 1990; Robinson, Heaton, Lehman, & Stilson, 1980). The task is appropriate for both children and adults (Chelune & Baer, 1986; Welsh, Pennington, & Groisser, 1991), with normative data available from ages 6 to 90 (Heaton, Chelune, Talley, Kay, & Curtiss, 1993).

Several computer programs for administering and scoring the WCST have been developed (Beaumont, 1981; Beaumont & French, 1987; Harris, 1990; Loong, 1990). Computer versions of this test are appealing, as they are less time-consuming to administer and score and provide greater accuracy in data collection. However, a recent study demonstrated that high-functioning autistic children performed significantly better on the computerized format than the standardly administered version of the test (Ozonoff, 1995a). This suggests that the two forms of the test may not be equivalent for the autistic population and may not measure the same deficits.

The *Trail Making Test* is also thought to measure, at least in part, mental flexibility (there is also a significant motor component to the test; Lezak, 1995).

In the critical "Part B" condition of this test, subjects must connect randomly arranged numbers and letters in alternating order (e.g., 1–A–2–B...), flexibly shifting back and forth between two strategies, numerical counting and alphabetic sequencing. Spreen and Strauss (1991) reported detailed administration and scoring instructions and normative data for both children and adults.

There are a number of other less widely used neuropsychological tasks that can be employed to measure flexibility. The *Alternate Uses Test* (Guilford, Christensen, Merrifield, & Wilson, 1978) requires subjects to generate as many uses for several common objects as possible. Frontal patients tend to perseverate on conventional uses of the objects, demonstrating difficulty switching from one principle of classification to others (Zangwill, 1966). Similarly, a number of *design fluency tasks* have been developed (see Lezak, 1995, for a discussion of several such tests), all of which measure the ability to generate different designs without repeating drawings or perseverating on design themes (e.g., specific details repeated in each drawing). Finally, the *Object Sorting Test* of Goldstein and Sheerer (1941) consists of a set of objects that can be grouped in a variety of ways, both conceptual (e.g., by function or by the setting in which they are normally found) and perceptual (e.g., by size, color, material). Subjects must flexibly shift back and forth between different sorting strategies. Decrements in performance have been documented in both frontal patients (Tow, 1955) and individuals with autism (Minshew *et al.*, 1992).

Tests of Planning and Organization

Planning involves identification and organization of the steps, skills, and materials needed to achieve a goal. In order to plan, one must be able to look ahead to the future, anticipate possible changes or problems, generate alternative courses of action, and weigh and make choices among the alternatives (Lezak, 1995). Planning also requires working memory (Baddeley, 1986), as it is necessary to hold the alternatives "on-line" while determining the most appropriate course of action.

The *Tower of Hanoi* and related *Tower of London* tests are thought to be primary measures of planning (Shallice, 1982). They consist of three pegs and three rings of different colors. Subjects must move the rings from an initial starting position to a specified goal state in the fewest moves possible. This places substantial demands on planning and organizational capacities. To successfully complete the task, subjects must plan a number of moves ahead, anticipating intermediate ring configurations, and determining the most efficient order of moves to achieve the goal state. These tasks are appropriate for use with both children and adults (Levin *et al.*, 1991; Welsh *et al.*, 1991). Deficits in planning have been demonstrated in frontal-damaged adults (Shallice, 1982) and, as reported above, individuals with autism and AS (Berthier, 1995; Ozonoff *et al.*, 1991a,b). Administration and scoring procedures are described by Borys *et al.* (1982) and Krikorian, Bartok, and Gay (1994).

Maze tasks are also thought to measure planning (Lezak, 1995). Subjects must find the most direct route from start to finish, making as few errors as possible. This requires planning several steps ahead in the route. Frontal patients typically display deficits on maze tests (Tow, 1955).

Finally, copying tasks, such as the *Rey–Osterrieth Complex Figure Test*, can be used to measure organizational ability. This figure consists of a base rectangle segmented by horizontal, vertical, and diagonal lines; it also contains numerous internal and external details. Subjects are asked first to copy the figure, then to reproduce it from memory approximately half an hour later. Two recently developed coding systems allow clinicians to assess how well a figure has been organized on the page and how well aligned the corners, sides, and intersecting lines are (Stern *et al.*, 1994; Waber & Holmes, 1985). This test is appropriate for use with children (Akshoomoff & Stiles, 1995a,b; Waber & Holmes, 1985, 1986).

Tests of Inhibition

The ability to inhibit both thoughts and actions when necessary is clearly important to learning and successful school performance. Tests exist that measure both the ability to inhibit the processing of irrelevant distractor stimuli (i.e., central or cognitive inhibition) and the ability to inhibit actions or behaviors (i.e., response inhibition). In general, as discussed above, inhibition is thought to be a relatively spared executive process in autism and AS.

Although the *Stroop Color Word Test* (Stroop, 1935) appears to measure a variety of different cognitive functions (Dempster, 1991; Mirsky, Anthony, Duncan, Ahearn, & Kellam, 1991), its primary clinical utility is as a measure of inhibition (Lezak, 1995). Subjects are given a list of color words printed in contrasting ink (e.g., BLUE printed in red ink) and instructed to name the color of the ink. This requires suppressing the prepotent tendency to read the word and focusing instead on a relatively less salient dimension of the stimulus. Norms for ages 16 and older are available (Golden, 1978). As discussed above, individuals with autism typically do not display deficits on this executive function task (Bryson, 1983; Eskes *et al.*, 1990).

The *Matching Familiar Figures Test* (Kagan, 1965), described above, also appears to tap inhibition. In this task, subjects are shown a complex picture (e.g., a cowboy wearing an elaborate outfit and accessories) and must select a target that matches exactly from among several distractors that look very similar. This test thus requires the control of impulsive responding.

The *Continuous Performance Test* (Halperin, Sharma, Greenblatt, & Schwartz, 1991; Klee & Garfinkel, 1983) also measures inhibition and distractibility, among other things (e.g., sustained attention). In this test, a list of letters, numbers, or other stimuli are presented on a computer and subjects are told to respond only when a prespecified target (e.g., an R) or pattern (e.g., an X only when it follows an A) appears. Both errors of omission (thought to indicate distractibility) and errors of commission (thought to indicate inhibitory dysfunction) can be scored. Poor performance on this test is often seen in children with attention problems, whereas individuals with autism typically do not show deficits on this task relative to controls (Buchsbaum *et al.*, 1992; Garretson, Fein, & Waterhouse, 1990).

Other Testing Considerations

It is often helpful to compare the results of executive function testing with results of other nonexecutive measures. For example, an appropriate intelligence test might be given to see if the child's executive functions are significantly worse than predicted by his or her general intellectual abilities. If both tests use standard scores (mean=100, standard deviation=15), then a discrepancy of either one or two standard deviations may be used to indicate significant impairment, depending on how conservative the examiner wishes to be in diagnosis. Similarly, other nonexecutive neuropsychological tests, such as measures of spatial processing or memory, might be contrasted with executive function scores to examine whether this neuropsychological domain represents a selective area of deficit relative to other cognitive functions.

Neuropsychological testing is not always as informative as it might be, however, for two reasons. First, many of the measures described above are not well-normed. Many rely on limited normative data collected in research studies that did not use random sampling or recruit large samples. Thus, it can be difficult to ascertain the degree of impairment in an individual case relative to population norms. Second, some children will perform adequately on paper-and-pencil measures of executive function when tested in a structured, quiet, one-on-one setting, yet demonstrate profound organizational, planning, or flexibility deficits in the less structured real world. Therefore, additional data must be collected in a complete executive function evaluation.

Behavioral Observations

Additional information about a child's executive functions can be obtained by observing qualitative aspects of performance during the assessment. Even on tests that do not explicitly tap the executive system, relevant information can be gleaned. For example, how a child uses space in drawings can be used to examine planning. Does the child leave enough room to fit a complete drawing on a piece of paper? Or is the drawing crammed in one corner or on one-half of the paper without utilizing all of the available space? Planning and organization can also be informally assessed by giving children a multistep task and observing how they complete it (Sohlberg & Mateer, 1989). For example, they might be asked to plan a family outing or organize a cupboard. Examiners can observe the approach the child takes during these tasks: aimless wandering, trial and error, or more systematic step-by-step approaches. Lezak (1995) also recommended asking the simple question, "What should you do before beginning something important?" and noting the level of planning evident in the response.

Most children with autism spectrum conditions demonstrate a tendency to perseverate on topics or stick rigidly to a familiar problem-solving strategy, even when it is clearly incorrect. When children do demonstrate such a tendency, the examiner should note the parameters of the perseveration. Is it apparent on all tests, only on certain types of items, or only when the child is fatigued or frustrated? Can the child recover from the perseveration on his or her own or is assistance needed from the examiner? What is the child's emotional response to perseveration? Surprisingly, in my clinical experience, many children with autism do not seem to notice or, perhaps, care that they have gotten stuck in a maladaptive problem-solving strategy. On the WCST, for example, many children with autism begin perseverating on the very first item of the test; consequently, they are told many times (sometimes hundreds of times) in a row that their answer is incorrect. Whereas normally developing children often become frustrated under such conditions, crying or refusing to continue, most autistic children continue the test, seemingly unaware or unconcerned that their method of sorting the cards is not the one the examiner is hoping for. Another interesting observation I have made during administrations of the WCST is that some children with autism appear aware of the correct sorting principle, yet fail to change their behavior accordingly. This is evidenced by the child who continues sorting cards by color, even when told this is incorrect (the correct sorting strategy has become shape), but who comments whenever the cards simultaneously match both color and shape, "This one is right." Such children seem to know that the strategy the examiner considers correct has changed, but are unwilling or unable to alter their behavior to match the new expectation.

Finally, examiners can observe children for evidence of inhibitory difficulties. Distractibility, restlessness, and motor overflow are usually only too obvious during testing. Additionally, examiners should note whether the child is bothered by extraneous stimuli, such as noise outside the testing room, a ticking clock, an interruption, or test materials scattered on the table. On nonexecutive cognitive tasks, such as multiple-choice tests, the examiner can also observe the extent to which the child is reflective in considering options and able to inhibit impulsive, prepotent responses.

Parent and Teacher Interviews

Finally, when evaluating children with autism or AS, it is necessary to obtain information from adults who know the child well. Individuals with autism spectrum disorders typically lack the self-awareness and insight to recognize problems in executive function or are unable, because of developmental, cognitive, or communicative limitations, to articulate the nature of the problems they are experiencing. Thus, parents and, if possible, teachers should be interviewed about home and classroom manifestations of cognitive inflexibility, disorganization, planning difficulties, distractibility, and inhibitory dysfunction.

For example, the examiner should ask specific questions about how well the child is able to organize his or her school- and homework. Does he or she take down homework assignments correctly? Does he or she recognize the materials needed for particular assignments and bring them home? Does the child budget the appropriate amount of time for assignments? Can he or she self-regulate, ignoring distractors in order to get work done? Can the child break large assignments into subcomponents and work sequentially at fulfilling subgoals? Does he or she remember to bring homework back to school and turn it in to receive credit? (See Denckla & Reader, 1993, for a discussion of these issues in children with Tourette's syndrome.)

Also ask parents and teachers to describe the child's organization of school materials and personal possessions at home. Many times, this will elicit a description of lockers and bedrooms filled to overflowing with old, unused, or irrelevant items (often "collectibles" related to a child's idiosyncratic interests). Is the child able to keep track of his or her items? Or is there a tendency to lose things or not be able to identify their whereabouts when needed?

THE IMPORTANCE OF REMEDIATION

Executive function deficits translate into a number of problems in the classroom. Many students with autism and AS have difficulty organizing and regulating themselves in class, resulting in failure to complete work on time, off-task behavior, and failure to bring home what is needed to complete homework assignments. The child often is unable to discriminate major tasks from minor details and allocate time and energy accordingly. Difficulties with self-regulation, goal selection, attentional control, and attention shifting may result in spells of daydreaming or absorption in inner thoughts and processes. The inflexibility and rigid problem-solving strategies of individuals with autism spectrum conditions also affect school performance, even when motivation and intellectual abilities are high. Such difficulties often extend to the home and other environments, affecting not only academic but everyday functioning as well.

Despite the seriousness and wide-ranging effects of these problems, both the public and professionals are much less aware of executive dysfunction than, say, reading disability or attention deficit disorder. Because executive problems are both more subtle and less well-understood than other learning disabilities, they rarely qualify a child for special education services. In fact, they are often viewed as voluntary (Mateer & Williams, 1991). Teachers and parents may find it difficult to understand how a child of average or above-average intelligence can "forget" about a long-planned field trip or fail to realize what materials are necessary for completion of a homework assignment. This can lead to misattributions of willfulness, laziness, or disobedience, with parents and teachers feeling that the child could do it *if he (or she) really wanted to.* This stands in contrast to a child with dyslexia, whose complicity in his or her reading problems is rarely suspected. Such misunderstanding can have profound negative effects on self-esteem (Denckla & Reader, 1993). Therefore, if the nature of executive function problems is not appreciated by teachers and parents, students with autism and AS may fail to receive the level of support necessary to succeed in school, despite average or better intelligence.

TREATMENT STRATEGIES FOR EXECUTIVE DYSFUNCTION

It has been mentioned several times in this chapter that disorders other than autism also involve executive dysfunction. For example, individuals with conduct disorder (Hurt & Naglieri, 1992; Lueger & Gill, 1990), obsessive-compulsive disorder (Head, Bolton, & Hymas, 1989), schizophrenia (Axelrod, Goldman, Tompkins, & Jiron, 1994; Beatty, Jocic, Monson, & Katzung, 1994), ADHD (Chelune et al., 1986), early-treated phenylketonuria (Diamond et al., 1993; Welsh, Pennington, Ozonoff, Rouse, & McCabe, 1990), fragile X syndrome (Mazzocco, Hagerman, Cronister-Silverman, & Pennington, 1992; Mazzocco, Pennington, & Hagerman, 1993), Parkinson's disease (Owen et al., 1995), and head injury (Jennett & Teasdale, 1981) demonstrate executive deficits similar to those described in autism spectrum conditions. This is mentioned here because many of the treatment strategies discussed below were taken from the rehabilitation literature on other disorders. Clinicians working with head-injured patients in particular are far ahead of those working with autistic individuals in the remediation of executive function disorders.

Medication Approaches

A number of approaches can be taken to manage executive function deficits. One approach is psychopharmacological intervention. This treatment strategy has been widely used with other disorders, such as ADHD. A number of studies have demonstrated that stimulant medications (e.g., methylphenidate, dextroamphetamine, pemoline) significantly improve attentional and cognitive performance in children with ADHD (Tannock, Schachar, Carr, Chajczyk, & Logan, 1989; van der Meere, Shalev, Borger, & Gross-Tsur, 1995; Werry & Aman, 1984). Only one investigation has evaluated the effectiveness of psychostimulant medications with autistic children, however (Quintana et al., 1995); this study found modest reductions in hyperactivity following administration of methylphenidate, but did not examine executive or other cognitive processes. Thus, if a child with autism or AS also has clear attentional problems or meets criteria for ADHD, a medication consultation may be indicated. Because the extent to which executive processes are responsive to pharmacological intervention in individuals with autism spectrum conditions has not yet been established, however, it is important in such cases to have both parents and clinicians carefully monitor the child's executive skills to see whether the medication is having the desired effect. Finally, although this approach may be a potentially helpful *adjunct* to the other interventions described below, it is probably not helpful when used in isolation to treat executive problems.

Cognitive–Behavioral Approaches

A second approach to remediating executive dysfunction is cognitive behavior management. This strategy, in which contingency-based programs are used to address self-regulation and attentional problems, has often been used with children with ADHD (Lerner, Lowenthal, & Lerner, 1995). A good example of this approach is self-management programs. This technique teaches individuals to monitor their own behavior, shifting control from external sources (e.g., parents or teachers) to the individual. A number of studies have demonstrated that such programs are effective in teaching autistic individuals to monitor their own functioning, successfully reducing undesired behavior while increasing target skills (Koegel & Koegel, 1990; Lagomarcino & Rusch, 1989; Sainato, Strain, LeFebvre, & Rapp, 1991). Self-management programs can be particularly helpful in teaching attending and on-task behaviors. An excellent resource for setting up such programs is Quinn, Swaggart, and Myles (1994).

Metacognitive strategies have also been suggested to improve organizational skills (Jordan & Powell, 1990; Sohlberg, Mateer, & Stuss, 1993). It can be helpful to teach students the learning strategies of self-questioning and self-instruction. For example, before starting a work assignment, they can be taught to ask themselves, "Do I have everything I need? What else might be required?" A self-reminding procedure termed *WSTC* (*W*hat am I supposed to be doing? *S*elect a strategy. *T*ry the strategy. *C*heck the strategy.) has been used successfully with head trauma patients to increase organization and problem-solving abilities (Sohlberg et al., 1993). See Jordan and Powell (1990) for a more extensive discussion of the use of metacognitive strategies with autistic children.

External Structuring

A third set of approaches involves modifications in the child's home and school environments to facilitate more independent executive functioning. Because children with autism and AS lack the internal structure for organizing, planning, and self-regulating, the environment or someone in it can supply external structure to assist the child with these skills.

Often, parents express confusion regarding how to have the environmental modifications and teaching strategies discussed below formally implemented in their child's classroom. Some mildly affected individuals with autism or AS do not qualify for special education services. Others will be provided with some special services, but still receive the majority of their education in regular classrooms. These students can be protected by Section 504 of the Americans with Disabilities Act (1990). A 504/ADA Plan is an individualized document that protects the rights of "individuals with handicaps in one or more major life activities, such as walking, seeing, speaking, breathing, or *learning*." One way to implement the accommodations discussed below is through a 504/ADA plan, which permits individualized treatment in the regular education setting.

Classroom Modifications

Lerner *et al.* (1995) identified a number of characteristics of teachers and classrooms where executive function disorders are successfully managed. These include:

- A well-planned classroom schedule
- Consistent classroom routines and rules
- Clear presentation of instructions
- Placement of the student near the teacher's desk
- Elimination of distractions, such as windows or high-use corridors, near the student
- Provision of a special work station for the student to use when noise or other classroom distractions disrupt the child's work
- Allocation of sufficient time for instructions, repetition of instructions, and individual student assistance
- Explicit identification of assignment goals and subgoals
- Consistent places that assignment materials are kept
- Frequent monitoring of student work pace and work product
- Directing questions toward the student to see that he or she understands the work and is attending
- Establishment of a consistent method of collecting assignments
- Immediate feedback on performance, including reinforcement for both effort and productivity

Direct Teaching of External Compensatory Systems

A number of organizational strategies that can be directly taught to children have been identified. Although many of these approaches were first described for individuals with disorders other than autism (e.g., ADHD, Tourette's syndrome, head trauma), in my clinical experience, such strategies are also enormously helpful with higher-functioning individuals with autism and AS. I refer the interested reader to the following original sources for further detail: Denckla and Reader (1993), Jordan and Powell (1990), Lerner *et al.* (1995), Mateer and Williams (1991), Siegel, Goldstein, and Minshew (1996), Sohlberg and Mateer (1989), Sohlberg *et al.* (1993).

One helpful organizational strategy is use of a weekly assignment log. This checklist is sent from school to home and back, keeping all parties informed of work due and progress on it. A description of the assignment and due date should be entered in the log by the child, often with the teacher's help. Teachers may need to check that the student has all homework assignments and associated materials before leaving school. Parents can then enter their initials in the log to indicate that the child has worked on the assignment at home and teachers can sign off when the assignment has been turned in. Teachers can indicate grades received, as well as the number of times that an assignment was not completed on time. Thus, in addition to organizing the child, assignment checklists are helpful in improving communication between home and school.

Assignment checklists can also be used to help the child break large, often overwhelming, tasks into manageable units. For example, the assignment checklist might also contain information about how to get started (e.g., "begin with item 7 on page 4"), how to recognize when the task is complete (e.g., "finish 10 math problems"), where to store or hand in the completed product (e.g., "a backpack near the door"), and a reminder to clean up. In addition, it may be necessary to provide the student with a list of materials needed for each assignment (e.g., calculator, specific assignment sheet, correct book, writing implement). Although this may seem obvious, students often fail to complete work because they do not have the appropriate materials at hand. Limit the list to only those items essential to the task.

Day planners or appointment books can also be used to organize the child. All events with a designated time should be entered in the day planner. This might include time to awaken, eat breakfast, and get to the bus stop, major school activities, after-school appointments, sports practice, and time to be home for dinner. It is very helpful, and children seem to enjoy it better, if an empty box is placed next to each item so that a check mark can be made in it once the activity has been completed. This provides a visual, concrete cue for the child to identify complete and incomplete activities. As day planners look relatively "normal" and do not make the child stand out from peers, they tend to be well-accepted. It may also be helpful for parents or teachers to adopt a day planner themselves, modeling its use for the child. Also, including preferred items, such as calculators, favorite writing implements, money, or small video games, in a pouch in the day planner can increase its relevance and worth to the child, reducing "forgetting."

"To do" lists can be made for tasks that need to get done, but do not have specific designated times (e.g., errands, telephone calls, chores, thank-you notes). Teach the child to cross out items as they are completed and, each evening, to transfer items that have yet to be finished to the next day's list. It may also be helpful to prioritize the most important items on the list with a color-coding system or rank-order the items by importance.

A kitchen timer can be placed on the student's desk or a watch with an alarm worn to help the child monitor work pace. This provides concrete cues for the beginning and end of each work activity.

Flexibility Training

Finally, some interesting work has been done with head trauma and schizophrenic patients, demonstrating that specific training exercises can increase flexibility in reasoning and problem-solving. As with the majority of the interventions discussed above, the effectiveness of these strategies with individuals with autism spectrum conditions has yet to be established.

The following exercises share the need to flexibly shift back and forth from one cognitive set or strategy to another. One task uses figure-ground reversal illusions (e.g., the classic pictures of a young woman versus a witch or a vase versus two faces in profile). Individuals are shown the picture and, if necessary, the two reversible figures are explicitly pointed out. Then the individual is prompted to switch back and forth from one figure to the other, describing certain details and answering specific questions about each figure to ensure that switching is actually taking place. This task has been used with non-autistic mentally retarded children (McKinney & Corter, 1971) and schizophrenic adults (Delahunty, Morice, & Frost, 1993); in both cases, such training exercises were successful in increasing flexibility on other executive-type tasks, such as the WCST (Delahunty et al., 1993).

Sorting tasks are also useful in promoting flexibility. In such tasks, the same set of objects is sorted into a number of different categorical sets. For example, children might be given a set of colored geometric forms that they first sort by shape and then, immediately afterward, by color. Or they might sort canned food items, first by brand (Green Giant, Del Monte, Libby's), then by size (8 oz, 16 oz, 64 oz), and finally by type (green versus waxed versus baked beans). Such exercises can even be incorporated into functional activities at home; for example, sorting laundry by color (whites versus dark colors), texture (delicates versus sturdy items), and type (shirts versus towels). Each requires flexibly shifting from a focus on one attribute to another. Sorting tasks have been used with nonautistic mentally retarded subjects (McKinney & Corter, 1971), schizophrenic adults (Delahunty et al., 1993), and autistic individuals (Bock, 1994). All three studies found that training on such exercises resulted in significant increases in flexibility on other executive function tasks.

Sohlberg and Mateer (1989) outlined several additional flexibility training exercises. In their Odd–Even Number Cancellation task, individuals are given a sheet of numbers and told to cross out all of the odd ones, until the therapist says "Change," at which point the subject is to cross out all of the even numbers; this switching goes back and forth until the entire page, containing approximately 250 numbers, has been completed. This task allows ample opportunity for practice in switching from one response set to another. Sohlberg and Mateer (1989) also recommended constructing Stroop-like materials (see above) that require individuals to switch from a prepotent response (i.e., reading) to a less salient response, such as identification of the color of the ink or the size of the letters (e.g., BIG, little, LITTLE, big, BIG, LITTLE, big, little, big). Training schizophrenic patients on these tasks has resulted in significant improvement on the WCST (Delahunty et al., 1993).

CONCLUSION

This chapter began with a review of the empirical evidence that individuals with autism and AS suffer from executive control problems. Research studies have consistently documented deficits in planning, flexibility, organization, and self-monitoring in autism spectrum disorders. In addition, parents and teachers frequently report such problems. It appears that, particularly in verbal, higher-functioning individuals, these deficits stand out in contrast to the many other areas in which the autistic individual has progressed. Yet these difficulties have received virtually no attention in the remediation literature on autism. Although a number of reports on treating executive problems have begun to appear for the head-injured, schizophrenic, and ADHD populations, there has been little clinical and even less research attention focused on those with autism. It is hoped that this chapter is a beginning step toward filling that gap. However, it is clear that numerous questions remain. Most prominently, there is, as yet, no empirical validation of the effectiveness of such interventions with autistic individuals, nor whether they generalize to settings, tasks, and materials that differ from those associated with training.

There has been a long debate about whether AS and high-functioning autism are, as Schopler (1996) recently put it, "different labels or different disabilities." In the research literature reviewed at the beginning of this chapter, it was clear that individuals with both autism and AS suffer from executive function difficulties. Most studies found that those with AS were just as impaired as those with autism on tests of executive function, performing less well than normally developing controls. Thus, from the executive function domain, there is little evidence that the two conditions differ, suggesting they may be different terms for the same disorder.

The interventions discussed in this chapter may appear to entail a great deal of adult assistance. Yet as time-consuming as they may be, they are preferable to hoping that children with autism will learn executive skills on their own. Executive impairment appears to be a core cognitive deficit of autism (Frith, 1989; Hughes *et al.*, 1994; Ozonoff, 1995b). Thus, it is more likely that such skills will not be acquired at all without explicit training. If we hope that our children will eventually function independently in the world, the capacities to plan, organize, flexibly solve problems, self-regulate, and achieve goals are critical. Integration of executive function interventions with social skills training, speech-language services, educational support, and other resources will permit each child with autism to achieve the greatest success possible.

REFERENCES

Akshoomoff, N. A., & Stiles, J. (1995a). Developmental trends in visuospatial analysis and planning: I. Copying a complex figure. *Neuropsychology, 9,* 364–377.

Akshoomoff, N. A., & Stiles, J. (1995b). Developmental trends in visuospatial analysis and planning: II. Memory for a complex figure. *Neuropsychology, 9,* 378–389.

American Psychiatric Association. (1994). *Diagnostic and statistical manual of mental disorders* (4th ed.). Washington, DC: Author.

Anderson, C. V., Bigler, E. D., & Blatter, D. D. (in press). Frontal lobe lesions, diffuse damage, and neuropsychological functioning in traumatic brain-injured patients. *Journal of Clinical and Experimental Neuropsychology.*

Axelrod, B. N., Goldman, R. S., Tompkins, L. M., & Jiron, C. C. (1994). Poor differential performance on the Wisconsin Card Sorting Test in schizophrenia, mood disorder, and traumatic brain injury. *Neuropsychiatry, Neuropsychology, and Behavioral Neurology, 7,* 20–24.

Baddeley, A. D. (1986). *Working memory.* Oxford: Clarendon Press.

Baron-Cohen, S. (1989). The autistic child's theory of mind: A case of specific developmental delay. *Journal of Child Psychology and Psychiatry and Allied Disciplines, 30,* 285–297.

Baron-Cohen, S., Leslie, A. M., & Frith, U. (1985). Does the autistic child have a "theory of mind"? *Cognition, 21,* 37–46.

Bauman, M., & Kemper, T. L. (1985). Histoanatomic observations of the brain in early infantile autism. *Neurology, 35,* 866–874.

Bauman, M., & Kemper, T. L. (1988). Limbic and cerebellar abnormalities: Consistent findings in infantile autism. *Journal of Neuropathology and Experimental Neurology, 47,* 369.

Beatty, W. W., Jocic, Z., Monson, N., & Katzung, V. M. (1994). Problem solving by schizophrenic and schizoaffective patients on the Wisconsin and California Card Sorting Tests. *Neuropsychology, 8,* 49–54.

Beaumont, J. G. (1981). A PASCAL program to administer a digit span test. *Current Psychological Reviews, 1,* 115–117.

Beaumont, J. G., & French, C. C. (1987). A clinical field study of eight automated psychometric procedures: The Leicester/DHSS project. *International Journal of Man–Machine Studies, 26,* 661–682.

Bennetto, L., Pennington, B. F., & Rogers, S. J. (1996). Impaired and intact memory functions in autism. *Child Development, 67,* 1816–1835.

Berthier, M. L. (1995). Hypomania following bereavement in Asperger's syndrome: A case study. *Neuropsychiatry, Neuropsychology, and Behavioral Neurology, 8,* 222–228.

Bock, M. A. (1994). Acquisition, maintenance, and generalization of a categorization strategy by children with autism. *Journal of Autism and Developmental Disorders, 24,* 39–51.

Borys, S. V., Spitz, H. H., & Dorans, B. A. (1982). Tower of Hanoi performance of retarded young adults and nonretarded children as a function of solution length and goal state. *Journal of Experimental Child Psychology, 33,* 87–110.

Bryson, S. E. (1983). Interference effects in autistic children: Evidence for the comprehension of single stimuli. *Journal of Abnormal Psychology, 92,* 250–254.

Buchsbaum, M. S., Siegel, B. V., Wu, J. C., Hazlett, E., Sicotte, N., Haier, R., Tanguay, P., Asarnow, R., Cadorette, T., Donoghue, D., Lagunas-Solar, M., Lott, I., Paek, J., & Sabalesky, D. (1992). Brief report: Attention performance in autism and regional brain metabolic rate assessed by positron emission tomography. *Journal of Autism and Developmental Disorders, 22,* 115–125.

Casey, B. J., Gordon, C. T., Mannheim, G. B., & Rumsey, J. M. (1993). Dysfunctional attention in autistic savants. *Journal of Clinical and Experimental Neuropsychology, 15,* 933–946.

Chelune, G. J., & Baer, R. A. (1986). Developmental norms for the Wisconsin Card Sorting Test. *Journal of Clinical and Experimental Neuropsychology, 8,* 219–228.

Chelune, G. J., Ferguson, W., Koon, R., & Dickey, T. O. (1986). Frontal lobe disinhibition in attention deficit disorder. *Child Psychiatry and Human Development, 16,* 221–234.

Courchesne, E., Akshoomoff, N. A., & Ciesielski, K. (1990). Shifting attention abnormalities in autism: ERP and performance evidence. *Journal of Clinical and Experimental Neuropsychology, 12,* 77.

Courchesne, E., Yeung-Courchesne, R., Press, G. A., Hesselink, J. R., & Jernigan, T. L. (1988). Hypoplasia of cerebellar vermal lobules VI and VII in autism. *New England Journal of Medicine, 318,* 1349–1354.

Damasio, A. R., & Maurer, R. G. (1978). A neurological model for childhood autism. *Archives of Neurology, 35,* 777–786.

Damasio, A. R., & Van Hoesen, G. W. (1983). Emotional disturbances associated with focal lesions of the limbic frontal lobe. In K. M. Heilman & P. Satz (Eds.), *The neuropsychology of human emotion* (pp. 85–110). New York: Guilford Press.

Dawson, G., Klinger, L. G., Panagiotides, H., Lewy, A., & Castelloe, P. (1995). Subgroups of autistic children based on social behavior display distinct patterns of brain activity. *Journal of Abnormal Child Psychology, 23,* 569–583.

Delahunty, A., Morice, R., & Frost, B. (1993). Specific cognitive flexibility rehabilitation in schizophrenia. *Psychological Medicine, 23,* 221–227.

Dempster, F. N. (1991). Inhibitory processes: A neglected dimension of intelligence. *Intelligence, 15,* 157–173.

Denckla, M. B., & Reader, M. J. (1993). Education and psychosocial interventions: Executive dysfunction and its consequences. In R. Kurlan (Ed.), *Handbook of Tourette's syndrome and related tic and behavioral disorders* (pp. 431–451). New York: Dekker.

Deutsch, G. (1992). The nonspecificity of frontal dysfunction in disease and altered states: Cortical blood flow evidence. *Neuropsychiatry, Neuropsychology, and Behavioral Neurology, 5,* 301–307.

Diamond, A., & Goldman-Rakic, P. S. (1986). Comparative development in human infants and infant rhesus monkeys on cognitive functions that depend on prefrontal cortex. *Society of Neuroscience Abstracts, 12,* 742.

Diamond, A., Hurwitz, W., Lee, E. Y., Bockes, T., Grover, W., & Minarcik, C. (1993, March 25–28). *Cognitive deficits on frontal cortex tasks in children with early-treated PKU: Results of two years of longitudinal study*. Paper presented at the meeting of the Society for Research in Child Development, New Orleans, LA.

Duncan, J. (1986). Disorganisation of behaviour after frontal lobe damage. *Cognitive Neuropsychology, 3*, 271–290.

Eskes, G. A., Bryson, S. E., & McCormick, T. A. (1990). Comprehension of concrete and abstract words in autistic children. *Journal of Autism and Developmental Disorders, 20*, 61–73.

Frith, U. (1989). *Autism: Explaining the enigma*. Oxford: Blackwell.

Garretson, H. B., Fein, D., & Waterhouse, L. (1990). Sustained attention in children with autism. *Journal of Autism and Developmental Disorders, 20*, 101–114.

George, M. S., Costa, D. C., Kouris, K., Ring, H. A., & Ell, P. J. (1992). Cerebral blood flow abnormalities in adults with infantile autism. *Journal of Nervous and Mental Disease, 180*, 413–417.

Gillberg, C. (1994, May 19 20). *Diagnostic issues in Asperger syndrome*. Paper presented at the 15th Annual TEACCH Conference, Chapel Hill, NC.

Golden, C. J. (1978). *Stroop Color and Word Test manual*. Los Angeles: Western Psychological Services.

Goldstein, K. H., & Sheerer, M. (1941). Abstract and concrete behavior: An experimental study with special tests. *Psychological Monographs, 53*, 239.

Grafman, J., Jonas, B., & Salazar, A. (1990). Wisconsin Card Sorting Test performance based on location and size of neuroanatomical lesion in Vietnam veterans with penetrating head injury. *Perceptual and Motor Skills, 71*, 1120–1122.

Grant, D. A., & Berg, E. A. (1948). A behavioral analysis of degree of reinforcement and ease of shifting to new responses in a Weigle-type card sorting problem. *Journal of Experimental Psychology, 32*, 404–411.

Guilford, J. P., Christensen, P. R., Merrifield, P. R., & Wilson, R. C. (1978). *Alternate Uses: Manual of instructions and interpretation*. Orange, CA: Sheridan.

Halperin, J. M., Sharma, V., Greenblatt, E., & Schwartz, S. T. (1991). Assessment of the Continuous Performance Test: Reliability and validity in a nonreferred sample. *Psychological Assessment, 3*, 603–608.

Harris, M. E. (1990). *Wisconsin Card Sorting Test: Computer version, research edition*. Odessa, FL: Psychological Assessment Resources.

Head, D., Bolton, D., & Hymas, N. (1989). Deficit in cognitive shifting ability in patients with obsessive–compulsive disorder. *Biological Psychiatry, 25*, 929–937.

Heaton, R. K. (1981). *Wisconsin Card Sorting Test manual*. Odessa, FL: Psychological Assessment Resources.

Heaton, R. K., Chelune, G. J., Talley, J. L., Kay, G. G., & Curtiss, G. (1993). *Wisconsin Card Sorting Test manual: Revised and expanded*. Odessa, FL: Psychological Assessment Resources.

Hermelin, B., & O'Connor, N. (1970). *Psychological experiments with autistic children*. Oxford: Pergamon.

Hughes, C., & Russell, J. (1993). Autistic children's difficulty with mental disengagement from an object: Its implications for theories of autism. *Developmental Psychology, 29*, 498–510.

Hughes, C., Russell, J., & Robbins, T. W. (1994). Evidence for executive dysfunction in autism. *Neuropsychologia, 32*, 477–492.

Hurt, J., & Naglieri, J. A. (1992). Performance of delinquent and nondelinquent males on planning, attention, simultaneous, and successive cognitive processing tasks. *Journal of Clinical Psychology, 48*, 120–128.

Jennett, B., & Teasdale, G. (1981). Management of head injuries. *Contemporary Neurology Series, 20*, 258–260.

Jordan, R., & Powell, S. (1990). Teaching autistic children to think more effectively. *Communication, 24*, 20–25.

Kagan, J. (1965). Individual differences in the resolution of response uncertainty. *Journal of Personality and Social Psychology, 2*, 154–160.

Kanner, L. (1943). Autistic disturbances of affective content. *Nervous Child, 2,* 217–250.

Klee, S. H., & Garfinkel, B. D. (1983). The computerized continuous performance task: A new measure of inattention. *Journal of Abnormal Child Psychology, 11,* 487–495.

Koegel, R. L., & Koegel, L. K. (1990). Extended reductions in stereotypic behavior of students with autism through a self-management treatment package. *Journal of Applied Behavior Analysis, 23,* 119–127.

Krikorian, R., Bartok, J., & Gay, N. (1994). Tower of London procedure: A standard method and developmental data. *Journal of Clinical and Experimental Neuropsychology, 16,* 840–850.

Lagomarcino, T. R., & Rusch, F. R. (1989). Utilizing self-management procedures to teach independent performance. *Education and Training in Mental Retardation, 24,* 297–305.

Lerner, J. W., Lowenthal, B., & Lerner, S. R. (1995). *Attention deficit disorders: Assessment and teaching.* Pacific Grove, CA: Brooks/Cole.

Levin, H. S., Culhane, K. A., Hartmann, J., Evankovich, K., Mattson, A. J., Harward, H., Ringholz, G., Ewing-Cobbs, L., & Fletcher, J. M. (1991). Developmental changes in performance on tests of purported frontal lobe functioning. Special Issue: Developmental consequences of early frontal lobe damage. *Developmental Neuropsychology, 7,* 377–395.

Lezak, M. D. (1995). *Neuropsychological Assessment* (3rd ed.). London: Oxford University Press.

Lhermitte, F. (1986). Human autonomy and the frontal lobes, part II: Patient behavior in complex and social situations: The "environmental dependency syndrome." *Annals of Neurology, 19,* 335–343.

Loong, J. W. K. (1990). *The Wisconsin Card Sorting Test, IBM version.* San Luis Obispo, CA: Wang Neuropsychological Laboratory.

Lord, C. (1988). Enhancing communication in adolescents with autism. *Topics in Language Disorders, 9,* 72–81.

Lovaas, O. I., Koegel, R. L., & Schreibman, L. (1979). Stimulus overselectivity in autism: A review of research. *Psychological Bulletin, 86,* 1236–1254.

Lueger, R. J., & Gill, K. J. (1990). Frontal-lobe cognitive dysfunction in conduct disorder adolescents. *Journal of Clinical Psychology, 46,* 696–706.

Luria, A. R. (1966). *The higher cortical functions in man.* New York: Basic Books.

MacLeod, C. M. (1991). Half a century of research on the Stroop effect: An integrative review. *Psychological Bulletin, 109,* 163–203.

Marriage, K. J., Gordon, V., & Brand, L. (1995). A social skills group for boys with Asperger's syndrome. *Australian and New Zealand Journal of Psychiatry, 29,* 58–62.

Mateer, C. A., & Williams, D. (1991). Effects of frontal lobe injury in childhood. Special Issue: Developmental consequences of early frontal lobe damage. *Developmental Neuropsychology, 7,* 359–376.

Mazzocco, M. M., Hagerman, R. J., Cronister-Silverman, A., & Pennington, B. F. (1992). Specific frontal lobe deficits among women with the fragile X gene. *Journal of the American Academy of Child and Adolescent Psychiatry, 31,* 1141–1148.

Mazzocco, M. M., Pennington, B. F., & Hagerman, R. J. (1993). The neurocognitive phenotype of female carriers of fragile X: Additional evidence for specificity. *Journal of Developmental and Behavioral Pediatrics, 14,* 328–335.

McEvoy, R. E., Rogers, S. J., & Pennington, B. F. (1993). Executive function and social communication deficits in young autistic children. *Journal of Child Psychology and Psychiatry and Allied Disciplines, 34,* 563–578.

McKinney, J. D., & Corter, H. M. (1971). Flexibility training with educable mentally retarded children. *Journal of School Psychology, 9,* 455–465.

Mesibov, G. B. (1984). Social skills training with verbal autistic adolescents and adults: A program model. *Journal of Autism and Developmental Disorders, 14,* 395–404.

Minshew, N. J., Goldstein, G., Muenz, L. R., & Payton, J. B. (1992). Neuropsychological functioning nonmentally retarded autistic individuals. *Journal of Clinical and Experimental Neuropsychology, 14,* 749–761.

Mirsky, A. F., Anthony, B. J., Duncan, C. C., Ahearn, M. B., & Kellam, S. G. (1991). Analysis of the elements of attention: A neuropsychological approach. *Neuropsychology Review*, 2, 109–145.

Mountain, M. A., & Snow, W. G. (1993). Wisconsin Card Sorting Test as a measure of frontal pathology: A review. *Clinical Neuropsychologist*, 7, 108–118.

Owen, A. M., Sahakian, B. J., Hodges, J. R., Summers, B. A., Polkey, C. E., & Robbins, T. W. (1995). Dopamine-dependent frontostriatal planning deficits in early Parkinson's disease. *Neuropsychology*, 9, 126–140.

Ozonoff, S. (1997a). Causal mechanisms of autism: Unifying perspectives from an information processing framework. In D. J. Cohen & F. R. Volkmar (Eds.), *Handbook of autism and pervasive developmental disorders* (2nd ed.) (pp. 868–879). New York: Wiley.

Ozonoff, S. (1997b). Components of executive function in autism and other disorders. In J. Russell (Ed.), *Executive functioning and autism* (pp. 179–211). London: Oxford University Press.

Ozonoff, S. (1995a). Reliability and validity of the Wisconsin Card Sorting Test in studies of autism. *Neuropsychology*, 9, 491–500.

Ozonoff, S. (1995b). Executive functions in autism. In E. Schopler & G. B. Mesibov (Eds.), *Learning and cognition in autism* (pp. 199–219). New York: Plenum Press.

Ozonoff, S., & McEvoy, R. E. (1994). A longitudinal study of executive function and theory of mind development in autism. *Development and Psychopathology*, 6, 415–431.

Ozonoff, S., & Miller, J. N. (1995). Teaching theory of mind: A new approach to social skills training for individuals with autism. *Journal of Autism and Developmental Disorders*, 25, 415–433.

Ozonoff, S., Pennington, B. F., & Rogers, S. J. (1991a). Executive function deficits in high-functioning autistic individuals: Relationship to theory of mind. *Journal of Child Psychology and Psychiatry and Allied Disciplines*, 32, 1081–1105.

Ozonoff, S., Rogers, S. J., & Pennington, B. F. (1991b). Asperger's syndrome: Evidence of an empirical distinction from high-functioning autism. *Journal of Child Psychology and Psychiatry and Allied Disciplines*, 32, 1107–1122.

Ozonoff, S., & Strayer, D. L. (1997). Inhibitory function in nonretarded children with autism. *Journal of Autism and Developmental Disorders*, 27, 59–77.

Ozonoff, S., Strayer, D. L., McMahon, W. M., & Filloux, F. (1994). Executive function abilities in autism and Tourette syndrome: An information processing approach. *Journal of Child Psychology and Psychiatry and Allied Disciplines*, 35, 1015–1032.

Pennington, B. F., & Ozonoff, S. (1996). Executive functions and developmental psychopathology. *Journal of Child Psychology and Psychiatry*, 37, 51–87.

Prior, M., & Hoffmann, W. (1990). Brief report: Neuropsychological testing of autistic children through an exploration with frontal lobe tests. *Journal of Autism and Developmental Disorders*, 20, 581–590.

Quinn, C., Swaggart, B. L., & Myles, B. S. (1994). Implementing cognitive behavior management programs for persons with autism: Guidelines for practitioners. *Focus on Autistic Behavior*, 9, 1–13.

Quintana, H., Birmaher, B., Stedge, D., Lennon, S., Freed, J., Bridge, J., & Greenhill, L. (1995). Use of methylphenidate in the treatment of children with autistic disorder. *Journal of Autism and Developmental Disorders*, 25, 283–294.

Ritvo, E. R., Freeman, B. J., Scheibel, A. B., Duong, T., Robinson, H., Guthrie, D., & Ritvo, A. (1986). Lower Purkinje cell counts in the cerebella of four autistic subjects: Initial findings of the UCLA–NSAC research report. *American Journal of Psychiatry*, 143, 862–866.

Robinson, A. L., Heaton, R. K., Lehman, R. A., & Stilson, D. W. (1980). The utility of the Wisconsin Card Sorting Test in detecting and localizing frontal lobe lesions. *Journal of Consulting and Clinical Psychology*, 48, 605–614.

Rumsey, J. M. (1985). Conceptual problem-solving in highly verbal, nonretarded autistic men. *Journal of Autism and Developmental Disorders*, 15, 23–36.

Rumsey, J. M., & Hamburger, S. D. (1988). Neuropsychological findings in high-functioning men with infantile autism, residual state. *Journal of Clinical and Experimental Neuropsychology, 10,* 201–221.

Rumsey, J. M., & Hamburger, S. D. (1990). Neuropsychological divergence of high-level autism and severe dyslexia. *Journal of Autism and Developmental Disorders, 20,* 155–168.

Sainato, D. M., Strain, P. S., LeFebvre, D., & Rapp, N. (1991). Effects of self-evaluation on the independent work skills of preschool children with disabilities. *Exceptional Children, 56,* 540–549.

Schneider, S. G., & Asarnow, R. F. (1987). A comparison of cognitive/neuropsychological impairments of nonretarded autistic and schizophrenic children. *Journal of Abnormal Child Psychology, 15,* 29–45.

Schopler, E. (1996). Are autism and Asperger syndrome different labels or different disabilities? *Journal of Autism and Developmental Disorders, 26,* 109–110.

Shallice, T. (1982). Specific impairments in planning. In D. E. Broadbent & L. Weiskrantz (Eds.), *The neuropsychology of cognitive function* (pp. 199–209). London: Royal Society.

Sherman, M., Nass, R., & Shapiro, T. (1984). Brief report: Regional cerebral blood flow in autism. *Journal of Autism and Developmental Disorders, 14,* 439–446.

Siegel, D. J., Goldstein, G., & Minshew, N. J. (1996). Designing instruction for the high-functioning autistic individual. *Journal of Developmental and Physical Disabilities, 8,* 1–19.

Sohlberg, M. M., & Mateer, C. A. (1989). *Introduction to cognitive rehabilitation: Theory and practice.* New York: Guilford Press.

Sohlberg, M. M., Mateer, C. A., & Stuss, D. T. (1993). Contemporary approaches to the management of executive control dysfunction. *Journal of Head Trauma Rehabilitation, 8,* 45–58.

Spreen, O., & Strauss, E. (1991). *A compendium of neuropsychological tests: Administration, norms, and commentary.* London: Oxford University Press.

Stern, R. A., Singer, E. A., Duke, L. M., Singer, N. G., Morey, C. E., Daughtrey, E. W., & Kaplan, E. (1994). The Boston Qualitative Scoring System for the Rey-Osterrieth Complex Figure: Description and interrater reliability. *Clinical Neuropsychologist, 8,* 309–322.

Stroop, J. R. (1935). Studies of interference in serial verbal reactions. *Journal of Experimental Psychology, 18,* 643–662.

Stuss, D. T., & Benson, D. F. (1986). *The frontal lobes.* New York: Raven Press.

Szatmari, P., Tuff, L., Finlayson, A. J., & Bartolucci, G. (1990). Asperger's syndrome and autism: Neurocognitive aspects. *Journal of the American Academy of Child and Adolescent Psychiatry, 29,* 130–136.

Tannock, R., Schachar, R. J., Carr, R. P., Chajczyk, D., & Logan, G. D. (1989). Effects of methylphenidate on inhibitory control in hyperactive children. *Journal of Abnormal Child Psychology, 17,* 473–491.

Tow, P. M. (1955). *Personality changes following frontal leucotomy.* London: Oxford University Press.

van der Meere, J., Shalev, R., Borger, N., & Gross-Tsur, V. (1995). Sustained attention, activation, and MPH in ADHD. *Journal of Child Psychology and Psychiatry, 36,* 697–703.

Waber, D. P., & Holmes, J. M. (1985). Assessing children's copy productions of the Rey-Osterrieth Complex Figure. *Journal of Clinical and Experimental Neuropsychology, 7,* 264–280.

Waber, D. P., & Holmes, J. M. (1986). Assessing children's memory productions of the Rey-Osterrieth Complex Figure. *Journal of Clinical and Experimental Neuropsychology, 8,* 563–580.

Wainwright-Sharp, J. A., & Bryson, S. E. (1993). Visual orienting deficits in high-functioning people with autism. *Journal of Autism and Developmental Disorders, 23,* 1–13.

Waterhouse, L., & Fein, D. (1982). Language skills in developmentally disabled children. *Brain and Language, 15,* 307–333.

Welsh, M. C., & Pennington, B. F. (1988). Assessing frontal lobe functioning in children: Views from developmental psychology. *Developmental Neuropsychology, 4,* 199–230.

Welsh, M. C., Pennington, B. F., & Groisser, D. B. (1991). A normative–developmental study of executive function: A window on prefrontal function in children. *Developmental Neuropsychology*, 7, 131–149.

Welsh, M. C., Pennington, B. F., Ozonoff, S., Rouse, B., & McCabe, E. R. B. (1990). Neuropsychology of early-treated phenylketonuria: Specific executive function deficits. *Child Development*, 61, 1697–1713.

Werry, J. S., & Aman, M. (1984). Methylphenidate in hyperactive and enuretic children. In B. Shopsin & L. Greenhill (Eds.), *The psychobiology of childhood* (pp. 183–195). Jamaica, NY: Spectrum.

Wing, L. (1981). Asperger's syndrome: A clinical account. *Psychological Medicine*, 11, 115–129.

World Health Organization. (1989). *International classification of diseases and disorders* (Draft 10th ed.). Geneva: Author.

Zangwill, O. L. (1966). Psychological deficits associated with frontal lobe lesions. *International Journal of Neurology*, 5, 395–402.

Zilbovicius, M., Garreau, B., Samson, Y., Remy, P., Barthelemy, C., Syrota, A., & Lelord, G. (1995). Delayed maturation of the frontal cortex in childhood autism. *American Journal of Psychiatry*, 152, 248–252.

V

Related Conditions

13

Repetitive Thoughts and Behavior in Pervasive Developmental Disorders
Phenomenology and Pharmacotherapy

CHRISTOPHER J. McDOUGLE

OVERVIEW

The repetitive thoughts and behavior of patients with pervasive developmental disorder(s) [PDD(s)] can be quite interfering, often disrupting educational and vocational opportunities, as well as general quality of life for the individual and family members. To date, results from studies designed to differentiate the nature of repetitive thoughts and behavior in specific subtypes of PDD, such as Asperger's disorder, have not been published. Recent data indicate that drugs that are potent inhibitors of serotonin [5-hydroxytryptamine (5-HT)] neuronal uptake may be effective for reducing repetitive thoughts and behavior in some children, adolescents, and adults with PDDs.

This chapter will begin with a discussion of the phenomenology of repetitive thoughts and behavior in individuals with PDD, including a definition of the terms *obsession* and *compulsion* and presentation of results from a study comparing the types and frequency of repetitive thoughts and behavior between adults with autistic disorder and obsessive-compulsive disorder (OCD). This section on the phenomenology of repetitive thoughts and behavior among

CHRISTOPHER J. McDOUGLE • Section of Child and Adolescent Psychiatry, Department of Psychiatry, Indiana University School of Medicine, Indianapolis, Indiana 46202.

Asperger Syndrome or High-Functioning Autism?, edited by Schopler *et al.* Plenum Press, New York, 1998.

patients with PDD will be followed by a review of the pharmacological treatment of these symptoms with potent serotonin uptake inhibitors (SUIs), including clomipramine, fluvoxamine, fluoxetine, and sertraline. The chapter will conclude with recommendations for future directions of research into the phenomenology and pharmacological management of repetitive thoughts and behavior in patients with PDD.

PHENOMENOLOGY

A half-century following Kanner's original description (Kanner, 1943), repetitive thoughts and behavior remain integral clinical characteristics of the classification of PPDs by the *Diagnostic and Statistical Manual of Mental Disorders* (DSM-IV) (American Psychiatric Association, 1994). Throughout the years, a plethora of terms have been used to describe these phenomena, including *automanipulation, gesturing, motility disturbances, perseverations, posturing, preoccupations, rituals, self-stimulatory behaviors, stereopathies,* and *stereotypies,* among others. Whereas some of these terms reflect strictly behavioral observations, others, such as *maintenance of sameness* and *resistance to change* assume a relationship between the behavior and a corresponding internal emotional or mental state.

In Kanner's (1943) original description of 11 autistic children, the repetitive natures of behavior, speech, and modes of social interaction were designated core common elements of the clinical presentation of the autistic syndrome. Verbal and motor rituals, obsessive questioning, a rigid adherence to routine, a preoccupation with details, and an anxiously obsessive desire for the maintenance of sameness and completeness were all noted. Interestingly, religious and somatic obsessions, repetitive handwashing, and tics were identified in family members. Prior and Macmillan (1973) referred to the repetitive phenomena of autism as *sameness behavior,* and found it to occur significantly more frequently in autistic children than in children with other developmental disabilities. Behaviors such as creating and maintaining patterns, lining things up in rows, insisting that furniture and other objects remain in the same place, and rituals in going to bed, dressing or eating, discriminated between the autistic and nonautistic groups. In a review of repetitive phenomena seen in normal development and in clinical populations, Hoder and Cohen (1983) described constant repetitive behavior including stereotyped walking, whirling, darting, sidewalking, lunging, hand flapping, head banging, and body rocking in patients with autism. In a follow-up study of 14 autistic men, 86% demonstrated stereotyped, repetitive movements, including characteristic arm shaking, tapping of table surfaces, and arranging objects (Rumsey, Rapoport, & Sceery, 1985). DSM-IV incorporates many elements of Kanner's (1943) description: Stereotyped and repetitive speech and body movements, encompassing preoccupation with one or more stereotyped and restricted patterns of interest, apparently inflexible adherence to specific, nonfunctional routines or rituals, and a persistent preoccupation with parts of objects, remain integral elements of the current diagnostic criteria for autistic disorder.

The terms *obsession* and *compulsion* have been used to describe the repetitive thoughts and behavior characteristic of PDD. In DSM-IV, obsessions are defined as recurrent and persistent thoughts, impulses, or images that are experienced, at some time during the disturbance, as intrusive and inappropriate and that cause marked anxiety or distress. The individual with the obsessions attempts to ignore, suppress, or neutralize these thoughts, impulses, or images with a compulsion, defined in DSM-IV as a repetitive behavior or mental act that is performed in response to an obsession, or according to rules that must be applied rigidly. Additional DSM-IV diagnostic criteria for OCD stipulate that, at some point during the course of the disorder, the person has recognized that the obsessions or compulsions are excessive or unreasonable, and that the obsessions or compulsions cause marked distress, are time-consuming, or significantly interfere with the person's normal routine, occupational (or academic) functioning, or usual social activities or relationships.

Implicit in these definitions is a great degree of dependence on the patient's subjective rating of his or her internal state. Accordingly, Baron-Cohen (1989) suggested that these two terms be applied cautiously with respect to the repetitive thoughts and behavior characteristic of individuals with PDD, because many of these patients cannot speak about their internal state of mind. On the other hand, an inability to articulate subjective states does not necessarily imply their absence. In particular, ascribing a sense of ego-syntonicity to the repetitive thoughts and behavior of individuals with PDD by default does not seem supportable.

Without verbal reports about their thoughts and internal states, it may be difficult to assess the incidence of obsessive-compulsive symptoms in patients with PDD. A possible means of determining if these individuals possess obsessions and compulsions would be to compare and contrast the content of the repetitive thoughts and behavior between patients with PDD and those with OCD (Baron-Cohen, 1989). Our group recently conducted a study designed to systematically investigate the nature of repetitive thoughts and behavior in adults with autistic disorder, and to compare them with those of adults with OCD using a case-controlled method (McDougle *et al.*, 1995).

Fifty consecutive patients (36 males and 14 females between the ages of 18 and 53) admitted to the Yale Adult Pervasive Developmental Disorders (Autism) Clinic with a principal DSM-III-R (and DSM-IV) diagnosis of autistic disorder and 50 age- and sex-matched adults (36 males and 14 females aged 19 to 47) with a primary DSM-III-R (and DSM-IV) diagnosis of OCD without a lifetime history of motor and/or phonic tics were compared. The mean age of the autistic group did not differ significantly from the OCD group (30.4±7.9 versus

30.1±7.2 years). The mean IQ of the autistic group was 69.7±27.2, which places the group as a whole into the range of Mild Mental Retardation. Thirty-five of the autistic patients met DSM-IV criteria for Mental Retardation (Mild, N=10; Moderate, N=10; Severe, N=8; Profound, N=0) or Borderline Intellectual Functioning (N=7), and 15 of these 35 autistic patients were mute. Thus, it was difficult to assess the presence or absence of obsessive thoughts, as well as the ego-syntonic versus ego-dystonic nature (degree of insight) of their repetitive thoughts and behavior. None of the OCD patients were mentally retarded or had borderline intellectual functioning, as this is an exclusion criterion for entry into the OCD Clinic. All patients were medication-free at the time of assessment.

The Yale–Brown Obsessive Compulsive Scale (Y–BOCS) Symptom Checklist (SCL) (Goodman, Price, Rasmussen, Mazure, Delgado, *et al.*, 1989; Goodman, Price, Rasmussen, Mazure, Fleischmann, *et al.*, 1989) was used to determine the presence of obsessive-compulsive symptoms. The DSM-III-R ego-dystonicity criterion for OCD ("With Poor Insight" in DSM-IV) was suspended so that repetitive thoughts and behavior could be equated with obsessions and compulsions. The patients were administered the Y–BOCS SCL in the presence of a parent or other primary caregiver who was most familiar with the patient's behavior and who assisted in completing the scale. Only current symptoms (those displayed within the past month) were determined. The symptoms are classified into subcategories according to thematic content (e.g., Contamination obsessions) or to behavioral manifestations (e.g., Cleaning/Washing compulsions). Because of the heterogeneous composition of the Miscellaneous obsessions and Miscellaneous compulsions categories, certain items from the original categories were selected to constitute new categories because clinical experience suggested that they were the most characteristic of patients with autism. Obsessive-compulsive symptomatology was assessed using eight categories of obsessions (Aggressive, Contamination, Sexual, Hoarding, Religious, Symmetry, Somatic, and Need to Know or Remember) and nine categories of compulsions [Cleaning, Checking, Repeating (routine activities), Counting, Ordering, Hoarding, Need to Tell or Ask, Need to Touch, Tap, or Rub, and Self-Damaging or Self-Mutilating behaviors].

Most patients of both diagnostic groups reported repetitive thoughts and behavior of multiple categories. Incidence and types of repetitive thoughts and behavior are displayed in Figure 13-1. Repetitive thoughts most commonly endorsed by the autistic group were, in descending order, Need to Know or Remember, Hoarding, and Contamination. The three most common types of obsessions present in the OCD group were Aggressive, Contamination, and Symmetry. Repetitive behavior most commonly reported by the autistic group involved Repeating, Need to Touch, Tap, or Rub, Ordering, and Hoarding. On the whole, the autistic patients endorsed more repetitive behavior than repetitive thoughts. The three most frequently reported compulsions in the OCD group were Checking, Cleaning, and Repeating. Eighteen of the autistic patients had

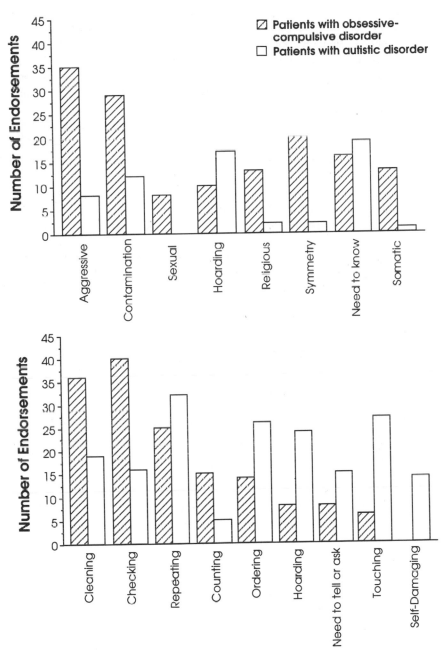

Fig. 13-1. Repetitive thoughts (top) and behavior (bottom) reported by autistic ($N = 50$) and obsessive-compulsive ($N = 50$) patients. From the *American Journal of Psychiatry, 152,* 772–777, 1995. Copyright 1995 by the American Psychiatric Association. Reprinted by permission.

repetitive behavior alone, 32 had both repetitive thoughts and behavior, and none had only repetitive thoughts. Of the 35 verbal patients, it was determined that only 8 patients made an active effort to suppress their thoughts and to resist their repetitive behavior. Forty-five of the OCD patients had both obsessions and compulsions, 4 had obsessions alone, and 1 had only compulsions. In 47 of the 50 cases, the obsessions and compulsions were experienced as excessive or unreasonable and the patient attempted to suppress the thoughts and resist the behavior.

Discriminant function analysis indicated that the autistic and OCD patients exhibited different patterns of repetitive thoughts and behavior (see Table 13-1). Two obsession variables (Aggressive and Symmetry) and five compulsion variables (Checking, Counting, Hoarding, Need to Touch, Tap, or Rub, and Self-Damaging or Self-Mutilating behaviors) together maximally separated the autism and OCD groups. The autism group was less likely to have Aggressive and Symmetry obsessions and Checking and Counting compulsions, and more likely to have compulsions categorized as Hoarding, Need to Touch, Tap, or Rub, and Self-Damaging or Self-Mutilating behaviors.

Table 13-1. Results of Direct Discriminant Function Analysis of Yale–Brown Obsessive Compulsive Scale Symptom Checklist Variables

Name of symptom category	Univariate F (1,98)	Univariate p	Relationship with autism group[a]
Repetitive thoughts			
Aggressive	41.49	0.0001	−
Contamination	13.30	0.0004	−
Sexual	9.33	0.003	−
Hoarding	2.5	0.12	+
Religious	10.28	0.002	−
Symmetry	22.81	0.0001	−
Need to know	0.39	0.53	+
Somatic	13.31	0.0004	−
Repetitive behavior			
Cleaning	12.96	0.0005	−
Checking	29.90	0.0001	−
Repeating	2.00	0.16	+
Counting	6.53	0.012	−
Ordering	6.26	0.014	+
Hoarding	13.07	0.0005	+
Need to tell or ask	2.79	0.098	+
Touching	24.42	0.0001	+
Self-damaging	19.06	0.0001	+

Note. From the *American Journal of Psychiatry*, *152*, 772–777, 1995. Copyright 1995 by the American Psychiatric Association. Reprinted by permission.
[a] −, inverse relationship with the autism group; +, positive relationship with the autism group.

SUMMARY AND DISCUSSION OF PHENOMENOLOGY

The results of this study indicate that adults with autistic disorder and OCD can be distinguished on the basis of their current types of repetitive thoughts and behavior. Compared with the OCD group, the autistic patients were significantly less likely to experience thoughts with Aggressive, Contamination, Sexual, Religious, Symmetry, and Somatic thematic content (Table 13-1). Repetitive Ordering, Hoarding, Telling or Asking (trend), Touching, Tapping, or Rubbing, and Self-Damaging or Self-Mutilating behaviors occurred significantly more frequently in the autistic patients, whereas Cleaning, Checking, and Counting behaviors were less common in the autistic group compared with the OCD patients (Table 13-1).

Not surprisingly, the autistic adults had more "compulsions" than "obsessions," and no autistic patient had "obsessions" alone. Similarly, a study of children with OCD found that compulsions rather than obsessions were more frequently the presenting complaint, and that "pure" obsessives were rare compared with the more frequent "pure" compulsives (Rapoport, Swedo, & Leonard, 1992). Whereas compulsions are a readily observable behavioral component, obsessions reflect an awareness of and ability to articulate intrusive thoughts and ideas. It may be that many autistic patients and children with OCD have not developed the cognitive capacity to perceive and describe repetitive thoughts. Indeed, the probable significant difference in full-scale IQ scores between the autistic and OCD patients in this study may account for some of the disparity in the incidence and types of repetitive thoughts and behavior that were identified.

The results of this study seem to confirm that the types of repetitive thoughts and behavior of autistic and OCD adults are significantly different. The repetitive behavior identified in the autistic group was, in general, less well organized and complex than that of the OCD patients. Functional gaps in cognitive abilities, level of awareness, or an ability to communicate well, might have contributed to the divergent clinical manifestations of repetitive thoughts and behavior between these two groups. The present findings will require cross-validation in new samples of patients in order to exclude the possibility that the observed differences in symptoms between groups were not unique to these particular samples. In addition, because the stereotyped behaviors of autistic patients have been shown to be more common in unstructured than structured settings (Volkmar, Hoder, & Cohen, 1985), this situational specificity is worthy of study in future investigations. Until additional studies are undertaken, caution should also be raised against generalizing these results to children with autism and OCD.

Because a DSM-IV diagnosis of OCD depends on the ego-dystonic quality of obsessive thoughts or compulsive behavior, in the absence of communication about a corresponding internal mental or emotional state, the repetitive actions of most autistic individuals currently do not meet criteria for OCD. For young children, however, DSM-IV waives the criterion that the person recognizes that his or her behavior is excessive or unreasonable. Perhaps the repetitive behavior of cognitively handicapped individuals, like many autistic patients, should be treated in a similar manner. Furthermore, preliminary data indicate that SUIs (McDougle, 1997) and behavior therapy (Lindley, Marks, Philpott, & Snowden, 1977), the mainstays of treatment for primary OCD (Foa, 1979; McDougle, Goodman, Leckman, & Price, 1993), may reduce the repetitive behavior of some autistic patients.

PHARMACOTHERAPY

Although little is definitively known regarding the pathophysiology of the syndrome of autism, abnormalities in the 5-HT neurotransmitter system have been identified in a subset of patients (Ciaranello & Ciaranello, 1995). Schain and Freedman (1961) were the first to report elevated levels of whole-blood 5-HT (WBS) in the peripheral vascular system of autistic children. Others have replicated this finding in groups of autistic children compared with normal controls (Anderson et al., 1987). Antibodies against human brain 5-HT receptors were identified in the blood and cerebrospinal fluid (CSF) of a child with autism (Todd & Ciaranello, 1985), although subsequent studies found no difference in the degree of immunoglobulin inhibition of binding of the 5-HT1A receptor agonist [^{3}H]-8-hydroxy-N,N-dipropyl-2-aminotetralin to 5-HT1A receptors between autistic patients and controls (Cook, Perry, Dawson, Wainwright, & Leventhal, 1993; Yuwiler et al., 1992). Blunted neuroendocrine responses to pharmacological probes of the 5-HT system have been observed in autistic children (Hoshino et al., 1984) and adults (McBride et al., 1989) compared with normal subjects. Finally, acute dietary depletion of the 5-HT precursor tryptophan has been associated with an exacerbation of behavioral symptoms in drug-free autistic adults (McDougle, Naylor, Cohen, Aghajanian, et al., 1996). Based on evidence implicating a dysregulation in 5-HT function in some patients with autism, drugs that affect this system have been studied (McDougle, 1997).

The clear efficacy of potent SUIs, such as clomipramine (Greist, Jefferson, Kobak, Katzelnick, & Serlin, 1995), fluvoxamine (Goodman, Price, Rasmussen, Delgado, et al., 1989), fluoxetine (Tollefson et al., 1994), sertraline (Greist, Chouinard, et al., 1995), and paroxetine (Wheadon, Bushnell, & Steiner, 1993), has been established in double-blind studies in adult patients with primary OCD. Consistent with these drug response data are the hypotheses that changes in 5-HT function are critical to the treatment of OCD and perhaps involved in the pathophysiology of at least some patients with the disorder (McDougle et al., 1993). The differential efficacy of the SUIs, when directly compared with agents that inhibit norepinephrine (NE) uptake (Goodman, Price, et al., 1990; Leonard,

Swedo, Rapoport, Coffey, & Cheslow, 1989; Zohar & Insel, 1987), supports the hypothesized importance of 5-HT in the treatment of obsessive-compulsive symptoms. Results from pharmacological challenge studies employing *m*-chlorophenylpiperazine (Hollander et al., 1991; Zohar, Insel, Zohar-Kadouch, Hill, & Murphy, 1988) and metergoline (Benkelfat *et al.*, 1989) in OCD patients improved following SUI treatment suggest that SUIs may "stabilize" dysregulated 5-HT neuronal function. Although inconsistent, a relationship between SUI-induced changes in biological markers of the 5-HT system and drug treatment response has been identified in some studies involving OCD patients (Flament, Rapoport, Murphy, Berg, & Lake, 1987; Thoren, Asberg, Cronholm, Jornestedt, & Traskman, 1980).

Based on the efficacy of SUIs in the treatment of obsessive-compulsive symptoms in patients with OCD, the high prevalence of interfering repetitive thoughts and behavior in patients with PDD, and the hypothesis that 5-HT may contribute to the pathophysiology of some patients with PDD, investigators have been examining the clinical response and side effect profile of SUIs in children, adolescents, and adults with PDD.

CLOMIPRAMINE

Clomipramine is a nonselective tricyclic agent that has been shown in double-blind, placebo-controlled trials to be efficacious in the treatment of OCD (Greist, Jefferson, *et al.*, 1995). Although clomipramine affects NE and dopamine (DA) neuronal uptake, its most potent action is to inhibit 5-HT uptake.

In the first published controlled study of clomipramine in autism, Gordon, State, Nelson, Hamburger, and Rapoport (1993) found clomipramine (152±56 mg/day) superior to the relatively selective NE uptake inhibitor desipramine (127+52 mg/day) and placebo in a 10-week (5 weeks on each drug or placebo), randomized, crossover study in children with autism (mean age, 9.6 years). In the comparison of clomipramine with placebo, significant improvement was found in the core symptoms of autism, anger/uncooperativeness, hyperactivity, and "obsessive-compulsive" symptoms. When clomipramine was compared with desipramine, significant changes in the core symptoms of autism, anger/uncooperativeness, and "obsessive-compulsive" symptoms were also observed. There was no significant difference between the two drugs in the treatment of hyperactivity. Adverse effects from clomipramine included prolongation of the corrected QT interval, tachycardia, and a grand mal seizure, whereas irritability, temper outbursts, and uncharacteristic aggression were seen with desipramine.

A number of open-label trials of clomipramine in children, adolescents, and adults with PDD have also been reported. The Yale group found that four of five young adults with a DSM-III-R diagnosis of autism presenting with disturbances in social relatedness, repetitive thoughts and behavior, and/or impulsive aggression had a significant improvement in symptomatology with open-label clomipramine treatment (McDougle *et al.*, 1992). The fifth patient remained unchanged. Up to 12 weeks of treatment with clomipramine was necessary in some cases before appreciable change occurred. The dose of clomipramine in the four responders ranged from 75 to 250 mg/day, with a mean dose of 185 mg/day. Other than dry mouth in two cases, the patients tolerated the drug well and had no adverse effects. Four patients showed a significant improvement in social interaction, three demonstrated a clinically meaningful decrease in aggression, and four had a significant reduction in repetitive behavior with clomipramine treatment.

In a study by Garber, McGonigle, Slomka, and Monteverde (1992) involving patients with mental retardation, autism, and cerebral palsy, 10 of 11 patients (age range 10–20 years) had a marked decrease in stereotypies and self-injurious behavior with clomipramine (mean dose 70±37 mg/day). Although 6 of the patients had histories of seizures (4 were maintained on anticonvulsants during clomipramine treatment), none had seizures during the trial. Side effects included hypomania, constipation, sedation, enuresis, worsening of stereotypy, new-onset aggression, and rash. Brasic *et al.* (1994) reported that clomipramine (200 mg/day) reduced repetitive behavior, including abnormal movements and compulsions, in 5 prepubertal boys with autistic disorder and severe mental retardation. A discussion of side effects was not included. In contrast, in a study by Sanchez *et al.* (1996), clomipramine led to significant clinical improvement in only 1 of 8 autistic children and was associated with significant untoward effects, including urinary retention, constipation, and behavioral toxicity. The authors suggested that autistic children may be more prone to develop side effects with clomipramine than older patients. We recently completed the first systematic study of clomipramine in adults with PDDs (Brodkin, McDougle, Naylor, Cohen, & Price, 1997). Thirty-five subjects (24 men and 11 women) who met DSM-IV criteria for PDD entered a 12-week open-label trial of clomipramine. The mean age of the group was 30.2 years (range 18–44 years). Fifteen of the patients had autistic disorder, 8 had Asperger's disorder, and 12 met criteria for PDD Not Otherwise Specified (NOS). Clomipramine was begun at 50 mg/day and dosage was increased by 50 mg/week to a maximum dose of 250 mg/day, based on clinical response and side effects. Behavioral measures of global improvement, repetitive thoughts and behavior, aggression, and social relatedness were obtained at baseline and then every 4 weeks throughout the trial.

Eighteen (55%) of the thirty-three adult patients with PDD who completed the trial were rated as responders after 12 weeks of open-label treatment with clomipramine. Clomipramine was effective in improving social relatedness, as measured by subscales II and V of the Ritvo–Freeman Scale (Freeman, Ritvo, Yokota, & Ritvo, 1986), and in reducing aggression and interfering repetitive thoughts and behavior. These improvements were not only detected by rating scales, but also led to an appreciable improvement in the quality of life for a substantial number of patients.

Some variability in symptom presentation between patients with different diagnostic categories of PDD was identified in this study. Those patients with Asperger's disorder had a higher mean total Y–BOCS score, a higher mean Y–BOCS obsession subscale score, and fewer symptoms of language impairment (as measured by subscale V of the Ritvo–Freeman Scale) relative to patients with autistic disorder and PDD-NOS. These findings may reflect the Asperger's disorder patients' relatively preserved language development and superior capability of reporting repetitive thoughts. As measured by the Ritvo–Freeman subscale II (Social Relationship to People), patients with Asperger's disorder were less impaired than those with autistic disorder and PDD-NOS. However, there were no significant differences among the three diagnostic subtypes in the pattern of symptomatic change or in global treatment response to clomipramine.

Clomipramine was well-tolerated by the majority of patients, with 22 of 35 patients having no significant side effects. However, 13 patients had clinically significant adverse effects. Three patients had seizures. Of these 3, 1 had tuberous sclerosis and an associated generalized seizure disorder. He was maintained on carbamazepine yet had a tonic–clonic seizure during the study. The second patient had an absence seizure disorder and was maintained on phenobarbital and carbamazepine. He had an increase in the frequency of absence seizures while receiving clomipramine (in addition to experiencing sedation and weight gain). The third patient had no previous history of seizures but had a tonic–clonic seizure during the study. The two patients with preexisting seizure disorders had the support of their neurologists and parents for participation in the trial, despite the risk of worsening seizures, because of the magnitude of their interfering behaviors. No adverse cardiovascular or extrapyramidal effects were observed.

Because of the potential efficacy and relative tolerability of clomipramine demonstrated in this study, controlled trials of clomipramine appear warranted in adults with PDDs. Close clinical monitoring for side effects should occur, however, particularly for those patients with known seizure disorders. These results should not be generalized to include children and adolescents with PDDs. Trials of tricyclic antidepressants in children should be undertaken only with caution because of the risk of cardiovascular toxicity (Gordon et al., 1993; Riddle, Geller, & Ryan, 1993). Based on a potentially better side effect profile, including no significant effects on the seizure threshold or on cardiac conduction, controlled studies of selective SUIs should be conducted in children, adolescents, and adults with PDDs.

FLUVOXAMINE

Fluvoxamine is a potent and selective SUI that has little or no affinity for 5-HT, DA, adrenergic, histaminic, or muscarinic receptors, and no known clinically active metabolites (Benfield & Ward, 1986). Its *in vitro* potency for blocking 5-HT uptake is equivalent to that of clomipramine, and it causes minimal inhibition of DA or NE uptake. Fluvoxamine has been shown to be effective in the treatment of refractory depression (Delgado, Price, Charney, & Heninger, 1988), and more efficacious than placebo (Goodman, Price, Rasmussen, Delgado, *et al.*, 1989) and desipramine (Goodman, Price, *et al.*, 1990) in the treatment of OCD. Importantly, a recent controlled study found fluvoxamine more effective than placebo in the treatment of social phobia (van Vliet, den Boer, & Westenberg, 1994), a disorder that may occur more frequently in first-degree relatives of autistic probands than in relatives of control probands (Smalley, McCracken, & Tanguay, 1995).

In the first report to describe the use of an SUI in autistic disorder, our group found fluvoxamine effective in the treatment of a 30-year-old man with autism and comorbid OCD (McDougle, Price, & Goodman, 1990). The patient had become obsessed with having the fingernails on each hand trimmed and manicured exactly the same as the corresponding nail on the opposite hand. He would typically spend up to 12 to 15 hours a day attending to his nails. If a hangnail or scab developed, the patient would gouge the opposite hand, to the point of bleeding, in order to "even it up." He realized that this behavior was excessive and irrational, but felt he had to perform the rituals in order to avoid the emergence of extreme anxiety. In addition, the patient had frequent aggressive outbursts, often resulting in physical injury to family members. He was extremely withdrawn socially and had no friends. After treatment with fluvoxamine up to 150 mg/day, the patient showed a significant reduction in obsessive-compulsive symptoms and aggressivity. His parents reported the emergence of a desire to pursue social relationships, improved interpersonal interaction, and less withdrawal from human contact.

We recently completed the first double-blind, placebo-controlled investigation of fluvoxamine in patients with autistic disorder (McDougle, Naylor, Cohen, Volkmar, *et al.*, 1996). The sample consisted of 27 men and 3 women aged 18–53 years (mean, 30.1 years) with a diagnosis of autistic disorder based on DSM-III-R, Autism Diagnostic Interview (Le Couteur *et al.*, 1989), and Autism Diagnostic Observation Schedule (Lord *et al.*, 1989) criteria. Each patient's symptoms were at least "moderate" in severity, as defined by global severity of illness rating on the Clinical Global Impression Scale (CGI) (Guy, 1976). The Autism Behavior Checklist (ABC) (Krug, Arick, & Almond, 1980) was completed with the parent or legal guardian of each patient to determine the patient's level of autistic behavior. Full-scale IQ was measured with the WAIS-R in the 26 verbal patients, whereas the Leiter International Performance Scale was used to assess IQ in the 4 nonverbal patients. Patients were psychotropic drug-free for at least 4 weeks prior to the start of the trial. One male patient had fragile X syndrome, whereas none of the other patients had a diagnosed genetic, metabolic, or neurological etiology for their syndrome.

After baseline behavioral ratings were obtained, patients were randomized to 12 weeks of double-blind treatment with fluvoxamine or placebo. The drug was started at 50 mg every night and the dosage was then increased by 50 mg daily every 3 or 4 days to a maximum dosage of 300 mg/day. Thus, the maximum dosage of fluvoxamine was attained within 3 weeks and patients received this dose for a minimum of 9 weeks.

Behavioral ratings were obtained every 4 weeks throughout the 12-week study. Repetitive thoughts and behavior were rated with a modified version of the Y–BOCS, a 10-item, semistructured, clinician-rated questionnaire that is valid and reliable for assessing the severity of obsessive-compulsive symptoms in patients with OCD. Based on previous findings (McDougle et al., 1995), the ego-dystonic-ity diagnostic criterion for OCD was eliminated in rating the repetitive thoughts and behavior of the autistic patients. Aggression was rated with a modified version of the Brown Aggression Scale, a 9-category instrument that assesses different aspects of aggressive behavior (Brown, Goodwin, Ballenger, Goyer, & Major, 1979). The Ritvo Freeman Real Life Rating Scale served as an in vivo observational measure of a variety of symptoms of autism, including sensory motor behaviors, social relationship to people, affectual reactions, sensory responses, and language. The Vineland Adaptive Behavior Scale (Sparrow, Balla, & Cicchetti, 1984) Maladaptive Behavior Subscales (Parts 1 and 2) were also administered at each assessment time point. Finally, the CGI global improvement item (7= "very much worse" to 1= "very much improved") was recorded at each rating session following the baseline period. Treatment response was determined by scores obtained at the end of the last week of the study on the global improvement item of the CGI. Patients with CGI scores of "much improved" or "very much improved" were categorized as responders. All 30 patients completed the 12-week study and were thus included in the efficacy analysis. Fifteen patients were randomized to fluvoxamine and 15 received placebo. There was no significant difference in dosage between patients random ized to fluvoxamine (276.7±41.7 mg/day) versus placebo (283.3±36.2 mg/day). The fluvoxamine group (age, 30.1±7.1 years) contained 2 women and 13 men, whereas the placebo group (age, 30.1±8.4 years) consisted of 1 woman and 14 men. There were no significant differences in age, gender distribution, ABC scores, or full-scale IQ scores between the two groups.

Ratings on the CGI showed fluvoxamine superior to placebo beginning at week 4 and continuing at weeks 8 and 12 (Figure 13-2). Eight out of fifteen (53%) of the fluvoxamine patients were categorized as responders compared with 0/15 in the placebo group. Treatment response was not correlated with age, level of autistic behavior, or full-scale IQ.

As measured by reduction in total Y–BOCS scores, fluvoxamine was superior to placebo in the treatment of repetitive thoughts and behavior beginning at week 8 and continuing at week 12 of treatment (Figure 13-3). Fluvoxamine was more effective than placebo in reducing Y–BOCS subscale scores for both repetitive thoughts and repetitive behavior.

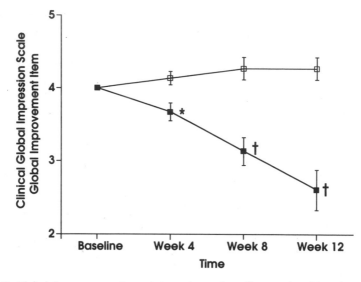

Fig. 13-2. Global improvement in autistic patients given fluvoxamine (closed squares) or placebo (open squares) for 12 weeks, as measured on the Clinical Global Impression Scale global improvement item. *p <.006, change from beginning of treatment trial, fluvoxamine versus placebo, Student's t test; [†]p <.0001, change from beginning of treatment trial, fluvoxamine versus placebo, Student's t test. Variance bars represent standard error.

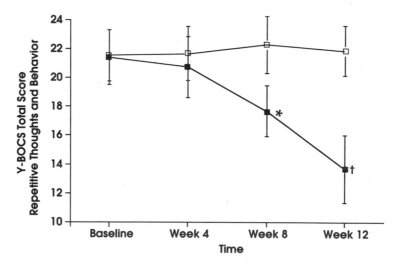

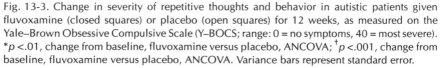

Fig. 13-3. Change in severity of repetitive thoughts and behavior in autistic patients given fluvoxamine (closed squares) or placebo (open squares) for 12 weeks, as measured on the Yale–Brown Obsessive Compulsive Scale (Y–BOCS; range: 0 = no symptoms, 40 = most severe). *p <.01, change from baseline, fluvoxamine versus placebo, ANCOVA; [†]p <.001, change from baseline, fluvoxamine versus placebo, ANCOVA. Variance bars represent standard error.

On the Vineland Maladaptive Behavior Subscales (Parts 1 and 2), fluvoxamine was more effective than placebo beginning at week 4 and continuing through weeks 8 and 12. As measured by total score on the Brown Aggression Scale, fluvoxamine was also superior to placebo in reducing aggression beginning at week 4 and continuing through weeks 8 and 12.

Fluvoxamine was superior to placebo in improving the behavioral symptoms of autistic disorder as measured by the Ritvo-Freeman Scale overall score. There was a trend for fluvoxamine to be superior to placebo beginning after 8 weeks. Following 12 weeks, fluvoxamine was significantly better than placebo. In particular, fluvoxamine was superior to placebo in improving language usage (subscale V) beginning at week 4 and continuing at weeks 8 and 12.

Fluvoxamine was well-tolerated, with no medically significant adverse events. Four patients reported nausea (three on active drug, one on placebo) during the first 2 weeks, but they developed tolerance and were able to continue. Three different patients developed moderate sedation (two on active drug, one on placebo), which also resolved. No anticholinergic side effects developed and no significant changes in pulse or sitting and standing blood pressure occurred. No laboratory or electrocardiographic changes could be attributed to fluvoxamine. No dyskinesias, adverse cardiovascular events, or seizures occurred. The lack of seizures with fluvoxamine is noteworthy, as nearly one-third of autistic patients develop seizures at some point in their lifetime (Volkmar & Nelson, 1990).

To date, there have been no published reports describing the use of fluvoxamine in autistic children and adolescents. Our preliminary experience suggests that fluvoxamine may be more effective for reducing interfering behaviors in adolescents than in prepubertal autistic children. In addition, our preliminary results indicate that fluvoxamine may be better tolerated by adolescents and adults with PDD than children.

FLUOXETINE

Fluoxetine is a potent and selective SUI that has been shown in double-blind, placebo-controlled investigations to be effective in the treatment of OCD (Tollefson et al., 1994). Preliminary open-label studies and case reports suggest that fluoxetine may be useful in the treatment of some patients with autistic disorder (Cook, Rowlett, Jaselskis, & Leventhal, 1992; Ghaziuddin, Tsai, & Ghaziuddin, 1991; Hamdan-Allen, 1991; Mehlinger, Scheftner, & Poznanski, 1990; Todd, 1991).

Mehlinger et al. (1990) reported that fluoxetine 20 mg every other day was useful in reducing ritualistic behavior and in improving mood in a 26-year-old autistic woman. Hamdan-Allen (1991) described marked improvement in trichotillomania (chronic hair-pulling) in an 18-year-old man with autism who had been resistant to a 6-month trial of imipramine at therapeutic blood levels. Todd (1991) reported that three of four patients with autism showed a significant reduction in ritualistic behavior or increased tolerance of changes in routine with fluoxetine treatment. Ghaziuddin *et al.* (1991) found fluoxetine 20–40 mg/day effective in reducing depressive symptoms in adolescents with autistic disorder, although many of the core features of autism remained unchanged.

In a larger open-label case series, Cook *et al.* (1992) found that fluoxetine in doses ranging from 20 mg every other day to 80 mg/day led to significant improvement in subjects with autistic disorder and in subjects with mental retardation without autism. The autistic subjects ranged in age from 7 to 28 years (mean, 15.9 years) and those with mental retardation ranged in age from 4.8 to 52 years (mean, 21 years). Subjects with autism and those with mental retardation had been treated with fluoxetine for approximately 6 months at the time of rating. In subjects with autistic disorder, fluoxetine led to an improvement in CGI severity scale scores in 15/23 subjects. Ten of sixteen mentally retarded subjects had an improvement of 1 point or more on CGI overall severity ratings including improvement in impulse control, attention span, and ability to tolerate frustration. Six of twenty-three subjects with autism and 3/16 subjects with mental retardation had side effects consisting primarily of restlessness, hyperactivity, agitation, decreased appetite, and insomnia.

SERTRALINE

Sertraline is a potent and selective SUI that has been shown in double-blind, placebo-controlled studies to be effective in the treatment of OCD (Greist, Chouinard, *et al.*, 1995). Results from our group suggest that sertraline may be useful for improving symptoms of aggression and repetitive behavior in some adults with PDDs, including autism (McDougle *et al.*, 1998). In an open-label study, 24/42 (57%) adults were rated as "much" or "very much improved" on the global improvement item of the CGI following 12 weeks of treatment with sertraline (50–200 mg/day). Five patients ended the trial prematurely because of the emergence of interfering anxiety (N=3), syncope (N=1), and noncompliance (N=1), respectively. No other significant side effects or adverse reactions occurred.

In an open-label study involving children (6–12 years old) with autism and transition-related behavioral deterioration, eight of nine patients showed a clinically significant improvement in response to sertraline (Steingard, Zimnitzky, DeMaso, Bauman, & Bucci, 1997). Dosages of sertaline were low in all cases (25–50 mg/day), and clinical response generally occurred within 2–8 weeks. Adverse effects were minimal (one child developed stomachaches), except for possible sertraline-induced behavioral worsening in two children when their doses were raised to 75 mg per day. In three children, the initial favorable clinical response appeared to diminish after 3–7 months of treatment.

SUMMARY AND DISCUSSION OF PHARMACOTHERAPY

Brain 5-HT has been hypothesized to be involved in modulating repetitive thoughts and behavior. Although the types, frequency, and quality of repetitive thoughts and behavior of age- and sex-matched adults with OCD and autistic disorder have been shown to be different (McDougle et al., 1995), these interfering symptoms often improve with SUI treatment in both diagnostic groups (McDougle, 1997; McDougle et al., 1993). Given the adaptive changes in receptor function that occur during chronic administration of SUIs, coupled with the delayed onset of improvement in repetitive thoughts and behavior in OCD (Goodman, Price, Rasmussen, Delgado, et al., 1989) and autistic patients (McDougle, Naylor, Cohen, Volkmar, et al., 1996), it is unclear what changes in 5-HT function are ultimately associated with improvement in these symptoms. It may be that variation in the time course of 5-HT receptor adaptation in neuroanatomical regions hypothesized to subserve repetitive thoughts and behavior contributes to this delayed response to SUIs. For example, El Mansari, Bouchard, and Blier (1994) showed that 8 but not 3 weeks of treatment with the selective SUI paroxetine enhanced 5-HT release, secondary to desensitization of the 5-HT autoreceptor, in the orbitofrontal cortex of guinea pigs. Alternatively, the SUIs may act indirectly on another system more closely tied to the pathophysiology of the disorders (e.g., DA), or they may compensate for dysfunction in one system by enhancing function of a different intact system (Goodman, McDougle, et al., 1990). In any case, central 5-HT appears to be significantly involved in the treatment of repetitive thoughts and behavior, if not the pathophysiology. A summary of results from available studies of potent SUIs in children, adolescents, and adults with PDDs, including relative efficacy and potential adverse effects, is presented in Table 13-2.

CONCLUSIONS

The purpose of this chapter was to describe the phenomenology of repetitive thoughts and behavior in individuals with PDD, and to review the pharmacological management of these often interfering symptoms. The results of a case-controlled study designed to determine the types and frequency of current repetitive thoughts and behavior in adults with autistic disorder and OCD were presented. The study revealed that adults with autism can be distinguished from those with OCD on the basis of their current types of repetitive thoughts and behavior. Studies designed to compare repetitive thoughts and behavior in children and adolescents with autism and OCD, as well as studies to determine the types and frequency of these phenomena in subtypes of PDD, such as Asperger's disorder, have not been published to date.

Table 13-2. Serotonin Uptake Inhibitors in Pervasive Developmental Disorders

Drug	Reference	Study design	N	Age (years)	Dose (mg/day)	Duration (weeks)	Efficacy	Adverse effects
Clomipramine (Anafranil®)	Gordon et al. (1993)	Double-blind crossover	12 vs. DMI; 12 vs. PLA	Range, 6–18; mean, 9.7	152 ± 56	5	CMI>DMI; CMI>PLA for stereotypies, anger, rituals; CMI = DMI>PLA for hyperactivity	Insomnia, constipation, sedation, twitching, EKG changes ($N = 1$), tachycardia ($N = 2$), grand mal seizure ($N = 1$)
	McDougle et al. (1992)	Open-label	5	Range, 13–33; mean, 25.2	185 ± 7	12	4/5 patients showed improved social relatedness and reduced repetitive behavior and aggression	Dry mouth
	Garber et al. (1992)	Open-label	11 (4 with autism)	Range, 10–20; mean, 15	70 ± 37	4–52	10/11 patients had 50% reduction in SIB and stereotypies	Hypomania, constipation, sedation, enuresis, aggression
	Brasic et al. (1994)	Open-label	5	Range, 6–12; mean, 9.4	200 ± 0.0	8–78	5/5 patients showed reduced "adventitious movements" and "compulsions"	Not reported

Drug	Reference	Study design	N	Age (years)	Dose (mg/day)	Duration (weeks)	Efficacy	Adverse effects
	Brodkin et al. (1997)	Open-label	35	Range, 18–44; mean, 30.2	139 ± 50	12	18/35 patients "much improved" or "very much improved," with reduced repetitive behavior, aggression, and echolalia	Constipation, sedation, weight gain, seizures ($N = 3$)
	Sanchez et al. (1996)	Open-label	8	Range, 3.5–8.7; mean, 6.4	103.6	5	7 patients worse, 1 moderately improved	Urinary retention, constipation, insomnia, sedation, aggression
Fluvoxamine (Luvox®)	McDougle et al. (1996)	Double-blind parallel groups	30	Range, 18–35; mean, 30.1	277 ± 42	12	8/15 patients "much improved" or very much improved" on fluvoxamine, 0/15 improved on placebo; reduced repetitive behavior and aggression and improved language usage	Nausea, sedation

(continued)

Table 13-2. (Continued)

Drug	Reference	Study design	N	Age (years)	Dose (mg/day)	Duration (weeks)	Efficacy	Adverse effects
Fluoxetine (Prozac®)	Cook et al. (1992)	Open-label	23	Range, 7.0–28.8; mean 15.9	28.3	26	15/23 patients had an improvement of 1 or more on CGI severity rating; reduced rituals and aggression, better eye contact	Agitation, hyperactivity, insomnia, "elated affect," decreased appetite, increased screaming
Sertraline (Zoloft®)	McDougle et al., (1998)	Open-label	42	Range, 18–39; mean, 26.1	122 ± 61	12	24/42 patients "much improved" or "very much improved"; improvement seen in repetitive behavior and aggression	Agitation, headaches, reduced appetite, sedation, weight gain
	Steingard et al. (1997)	Open-label	9	Range, 6–12; mean, 8.6	55.6	2–52	8/9 patients showed some degree of positive response; improvement seen in anxiety, depressed mood, explosive outbursts, and social interaction	Agitation, mild stomach discomfort

Note. N, number of subjects; CMI, clomipramine; DMI, desipramine; PLA, placebo; SIB, self-injurious behavior; CGI, Clinical Global Impression Scale.

The efficacy of potent SUIs, including clomipramine, fluvoxamine, fluoxetine, sertraline, and paroxetine, has clearly been established in patients with primary OCD. Preliminary investigations suggest that this class of drugs may also be effective in reducing interfering thoughts and behavior in some patients with PDD. Some of these studies indicate that the SUIs may be more efficacious and better tolerated in adolescents and adults with PDD than in children. These clinical observations of developmental differences in drug treatment response and tolerability may be reflective of the significant changes in 5-HT function that occur during ongoing brain development. Future research should include double-blind, placebo-controlled studies of the SUIs in prepubertal versus postpubertal individuals with PDD, as well as studies designed to determine the effect of these drugs on the repetitive thoughts and behavior of patients with different subtypes of PDD, including Asperger's disorder.

REFERENCES

American Psychiatric Association. (1994). *Diagnostic and statistical manual of mental disorders* (4th ed.). Washington, DC: Author.

Anderson, G. M., Freedman, D. X., Cohen, D. J., Volkmar, F. R., Hoder, E. L., McPhedran, P., Minderaa, R. B., Hansen, C. R., & Young, J. G. (1987). Whole blood serotonin in autistic and normal subjects. *Journal of Child Psychology and Psychiatry, 28*, 885–900.

Baron-Cohen, S. (1989). Do autistic children have obsessions and compulsions? *British Journal of Clinical Psychology, 28*, 193–200.

Benfield, P., & Ward, A. (1986). Fluvoxamine: A review of its pharmacodynamic and pharmacokinetic properties, and therapeutic efficacy in depressive illness. *Drugs, 32*, 313–334.

Benkelfat, C., Murphy, D. L., Zohar, J., Hill, J. L., Grover, G., & Insel, T. R. (1989). Clomipramine in obsessive–compulsive disorder: Further evidence for a serotonergic mechanism of action. *Archives of General Psychiatry, 46*, 23–28.

Brasic, J. R., Barnett, J. Y., Kaplan, D., Sheitman, B. B., Aisemberg, P., Lafargue, R. T., Kowalik, S., Clark, A., Tsaltas, M. O., & Young, J. G. (1994). Clomipramine ameliorates adventitious movements and compulsions in prepubertal boys with autistic disorder and severe mental retardation. *Neurology, 44*, 1309–1312.

Brodkin, E. S., McDougle, C. J., Naylor, S. T., Cohen, D. J., & Price, L. H. (1997). Clomipramine in adults with pervasive developmental disorders: A prospective open-label investigation. *Journal of Child and Adolescent Psychopharmacology, 7*, 109–121.

Brown, G. L., Goodwin, F. K., Ballenger, J. C., Goyer, P. F., & Major, L. F. (1979). Aggression in humans correlates with cerebrospinal fluid amine metabolites. *Psychiatry Research, 1*, 131–139.

Ciaranello, A. L., & Ciaranello, R. D. (1995). The neurobiology of infantile autism. *Annual Review of Neuroscience, 18*, 101–128.

Cook, E. H., Jr., Perry, B. D., Dawson, G., Wainwright, M. S., & Leventhal, B. L. (1993). Receptor inhibition by immunoglobulins: Specific inhibition by autistic children, their relatives, and control subjects. *Journal of Autism and Developmental Disorders, 23*, 67–78.

Cook, E. H., Jr., Rowlett, R., Jaselskis, C., & Leventhal, B. L. (1992). Fluoxetine treatment of children and adults with autistic disorder and mental retardation. *Journal of the American Academy of Child and Adolescent Psychiatry, 31*, 739–745.

Delgado, P. L., Price, L. H., Charney, D. S., & Heninger, G. R. (1988). Efficacy of fluvoxamine in treatment-resistant depression. *Journal of Affective Disorders, 15*, 55–60.

El Mansari, M., Bouchard, C., & Blier, P. (1994). Alteration of serotonin release in the orbito-frontal cortex by paroxetine. Relevance to obsessive–compulsive disorder. *Proceedings of the Society for Neuroscience, 20*(1), 226.

Flament, M. F., Rapoport, J. L., Murphy, D. L., Berg, C. J., & Lake, C. R. (1987). Biochemical changes during clomipramine treatment of childhood obsessive–compulsive disorder. *Archives of General Psychiatry, 44*, 219–225.

Foa, E. B. (1979). Failures in treating obsessive–compulsives. *Behavioral Research and Therapy, 7*, 169–176.

Freeman, B. J., Ritvo, E. R., Yokota, A., & Ritvo, A. (1986). A scale for rating symptoms of patients with the syndrome of autism in real life settings. *Journal of the American Academy of Child and Adolescent Psychiatry, 25*, 130–136.

Garber, H. J., McGonigle, J. J., Slomka, G. T., & Monteverde, E. (1992). Clomipramine treatment of stereotypic behaviors and self-injury in patients with developmental disabilities. *Journal of the American Academy of Child and Adolescent Psychiatry, 31*, 1157–1160.

Ghaziuddin, M., Tsai, L., & Ghaziuddin, N. (1991). Fluoxetine in autism with depression [Letter]. *Journal of the American Academy of Child and Adolescent Psychiatry, 30*, 3.

Goodman, W. K., McDougle, C. J., Price, L. H., Riddle, M. A., Pauls, D. L., & Leckman, J. F. (1990). Beyond the serotonin hypothesis: A role for dopamine in some forms of obsessive compulsive disorder? *Journal of Clinical Psychiatry, 51*(Suppl. 8), 36–43.

Goodman, W. K., Price, L. H., Delgado, P. L., Palumbo, J., Krystal, J. H., Nagy, L. M., Rasmussen, S. A., Heninger, G. R., & Charney, D. S. (1990). Specificity of serotonin reuptake inhibtors in the treatment of obsessive compulsive disorder: Comparison of fluvoxamine and desipramine. *Archives of General Psychiatry, 47*, 577–585.

Goodman, W. K., Price, L. H., Rasmussen, S. A., Delgado, P. L., Heninger, G. R., & Charney, D. S. (1989). Efficacy of fluvoxamine in obsessive–compulsive disorder: A double-blind comparison with placebo. *Archives of General Psychiatry, 46*, 36–43.

Goodman, W. K., Price, L. H., Rasmussen, S. A., Mazure, C., Delgado, P., Heninger, G. R., & Charney, D. S. (1989). The Yale–Brown Obsessive Compulsive Scale (Y–BOCS): Part II. Validity. *Archives of General Psychiatry, 46*, 1012–1016.

Goodman, W. K., Price, L. H., Rasmussen, S. A., Mazure, C., Fleischmann, R., Hill, C., Heninger, G. R., & Charney, D. S. (1989). The Yale–Brown Obsessive Compulsive Scale (Y–BOCS): Part I. Development, use, and reliability. *Archives of General Psychiatry, 46*, 1006–1011.

Gordon, C. T., State, R. C., Nelson, J. E., Hamburger, S. D., & Rapoport, J. L. (1993). A double-blind comparison of clomipramine, desipramine, and placebo in the treatment of autistic disorder. *Archives of General Psychiatry, 50*, 441–447.

Greist, J., Chouinard, G., DuBoff, E., Halaris, A., Kim, S. W., Koran, L., Liebowitz, M., Lydiard, R. B., Rasmussen, S., White, K., & Sikes, C. (1995). Double-blind parallel comparison of three dosages of sertraline and placebo in outpatients with obsessive–compulsive disorder. *Archives of General Psychiatry, 52*, 289–295.

Greist, J. H., Jefferson, J. W., Kobak, K. A., Katzelnick, D. J., & Serlin, R. C. (1995). Efficacy and tolerability of serotonin transport inhibitors in obsessive–compulsive disorder. *Archives of General Psychiatry, 52*, 53–60.

Guy, W. (1976). *ECDEU assessment manual for psychopharmacology* (Publication 76–338). Washington, DC: U. S. Department of Health, Education, and Welfare.

Hamdan-Allen, G. (1991). Brief report: Trichotillomania in an autistic male. *Journal of Autism and Developmental Disorders, 21*, 79–82.

Hoder, E. L., & Cohen, D. J. (1983). Repetitive behavior patterns of childhood. In M. Levine & W. Carey (Eds.), *Developmental–behavioral pediatrics* (pp. 607–622). Philadelphia: Saunders.

Hollander, E., DeCaria, C., Gully, R., Nitescu, A., Suckow, R. F., Gorman, J. M., Klein, D. F., & Liebowitz, M. R. (1991). Effects of chronic fluoxetine treatment on behavioral and neuroendocrine responses to metachlorophenylpiperazine in obsessive compulsive disorder. *Psychiatry Research*, *36*, 1–17.

Hoshino, Y., Tachibana, J. R., Watanabe, M., Murata, S., Yokoyama, F., Kaneko, M., Yashima, Y., & Kumoshiro, H. (1984). Serotonin metabolism and hypothalamic pituitary function in children with infantile autism and minimal brain dysfunction. *Japanese Journal of Psychiatry and Neurology*, *26*, 937–945.

Kanner, L. (1943). Autistic disturbances of affective contact. *Journal of Nervous Child*, *2*, 217–250.

Krug, D. A., Arick, J. R., & Almond, P. J. (1980). *Autism screening instrument for education planning* Portland, OR: ASIEP Educational Co.

Le Couteur, A., Rutter, M., Lord, C., Rios, P., Robertson, S., Holdgrafer, M., & McLennan, J. (1989). Autism Diagnostic Interview: A standardized investigator-based instrument. *Journal of Autism and Developmental Disorders*, *19*, 363–387.

Leonard, H. L., Swedo, S. E., Rapoport, J. L., Coffey, M., & Cheslow, D. (1989). Treatment of obsessive–compulsive disorder with clomipramine and desipramine in children and adolescents: A double-blind crossover comparison. *Archives of General Psychiatry*, *46*, 1088–1092.

Lindley, P., Marks, I., Philpott, R., & Snowden, J. (1977). Treatment of obsessive–compulsive neurosis with history of childhood autism. *British Journal of Psychiatry*, *130*, 592–597.

Lord, C., Rutter, M., Goode, S., Heemsbergen, J., Jordan, H., Mawhood, L., & Schopler, E. (1989). Autism Diagnostic Observation Schedule: A standardized observation of communicative and social behavior. *Journal of Autism and Developmental Disorders*, *19*, 185–212.

McBride, P. A., Anderson, G. M., Hertzig, M. E., Sweeney, J. A., Kream, J., Cohen, D. J., & Mann, J. J. (1989). Serotonergic responsivity in male young adults with autistic disorder. Results of a pilot study. *Archives of General Psychiatry*, *46*, 213–221.

McDougle, C. J. (1997). Psychopharmacology. In D. J. Cohen & F. R. Volkmar (Eds.), *Handbook of autism and pervasive developmental disorders* (2nd ed.), (pp. 707–729). New York: Wiley.

McDougle, C. J., Brodkin, E. S., Naylor, S. T., Carlson, D., Cohen, D. J. & Price, L. H. (1998). Sertraline in adults with pervasive developmental disorders: A prospective open-label investigation. *Journal of Clinical Psychopharmacology*, *18*, 62–66.

McDougle, C. J., Goodman, W. K., Leckman, J. F., & Price, L. H. (1993). The psychopharmacology of obsessive compulsive disorder: Implications for treatment and pathogenesis. In D. L. Dunner (Ed.), *Psychopharmacology II* (*Clinics of North America*, Vol. 16) (pp. 749–766). Philadelphia: Saunders.

McDougle, C. J., Kresch, L. E., Goodman, W. K., Naylor, S. T., Volkmar, F. R., Cohen, D. J., & Price, L. H. (1995). A case-controlled study of repetitive thoughts and behavior in adults with autistic disorder and obsessive compulsive disorder. *American Journal of Psychiatry*, *152*, 772–777.

McDougle, C. J., Naylor, S. T., Cohen, D. J., Aghajanian, G. K., Heninger, G. R., & Price, L. H. (1996). Effects of tryptophan depletion in drug-free adults with autism. *Archives of General Psychiatry*, *53*, 993–1000.

McDougle, C. J., Naylor, S. T., Cohen, D. J., Volkmar, F. R., Heninger, G. R., & Price, L. H. (1996). A double-blind, placebo-controlled study of fluvoxamine in adults with autistic disorder. *Archives of General Psychiatry*, *53*, 1001–1008.

McDougle, C. J., Price, L. H., & Goodman, W. K. (1990). Fluvoxamine treatment of coincident autistic disorder and obsessive compulsive disorder: A case report. *Journal of Autism and Developmental Disorders*, *20*, 537–543.

McDougle, C. J., Price, L. H., Volkmar, F. R., Goodman, W. K., Ward-O'Brien, D., Nielsen, J., Bregman, J., & Cohen, D. J. (1992). Clomipramine in autism: Preliminary evidence of efficacy. *Journal of the American Academy of Child and Adolescent Psychiatry*, *31*, 746–750.

Mehlinger, R., Scheftner, W. A., & Poznanski, E. (1990). Fluoxetine and autism [Letter]. *Journal of the American Academy of Child and Adolescent Psychiatry*, *29*, 1985.

Prior, M., & Macmillan, M. B. (1973). Maintenance of sameness in children with Kanner's syndrome. *Journal of Autism and Childhood Schizophrenia, 3,* 154–167.

Rapoport, J. L., Swedo, S. E., & Leonard, H. L. (1992). Childhood obsessive–compulsive disorder. *Journal of Clinical Psychiatry, 53,* 11–16.

Riddle, M. A., Geller, B., & Ryan, N. (1993). Another sudden death in a child treated with desipramine. *Journal of the American Academy of Child and Adolescent Psychiatry, 32,* 792–797.

Rumsey, J. M., Rapoport, J. L., & Sceery, W. R. (1985). Autistic children as adults: Psychiatric, social, and behavioral outcomes. *Journal of the American Academy of Child and Adolescent Psychiatry, 24,* 465–473.

Sanchez, L. E., Campbell, M., Small, A. M., Cueva, J. E., Armenteros, J. L., & Adams, P. B. (1996). A pilot study of clomipramine in young autistic children. *Journal of the American Academy of Child and Adolescent Psychiatry, 35,* 537–544.

Schain, R. J., & Freedman, D. X. (1961). Studies on 5-hydroxyindole metabolism in autistic and other mentally retarded children. *Journal of Pediatrics, 58,* 315–320.

Smalley, S. L., McCracken, J., & Tanguay, P. (1995). Autism, affective disorders, and social phobia. *American Journal of Medical Genetics (Neuropsychiatric Genetics), 60,* 19–26.

Sparrow, S. S., Balla, D. A., & Cicchetti, D. V. (1984). *Vineland Adaptive Behavior Scales (A revision of the Vineland Social Maturity Scale by Edgar A. Doll).* Circle Pines, MN: American Guidance Service.

Steingard, R. J., Zimnitzky, B., DeMaso, D. R., Bauman, M. L., & Bucci, J. P. (1997). Sertraline treatment of transition-associated anxiety and agitation in children with autistic disorder. *Journal of Child and Adolescent Psychopharmacology, 7,* 9–15.

Thoren, P. M., Asberg, M., Cronholm, B., Jornestedt, L., & Traskman, L. (1980). Clomipramine treatment of obsessive–compulsive disorder, I: A controlled clinical trial. *Archives of General Psychiatry, 37,* 1281–1285.

Todd, R. D. (1991). Fluoxetine in autism [Letter]. *American Journal of Psychiatry, 148,* 1089.

Todd, R. D., & Ciaranello, R. D. (1985). Demonstration of inter- and intraspecies differences in serotonin binding sites by antibodies from an autistic child. *Proceedings of the National Academy of Sciences USA, 82,* 612–616.

Tollefson, G. D., Rampey, A. H., Jr., Potvin, J. H., Jenike, M. A., Rush, A. J., Dominguez, R. A., Koran, L. M., Shear, M. K., Goodman, W., & Genduso, L. A. (1994). A multicenter investigation of fixed-dose fluoxetine in the treatment of obsessive–compulsive disorder. *Archives of General Psychiatry, 51,* 559–567.

van Vliet, I. M., den Boer, J. A., & Westenberg, H. G. M. (1994). Psychopharmacological treatment of social phobia: A double-blind placebo-controlled study with fluvoxamine. *Psychopharmacology, 115,* 128–134.

Volkmar, F. R., Hoder, E. L., & Cohen, D. J. (1985). Compliance, 'negativism,' and the effects of treatment structure in autism: A naturalistic, behavioral study. *Journal of Child Psychology and Psychiatry, 26,* 865–877.

Volkmar, F. R., & Nelson, D. S. (1990). Seizure disorders in autism. *Journal of the American Academy of Child and Adolescent Psychiatry, 1,* 127–129.

Wheadon, D. E., Bushnell, W. D., & Steiner, M. (1993). A fixed-dose comparison of 20, 40 or 60 mg paroxetine to placebo in the treatment of obsessive–compulsive disorder. *Proceedings of the American College of Neuropsychopharmacology Annual Meeting.*

Yuwiler, A., Shih, J. C., Chen, C.-H., Ritvo, E. R., Hanna, G., Ellison, G.-W., & King, B. H. (1992). Hyperserotoninemia and antiserotonin antibodies in autism and other disorders. *Journal of Autism and Developmental Disorders, 82,* 612–616.

Zohar, J., & Insel, T. R. (1987). Obsessive–compulsive disorder: Psychobiological approaches to diagnosis, treatment, and pathophysiology. *Biological Psychiatry, 22,* 667–687.

Zohar, J., Insel, T. R., Zohar-Kadouch, R. C., Hill, J. L., & Murphy, D. L. (1988). Serotonergic responsivity in obsessive–compulsive disorder: Effects of chronic clomipramine treatment. *Archives of General Psychiatry, 45,* 167–172.

14

Learning Characteristics of Individuals with Asperger Syndrome

STEPHEN R. HOOPER and MYRA BETH BUNDY

INTRODUCTION

Over 50 years ago Asperger (1944) described a group of children and adolescents whose primary difficulties involved establishing friendships and, more generally, relating to others. Although overshadowed for decades by Kanner's (1943) description of a similar group of children 1 year earlier (i.e., Autism Disorder), Asperger syndrome (AS) was "rediscovered" by Wing (1981) nearly 40 years later. In her recounting of the earlier description, she presented many of the key diagnostic features of AS, and complemented this discussion with clinical cases to illustrate the manifestations of this syndrome. Since that time, there has been increased interest in determining the validity of this taxon. Indeed, as a testament to the current volume, keen interest has been focused on AS and its relationship to autism. To date, the debate continues with respect to the uniqueness and general clinical validity of AS, with emergent evidence suggesting that there could be subtle, yet distinctive differences between AS and autism (e.g., Eaves, Ho, & Eaves, 1994; Goodman, 1989; Ozonoff, Rogers, & Pennington, 1991).

STEPHEN R. HOOPER • Department of Psychiatry and The Clinical Center for the Study of Development and Learning, University of North Carolina School of Medicine, Chapel Hill, North Carolina 27599-7255.   MYRA BETH BUNDY • Department of Psychology, Eastern Kentucky University, Richmond, Kentucky 40475.

Asperger Syndrome or High-Functioning Autism?, edited by Schopler *et al.* Plenum Press, New York, 1998.

In this regard, the learning characteristics and learning problems of individuals with AS remain an ongoing area of concern. What do we know about the specific learning characteristics of individuals with AS? Are these characteristics unique to AS, or are they similar to those of individuals with other types of developmental disorders? Although the psychoeducational characteristics of individuals with high-functioning autism (HFA) have been discussed by a number of investigators (Goldstein, Minshew, & Siegel, 1994; Minshew, Goldstein, Taylor, & Siegel, 1994; Shea & Mesibov, 1985; Siegel, Minshew, & Goldstein, 1996), with a number of specific learning impediments being described (e.g., Bennetto, Pennington, & Rogers, 1996; Minshew & Goldstein, 1993; Minshew, Goldstein, Muenz, & Payton, 1992; Minshew, Goldstein, & Siegel, 1995), the learning characteristics of individuals with AS are just starting to be uncovered.

This chapter provides a review of the available studies describing the learning characteristics of individuals with AS. In addition to discussing this literature, one of the tasks of this chapter will be to make comparisons to the learning characteristics documented in individuals with HFA. Two models of learning disabilities are also presented which may prove useful when attempting to describe the learning characteristics of individuals with AS, particularly when making comparisons to such characteristics of individuals with HFA. Finally, selected clinical and research issues are discussed, with a particular emphasis on definitional issues, and future directions are suggested for ongoing work with individuals with AS.

STUDIES EXAMINING THE LEARNING CHARACTERISTICS OF INDIVIDUALS WITH ASPERGER SYNDROME

A review of the literature produced approximately 20 studies that have primarily or secondarily examined the learning characteristics of individuals diagnosed with AS. In each of these studies, the diagnosis of AS was asserted via one of the major classification systems (i.e., ICD-10 or DSM-IV) or via operational criteria proposed by Asperger (1944) or Wing (1981). Given the task of comparing the learning characteristics of individuals with AS versus those with HFA, it is important to note that 9 of the studies used individuals with autism or HFA as one of the comparison groups. Six of the studies utilized a case study presentation, 9 studies used patients with various kinds of psychiatric disorders for comparison, and 1 study included a comparison group comprised of individuals with mild learning disabilities. All of the studies have been conducted over the past decade and in tandem with a broad conceptualization of learning disabilities — which includes a variety of social and learning impediments (Interagency Committee on Learning Disabilities, 1987; Pennington, 1991).

Studies were selected that focused on psychoeducational, neuropsychological, and social–emotional facets of this disorder. A synopsis of these studies, listed in chronological order, is presented in Table 14-1.

Psychoeducational

To date, several studies have examined the psychoeducational functioning of individuals with AS. Szatmari, Bartolucci, and Bremner (1989) provided some of the first information pertaining to the educational characteristics of individuals with AS. Using parent and child interviews along with a school history form, these investigators noted that their group of individuals with AS ($N = 28$) required less time in special education classes than their HFA group ($N = 25$). Further, Wing (1991) noted that most individuals with AS tend to function in the average range of intelligence, although some reportedly fall within the mild range of mental retardation. Similarly, Fine, Bartolucci, Szatmari, and Ginsberg (1994) found their sample of individuals with AS to have overall low average abilities, with no difference between their verbal and nonverbal abilities. Fine *et al.* also found no differences between the level and pattern of intellectual functioning in their AS group compared with individuals with HFA, but the AS group did perform at a lower level than an outpatient psychiatric comparison group.

In a study examining intellectual and academic achievement, Szatmari, Tuff, Finlayson, and Bartolucci (1990) found their group with AS to be indistinguishable from those with autism. In general, the former group had intellectual test profiles that varied in accordance with their developmental level, with the bulk of their sample falling well within the low average to average range. They noted that for individuals exhibiting Full Scale IQ scores > 85, there did not seem to be the Verbal IQ < Performance IQ discrepancy typically observed in individuals with Full Scale IQ < 85. Academic achievement skills were not impaired and, in fact, were at least commensurate with the low average to average intellectual functioning demonstrated by this sample. It was noted, however, that their arithmetic skills were somewhat lower than their reading decoding skills.

More recently, Klin, Volkmar, Sparrow, Cicchetti, and Rourke (1995) found their AS group to demonstrate average overall intellectual abilities, and this level of functioning was similar to the comparison group of HFA individuals. However, the AS group had higher Verbal IQ than Performance IQ scores, which was not a pattern demonstrated by the HFA group. In the Klin *et al.* sample, this pattern was universally observed across all AS subjects. A similar level and pattern of intellectual findings were seen by Ozonoff *et al.* (1991), with this pattern of abilities significantly separating their AS group from those with HFA. Further, although a significant number of individuals in the AS group exhibited reading decoding (36.8%), reading comprehension (52.6%), and arithmetic

Table 14-1. Studies Examining Specific Learning Characteristics of Individuals Diagnosed with Asperger Syndrome

Study	N	Sample characteristics	Diagnoses	Control/ comparison group	Measurement	Variables measured	Learning characteristics and findings
Barrows (1988)	6	Children	AS	No	Case history	Behavioral indicators of sensory integration deficits	Deficit in intersensory integration which disrupts perceptions of objective reality, and the feelings and behavior of others.
Gillberg (1989)	46	5–18 years; M:F = 10:1; < 10% MR; 17% above-average IQ; age and IQ matched	N = 23 AS N = 23 autism	Yes	Case exam	Clinical and neurological history	No clear distinction between the two groups, except for more motor clumsiness in the AS group and reduced optimality in the pre- and perinatal history of the autistic group.
Szatmari, Bartolucci, & Bremner (1989)	95	AS mean age = 14.3; FSIQ = 88.5; M:F = 4.6:1 HFA mean age = 23.3; FSIQ = 85.0; M:F = 4.3:1 Inpatient mean age = 13.7; FSIQ = 101.5; M:F = 4.3:1	N = 28 AS N = 25 HFA N = 42 psychiatric inpatients	Yes	Parent interview; child interview; school history	History of behavioral symptoms	HFA group showed more social impairment, higher frequency of echolalia and pronoun reversal, and more restricted range of activities. HFA had more time in special education than AS, but fewer psychiatric symptoms. Suggested differences are not substantial enough to separate autism and AS diagnoses.

Study	N	Sample characteristics	Diagnoses	Control/comparison group	Measurement	Variables measured	Learning characteristics and findings
Szatmari, Bremner, & Nagy (1989)	56	8–18 years	N = 28 AS N = 28 POC	Yes	Case history	Demographics, family history, neurological status, and social impairments	AS group showed more social isolation, one-sided social interactions, difficulty using verbal and nonverbal communication strategies, flat affect, and abnormalities in inflection.
Berthier, Starkstein, & Leiguarda (1990)	2	Right-handed; 17-year-old males	AS	No	Review of records; MRI; CT	Behavioral and cognitive symptomatology; brain structure	Observed left-sided neurological signs and cognitive impairments compatible with RH dysfunction. Neuroimaging showed bilateral areas of abnormal micropolygyri.
Jones & Kerwin (1990)	1	34-year-old	AS	No	CT; EEG WAIS-R	Brain structure and brain activity; IQ	Healthy adult with evidence of left temporal lobe damage and atrophy. EEG was normal. IQ was average, with VIQ > PIQ.

(continued)

Table 14-1. (Continued)

Study	N	Sample characteristics	Diagnoses	Control/comparison group	Measurement	Variables measured	Learning characteristics and findings
Szatmari, Tuff, Finlayson, & Bartolucci (1990)	89	AS ages = 8–18; M:F = 4.6:1; mean FSIQ = 86.6; HFA ages = 7–32 yrs.; M:F = 3.3:1; mean FSIQ = 82.2; POC ages = 7–17 yrs.; M:F = 5:1; mean FSIQ = 101.5	N = 28 AS; N = 25 HFA; N = 36 POC	Yes	WISC-R/WAIS-R; WRAT-R; Children's Token Test; Children's Word Finding Test; Benton Test of Facial Recognition; VMI; WCST; Grooved Pegboard	Intelligence, school achievement, auditory comprehension and memory, verbal problem solving, facial recognition, graphomotor construction, cognitive flexibility, manual speed and dexterity	AS and HFA groups did not differ significantly from each other, but differed from POC on all measures.
Tantam, Evered, & Hersov (1990)	3	F = 2 children M = 1 adult	AS	No	Record review	Marfan-like disorder of connective tissue	Connective tissue disorder led to anomalous development of midline brain structures with consequent social handicaps.
Fine, Bartolucci, Ginsberg, & Szatmari (1991)	78	AS mean age = 14 HFA = FSIQ > 70 POC mean age = 13.7	N = 23 AS N = 19 HFA N = 36 POC	Yes	Coding of intonation boundaries from audio recordings of 10-minute loosely structured interview	Rates of intonation types relative to the amount of speech produced	AS subjects did not differ from POC, but showed more "useful" patterns of intonation for communication than HFA.

Study	N	Sample characteristics	Diagnoses	Control/ comparison group	Measurement	Variables measured	Learning characteristics and findings
Ozonoff, Rogers, & Pennington (1991)	43	HFA mean age = 11.8; mean FSIQ = 87.2 AS mean age = 12.4; FSIQ = 92.6	N = 13 HFA N = 10 AS N = 20 matched, nonautistic controls	Yes	Emotion perception task; picture sequencing; appearance–reality task; mental–physical distinction task; brain function task; second-order belief attribution task; Tower of Hanoi; WCST; BSRT; CEFT	Executive functioning, theory of mind, verbal memory, visuospatial ability, attention to perceptual detail, school history	Both HFA and AS groups were impaired on executive functioning, emotional perception, and spatial abilities relative to controls; HFA group demonstrated relative deficits in theory of mind, verbal memory, and VIQ compared with AS.
Bowler (1992)	45	Adults; AS M:F = 13:2 Schizophrenic M:F = 7:8 Nonhandicapped M:F = 7:8	N = 15 AS N = 15 chronic schizophrenia N = 15 nonhandicapped	Yes	Written problems designed by authors, e.g., "Peter thinks that Jane thinks that ..."	Ability to use second-order theory of mind	AS solved problems designed to assess ability to use second-order theory of mind, but did not use mental state terms to explain their solutions. This did not differ from comparison groups.

(continued)

Table 14-1. *(Continued)*

Study	N	Sample characteristics	Diagnoses	Control/comparison group	Measurement	Variables measured	Learning characteristics and findings
Berthier, Bayes, & Tolosa (1993)	16	Early 20s; average education < 12th grade	N = 7 TS with AS; N = 9 TS	Yes	MRI; neurological exam; neuropsychological battery	Brain structure and function	5 of the 7 TS with AS showed brain abnormality versus 1 of the 9 TS; 15 W/AS had deficits in complex problem solving, spatial abilities, and more neurological soft signs than TS group. No differences between groups on IQ, memory, language functions.
David, Wacharasindhu, & Lishman (1993)	7		N = 4 psychotic symptoms; N = 1 schizophrenia; N = 1 personality disorder; N = 1 AS	No	Record review	Brain structure (developmental defects of the corpus callosum)	Discussed the importance of these defects to interhemispheric information transfer and related clinical manifestations.

Study	N	Sample characteristics	Diagnoses	Control/comparison group	Measurement	Variables measured	Learning characteristics and findings
Tantam, Holmes, & Cordess (1993)	18	*Experiment 1* AS mean age = 24 VIQ = 105.4, PIQ = 98.6 *Experiment 2* 12 Schizophrenic mean age = 23.3 VIQ = 107.4, PIQ = 117.2 AS mean age = 26.8 VIQ = 100.7, PIQ = 90	*N* = 9 AS *N* = 9 normals *N* = 6 schizoid personality disorder *N* = 6 AS	Yes	Ratings of videotapes of short, unstructured interactions between a volunteer interviewer and each group of subjects	Nonverbal expression	AS subjects looked less at the other person, made more self-stimulatory gestures, and looked at interviewer less than normals, and less than schizoid subjects when interviewer was vocalizing. No such differences when the interviewer was listening.
Berthier (1994)	19	Ages 13–37 FSIQ = 72–127	AS with TS	No	MRI	Brain structure	MRI was abnormal in 10 patients; 3 showed enlarged lateral ventricles; 7 showed polymicrogyri and increased sulcial width in posterior superior parietal lobe, opercular region, and left parietal–occipital region; posterior body of corpus callosum showed thinning.

(continued)

Table 14-1. *(Continued)*

Study	N	Sample characteristics	Diagnoses	Control/comparison group	Measurement	Variables measured	Learning characteristics and findings
Bowler & Worley (1994)	27	Young adults	N = 8 AS N = 10 nonhandicapped N = 9 mild LD	Yes	Asch's (1951) line judgment experimental procedure	Social influence on line judgment	AS subjects showed less conformity to incorrect judgments of others than either control group.
Davies, Bishop, Manstead, & Tantam (1994)	40	Age = 11–16 *Experiment 1*	N = 10 HFA or AS N = 10 low-ability autism N = 20 verbal mental age-matched, nonautistic controls	Yes	Facial and social–emotional tasks	Ability to process facial and nonfacial stimuli for emotion and recognition	No difference between low-ability autistic subjects and low-ability controls; but HFA and AS subjects performed significantly more poorly than controls across all tasks.
	50	*Experiment 2*	N = 9 HFA N = 11 high-ability nonautistic controls N = 10 low-ability autistic N = 20 MR controls				
Fine, Bartolucci, Szatmari, & Ginsberg (1994)	75	Ages 8–18	N = 18 HFA N = 23 AS N = 34 POC	Yes	Observation/coding of 10-minute conversation	Natural spontaneous conversation content	AS group did not differ from POC; HFA group referred less to previous conversation and more to physical environment than controls.

Study	N	Sample characteristics	Diagnoses	Control/comparison group	Measurement	Variables measured	Learning characteristics and findings
Ghaziuddin, Butler, Tsai, & Ghaziuddin (1994)	20	AS mean age = 13.6, HFA mean age = 12.9	N = 11 AS, N = 9 HFA	Yes	Bruininks–Oseretsky	Gross- and fine-motor skills	Both groups showed coordination problems, but no group differences noted.
Kracke (1994)	1	19-year-old male	AS	No	Observation, record review of case and family history	Facial recognition	Subject was unable to recognize faces; mild forms of AS and prosopagnosia were present in family history.
Klier, Volkmar, Sparrow, Cicchetti, & Rourke (1995)	40	N = 21 AS, N = 19 HFA, Samples were similar on age, sex, FSIQ	AS, HFA	Yes	Wechsler IQ, neuropsychological battery tapping 22 domains	IQ, fine motor, gross motor, visual-motor, visual-spatial, auditory perception, hand material, rote material, verbal and visual memory, verbal and nonverbal concept formation, articulation, vocabulary, verbal output, verbal content, prosody, pragmatics, word decoding, reading comprehension, arithmetic, social and emotional competence	Although FSIQ was comparable, AS group showed VIQ > PIQ patterns more frequently than the HFA group. Groups also differed on 11 neuropsychological domains, with AS group showing a profile consistent with expectations from the NVLD model.

Note. M = Male; F = female; AS = Asperger syndrome; HFA = high-functioning autism; MR = mental retardation; POC = psychiatric outpatient controls; RH = right hemisphere; WCST = Wisconsin Card Sorting Test; WISC-R = Wechsler Intelligence Scale for Children-Revised; WAIS-R = Wechsler Adult Intelligence Scale-Revised; WRAT-R = Wide Range Achievement Test-Revised; VMI = Developmental Test of Visual-Motor Integration; FSIQ = Full Scale Intelligence Quotient; MRI = magnetic resonance imaging; CT = computerized tomography; EEG = electroencephalogram; BSRT = Buschke Selective Reminding Test; CEFT = Children's Embedded Figures Test; TS = Tourette's syndrome.

problems (42.1%), these rates were not radically different from those of the HFA group.

Neuropsychological

A number of studies have addressed the issue of learning characteristics as defined by neuropsychological mechanisms and associated constructs. Using case study methodology, Barrows (1988) was perhaps one of the first to describe intersensory integration deficits in AS individuals. He suggested that the deficit in intersensory integration seriously disrupts such individuals' perceptions of objective reality, as well as their perceptions of the feelings and behaviors of others. Gillberg (1989) used a clinical history to suggest the presence of greater motor clumsiness in the AS group relative to a group of individuals with autism; however, outside of increased neurological vulnerability in the pre- and perinatal periods for individuals with autism, Gillberg found few differences between the groups.

Whereas some investigators have uncovered few neuropsychological differences between AS and HFA (Szatmari et al., 1990), particularly on tasks tapping diagnostic criteria pertaining to clumsiness and motor coordination (Ghaziuddin, Butler, Tsai, & Ghaziuddin, 1994), other investigators have begun to show subtle but unique neuropsychological characteristics in the AS population. For example, Ozonoff et al. (1991) found few differences between AS and HFA groups on measures of executive functioning, although both groups were significantly impaired relative to nonautistic controls; however, AS individuals demonstrated relatively intact functioning in theory of mind and verbal memory tasks whereas their HFA counterparts did not.

In one of the better-controlled studies conducted in this area, Klin, Volkmar, et al. (1995) used stringent diagnostic criteria based on the ICD-10 to ascertain groups of individuals manifesting AS and HFA. Once identified, the investigators compared these two groups on a comprehensive neuropsychological battery. Findings revealed significant differences between the groups, with the AS group performing more poorly on tasks tapping fine-motor skills, visual-motor integration, visual-spatial perception, nonverbal concept formation, gross motor skills, and visual memory. Additional deficits were noted in prosody, social competence, and emotional competence, although the two groups did not differ in these latter domains. Based on these findings, the authors suggested a significant convergence of AS with manifestations seen in individuals having nonverbal learning disabilities.

Similar findings also were reported by Berthier, Bayes, and Tolosa (1993), who documented significant differences between their AS groups with and without Tourette's syndrome on a variety of neuropsychological variables. Specific differences were noted on motor functioning and executive functions, in favor of the non-AS Tourette's syndrome group. A further inspection of the findings revealed that the AS group scored lower on all of the neuropsychological measures.

From a neurological perspective, a number of investigators have reported neurostructural differences and abnormalities in AS subjects. Tantam, Evered, and Hersov (1990) found connective tissue disorder in their three AS subjects. Although it remains unclear whether this is a neurological manifestation of AS, the authors did suggest that the connective tissue disorder may be responsible for the anomalous development of midline brain structures and the associated social deficits.

Berthier et al. (1993) found anomalies involving a variety of cortical regions in a sample of individuals having AS and Tourette's syndrome. Specifically, two patients showed right central perisylvian involvement, hypoplasia of the right temporal–occipital cortex, polymicrogyri in the posterior parietal lobes, and enlargement of the right lateral ventricle. David, Wacharasindhu, and Lishman (1993) and Berthier (1994) noted that defects in the corpus callosum also may play a role in the learning and social characteristics typically seen in AS. Berthier, Starkstein, and Leiguarda (1990) also reported abnormal neurological signs in two AS subjects. Specifically, they described left-sided neurological signs and cognitive impairments indicative of right hemisphere dysfunction. Further, neuroimaging procedures via magnetic resonance imaging and computerized tomography showed bilateral areas of abnormal micropolygyri.

Other investigators have implicated the left temporal lobe as being etiologically related to the behaviors typically seen in AS (Jones & Kerwin, 1990). Although of critical interest to the neurobiological basis of AS, particularly given findings suggesting that approximately 90% of individuals in the autism spectrum may have indications of brain damage or dysfunction (Steffenburg, 1991), the significance of these findings with respect to specific learning, behavioral, and social-emotional manifestations in AS remains to be determined.

Social–Emotional

For this overview of the learning characteristics of AS individuals, social–emotional difficulties also have been subsumed under a more liberal definition of learning disabilities. The inclusion of these characteristics is bolstered by the evolution of specific models that have attempted to account for selected social–emotional manifestations in individuals with learning disabilities (e.g., nonverbal learning disabilities model). To date, studies have addressed actual social functioning as well as the processing of social–emotional information. In fact, even a case study of prosopagnosia (i.e., inability to recognize faces) has been reported (Kracke, 1994), although the majority of studies have examined more specific aspects of social–emotional functioning.

Szatmari, Bremner, and Nagy (1989) compared their AS group (28 children and adolescents) with psychiatric outpatient controls across a variety of measures, including social functioning. The individuals with AS demonstrated a range of social impairments that were significantly different from the comparison group. In particular, the AS group tended to manifest increased social isolation, show poor nonverbal communication and inept social interactions, and maintain poor social relations.

Bowler (1992) and Bowler and Worley (1994) examined other facets of social relatedness in AS. Bowler (1992) studied the ability to use second-order theory of mind (i.e., second-order attribution of beliefs; "John thinks that Mary thinks...") in a sample of 15 individuals with AS, 15 individuals with chronic schizophrenia, and 15 nondisabled controls. On written problems designed to tap second-order theory of mind, the AS group did not use mental state terms to explain their solutions to the presented problems; however, this did not differ from the comparison groups. Bowler and Worley (1994) also examined the ease with which AS individuals could be influenced by social pressures. Using the classic Asch (1951) line judgment experimental paradigm, these investigators found that AS subjects showed less conformity to the incorrect judgments of others than either a group of young adults with mild learning disabilities or a group of nondisabled controls.

In addition to exploring social functioning in AS, a number of studies have examined the ability of such individuals to process social and emotional information. Fine, Bartolucci, Ginsberg, and Szatmari (1991) found that AS individuals did not differ significantly from a group of psychiatric outpatient controls in their vocal intonation patterns; however, they employed more "useful" patterns of intonation in their communication attempts than did HFA. Similar findings were noted by Fine et al. (1994) using 10 minutes of natural conversation. Their HFA group referred more to physical environmental qualities and less to previous conversational points in their discussions, but the AS group did not differ from a comparison group of individuals with nonspecific social problems.

Davies, Bishop, Manstead, and Tantam (1994) investigated the ability of AS individuals to process facial and nonfacial emotional stimuli for recognition. They found no differences between low-ability subjects with autism and low-ability controls; however, individuals with AS and with HFA performed more poorly than controls across all tasks. Tantam, Holmes, and Cordess (1993) explored the nonverbal expression capabilities of AS individuals. Using videotapes of short, unstructured interactions between a volunteer and each group of subjects, AS subjects tended to look less at the interviewer and to make more self-stimulatory gestures than normal controls and individuals with schizophrenia. This was especially obvious when the interviewer was talking, but there were no such differences when the interviewer was listening.

SELECTED MODELS OF LEARNING DISABILITIES AND THEIR UTILITY FOR UNDERSTANDING ASPERGER SYNDROME

Several models that have evolved out of the learning disability literature seem to hold much promise for increasing our understanding of learning and social–emotional functioning in AS. Two of these models, the Nonverbal Learning Disability Model and the Social–Emotional Learning Disability Model, not only describe many of the characteristics of AS *a priori*, but also provide neurobiological underpinnings for these learning and social problems. Both models are robust with respect to accounting for the variable presentation of individuals with AS, and they also may assist in explaining some of the similarities and differences in the learning characteristics of individuals with AS versus HFA (Siegel *et al.*, 1996). Further, these models provide specific avenues for assessment and intervention. Although their basic components appear quite similar in makeup, some differences between the models are to be noted.

Nonverbal Learning Disability Model

Although Rourke (1989) has popularized the nonverbal learning disability model, Johnson and Myklebust (1971) provided detailed depictions of these individuals over 25 years ago. They found that individuals with nonverbal learning disabilities typically were unable to comprehend the significance of many aspects of the environment, could not pretend and anticipate, and failed to learn and appreciate the implications of actions such as gestures, facial expressions, caresses, and other elements of emotion. Johnson and Myklebust noted that this disorder constituted a fundamental distortion of the total perceptual experience of the individual. They labeled this a social perception disability, and Myklebust (1975) later coined the term *nonverbal learning disability*. These observations were consistent with findings of Borod, Koff, and Caron (1983) as well as Ross and Mesulam (1979) in their study of right-brain-damaged adults, and Denckla (1983) extended this thinking to children in her description of a social (emotional) learning disability.

Consistent with these earlier notions, Rourke (1989) proposed a model that is psychometrically rather than neurologically derived. It is based on selected aspects of neuropsychologically based learning disability subtypes, and on a theory of differential hemispheric functioning advanced by Goldberg and Costa (1981). Relying primarily on data and speculative evidence derived from adult samples, Goldberg and Costa asserted that the right hemisphere is relatively more specialized for intermodal integration, whereas the left hemisphere is more specialized for intramodal integration. Neuroanatomically, these investigators postulated that intramodal integration may be related to a higher ratio of gray matter (i.e., neuronal mass and short nonmyelinated fibers) to white matter (i.e., long myelinated fibers) characteristic of the left hemisphere, whereas intermodal integration may be related to a higher ratio of white matter to gray matter characteristic of the right hemisphere.

Rourke extended this model by applying a developmental perspective and, given his previous findings with respect to learning disability subtypes (see Rourke, 1985), extended it to account for nonverbal learning disabilities. He hypothesized that involvement of the white matter of the right hemisphere (i.e., lesioned, excised, or dysfunctional white matter) interacts with developmental parameters, resulting in nonverbal learning disabilities. He reasoned that, although a significant lesion in the right hemisphere may be sufficient to produce a nonverbal learning disability, it is the destruction of white matter (i.e., matter associated with intermodal functions) that is necessary to produce these types of learning disabilities. Generally, the nonverbal learning disability syndrome would be expected to develop under any circumstance that significantly inter-feres with the functioning of right hemispheric systems or with access to those systems (e.g., agenesis of the corpus callosum). Functionally, the characteristics of such an individual, which Rourke noted should be observable by approxi-mately ages 7 to 9 years (Rourke, 1988, Rourke, Young, & Leenaars, 1989), implicate neuropsychological academic, and social–emotional/adaptive do-mains in a fashion similar to the emergent learning characteristics seen in individuals with AS.

Neuropsychologically, individuals with nonverbal learning disabilities tend to present a distinct profile of strengths and weaknesses. Relative strengths include auditory perception, simple motor functions, and intact rote verbal learning. Selective auditory attention, phonological skills, and auditory-verbal memory also appear intact. Neuropsychological deficits include bilateral tactile-perception problems and motor difficulties that usually are more marked on the left than on the right side of the body, visual-spatial organization problems, and nonverbal problem-solving difficulties. Paralinguistic aspects of language also are impaired (e.g., prosody, pragmatics).

Academically, these individuals evidence adequate word decoding and spelling, with most spelling errors reflecting good phonetic equivalents. Grapho-motor skills eventually can be age-appropriate, but are delayed early in devel-opment. Marked academic deficits tend to be manifested in mechanical arithmetic, mathematical reasoning, and reading comprehension. Academic sub-ject areas, such as science, also tend to be impaired, largely because of reading comprehension deficiencies and deficits in nonverbal problem solving.

Perhaps one of the most interesting aspects associated with this syndrome is that there appears to be a strong relationship with social–emotional and adaptive behavior deficits. These individuals present great difficulty adapting to novel situations, and manifest poor social perception and judgment. These difficulties, in turn, result in poor social interaction skills. There appears to be a marked tendency for these individuals to engage in social withdrawal and social isolation as age increases, and consequently, they are at risk for internalized forms of psychopathology such as depression and anxiety. In fact, Rourke *et al.* (1989) and Bigler (1989) noted the increased risk that these individuals have for depression and suicide. It will be interesting to see if these affective components of the model apply to individuals with AS.

Rourke proposed this model as an approximation of a developmental neuropsychological model for nonverbal learning disabilities. Given the associated features, a number of investigators have attempted to employ this model to gain an increased understanding of AS, and this conjecture has begun to receive empirical support (e.g., Klin, Volkmar, *et al.*, 1995). The model is noteworthy as it may contribute not only to conceptualizations of differential diagnosis of specific learning problems in AS, but also to issues of severity (e.g., how intact or impaired selected functions are will contribute to issues of severity). Ongoing examination of this association is required, but the model provides the opportunity to study the interaction between neurological and neuropsychological factors that may be contributing, directly and/or indirectly, to behavioral manifestations in AS.

Social–Emotional Learning Disabilities Model

Although the nonverbal learning disabilities model begins to approximate a developmentally based neuropsychological framework for the association between various learning characteristics, including learning disabilities and AS, it is less specific about the genesis of the deficient processing of social and emotional information. Over 10 years ago, Voeller (1986) described 15 children exhibiting visual-spatial deficits, math disabilities, and chronic social problems. All of the children had left-sided neurological signs, implying right hemispheric dysfunction, and all but one had attentional disturbances. Similar kinds of children have been described by Denckla (1983), Weintraub and Mesulam (1983), and other researchers (see Semrud-Clikeman & Hynd, 1990, for a review). Not surprisingly, given the emphasis on neuropsychologically based deficits in nonverbal affective communication, they proposed the term *social–emotional learning disabilities* (SELD), borrowed from Denckla, for children presenting with these symptoms.

A growing body of evidence suggests that defects in communicating facial affect (Blonder, Bowers, & Heilman, 1991) and emotional speech prosody (Ross & Mesulam, 1979) may be localizable to the right temporal–parietal cortex, in contrast to language functions, which are lateralized largely to the left temporal–parietal cortex (Pennington, 1991). In adults, recognition of facial affect is separable from the recognition of facial identity. Similarly, recognition of emotional content is separable from recognition of ideational content in written or oral language (Blonder *et al.*, 1991; Voeller, Hanson, & Wendt, 1988). Moreover, the receptive and expressive aspects of affective facial, gestural, and prosodic communication also appear to be dissociable (Bowers *et al.*, 1985). Impairments in processing affective signals place individuals at high risk for social dysfunction, such as those problems witnessed in AS. These social dysfunctions could include disturbances in attachment and peer interactions, which, in turn, may increase the risk for internalizing psychopathology (Pennington, 1991; Szatmari, Bremnar, *et al.*, 1989).

COMPARISON OF THE LEARNING CHARACTERISTICS OF INDIVIDUALS WITH ASPERGER SYNDROME VERSUS HIGH-FUNCTIONING AUTISM

This overview of the literature provides clear indications of learning problems and, perhaps, specific learning disabilities in individuals with AS across psychoeducational, neuropsychological, and social–emotional domains of functioning. Most of the studies suggested the presence of at least low average to average intellectual capabilities, with Wing (1991) suggesting a lower occurrence of mental retardation than typically found in individuals with autism. Further, whereas individuals with HFA can manifest a wide range of levels and patterns of intellectual ability (Siegel *et al.*, 1996), the literature remains mixed in this regard for individuals with AS. Several studies noted few, if any, differences between AS and HFA in terms of the level and pattern of intellectual functioning. Similarly, few, if any, differences were noted between these two groups in terms of academic achievement. Several other studies, however, suggested that many AS individuals may show significantly higher verbal abilities than nonverbal abilities, with one study suggesting the existence of this pattern largely in individuals with below-average intellectual capabilities (i.e., Full Scale IQ < 85). The reliability of this finding in this population remains to be seen, but it is important to note that this pattern would be consistent with the nonverbal learning disability model. Additionally, AS individuals may require less special education services than HFA children, despite selected learning and academic performance difficulties, but their unusual behavioral presentation may cause them to be misdiagnosed and/or underserved.

From a neuropsychological perspective, outside of suspected neurostructural anomalies (e.g., corpus callosum) and left-sided neurological findings in some individuals — findings that may or may not be unique to AS — several studies have found specific neuropsychological deficits distinguish AS from HFA. Specifically, fine and gross motor deficits, poor visual-motor abilities, difficulties with visual-spatial tasks, deficient visual memory, and poorly evolved nonverbal concept formation seem to be relatively unique to AS versus

HFA. Further, AS individuals showed higher verbal memory skills and more intact theory of mind functions than HFA individuals. This evolving profile of abilities likely contributes to learning differences, if not learning disabilities, in selected academic domains (e.g., writing, math), as well as in social functioning. Deficits in intersensory integration, motor clumsiness, executive functions, and prosody also have been described, but these qualities do not seem to distinguish them from AS individuals with HFA.

Lastly, individuals with AS have been described as having problems and differences in their processing of social and emotional information — another characteristic that would be consistent with the nonverbal learning disability model as well as the social–emotional learning disability model. However, it remains to be seen if these differences are distinct from those in HFA. Despite the reported social–emotional difficulties exhibited by AS individuals, the available literature suggests that such individuals tend to exhibit better conversational skills and more appropriate vocal intonation patterns than their HFA counterparts.

Taken together, it does seem that there are emergent findings suggesting subtle differences in the learning characteristics between AS and HFA. Although the level and, to some extent, the pattern of psychoeducational abilities appear roughly similar, there is some suggestion that AS individuals will show higher verbal than nonverbal abilities, particularly in individuals with lower IQs. The association of such a distinct pattern of intellectual abilities with HFA is simply not the case. The possibility of higher verbal abilities may help explain why these individuals require less special education services than HFA individuals, although this also remains to be validated. A variety of specific deficits in neuropsychological functioning have been documented relative to individuals with HFA, but those with AS seem to have higher theory of mind functions, evidence intact verbal memory, and demonstrate better verbal communication abilities.

ONGOING ISSUES AND FUTURE DIRECTIONS

From this review of the literature, a number of issues require continued examination. Much of the emergent literature on the learning characteristics seen in AS implicates this disorder as relatively unique in the larger spectrum of Pervasive Developmental Disorders (PPD), and this view has been at least partly legitimized by the tentative distinction between these various taxa as presented in the DSM-IV. Some data continue to surface, however, suggesting that AS is little more than a variant of HFA and, at least with respect to its learning characteristics, this will require further study.

Despite initial efforts to define AS in the current psychiatric nosologies, one of the biggest stumbling blocks with respect to learning about AS continues to be the lack of a singular *operational* definition. In fact, the two major diagnostic systems that include PPD — ICD-10 (WHO, 1990) and the DSM-IV (APA, 1994) — propose similar although slightly different definitions of AS. Further, some of the characteristics typically reported in diagnosed individuals, primarily motor clumsiness, remain poorly operationalized and poorly validated (Ghaziuddin *et al.*, 1994). Unfortunately, these slight differences in definition and the lack of operationalization of selected components undoubtedly will contribute to ongoing confusion in the interpretation of research pertaining to this disorder and, ultimately, to continued confusion regarding its validity.

At present, individuals with AS may be distinguished from those with other PPD (e.g., Rett's syndrome, Childhood Disintegrative Disorder, PDD — Not Otherwise Specified) on the basis of their higher intellectual functioning and the outstanding nature of their social and communication deficits relative to this higher level of functioning; however, its distinction from HFA remains unclear (Volkmar *et al.*, 1994). This has created inconsistent usage of the diagnosis by clinicians and researchers, with particular confusion with the HFA diagnosis. With an agreed-upon operational definition, guidelines for subject ascertainment could be consistent from one study to another and, consequently, interpretation of results could be generalized. Until this issue is addressed, the debate on the similarities and differences between AS and HFA will continue. Many of the studies reviewed in Table 14-1 (e.g., Klin, Volkmar, *et al.*, 1995) are noteworthy for directly comparing individuals in these two groups.

These definitional issues are compounded when one examines current definitions of learning disabilities. Learning disabilities traditionally have been defined by unexpected low achievement in basic academic domains (e.g., reading, arithmetic, writing), with numerous attempts to operationalize this concept via various discrepancy formulas (Hooper & Willis, 1989); however, little difference has been noted between many of these formulas in identifying children with learning disabilities (e.g., Francis, Shaywitz, Stuebing, Shaywitz, & Fletcher, 1996). Further, the application of these discrepancy formulas to individuals with AS also remains to be validated. Given the unusual learning styles that can be exhibited by many individuals with AS, it is likely that many of these formulas for uncovering specific learning problems simply will not work. For example, an individual with AS, or many other developmental disorders for that matter, may or may not show an ability–achievement discrepancy, but still manifest significant psychoeducational, neuropsychological, and social–emotional problems. The psychoeducational assessment strategies that have been employed to capture this discrepancy (e.g., tests of intellectual functioning and academic skills) may be too basic to uncover the specific learning characteristics of many individuals with AS. Indeed, such assessment actually may test the weaknesses of many of these individuals. This is where a more detailed approach to assessment (e.g., neuropsychological assessment) can provide more specific information about an individual's learning abilities, styles, and disabilities.

If an ability–achievement discrepancy model of learning disabilities is applied to individuals with AS, then consideration should be given to examining other types of "ability–achievement" discrepancies, perhaps with specific consideration being given to the target behaviors of concern. For example, instead of using IQ as the ability component when trying to examine social functioning, perhaps using the individual's social knowledge would be a better starting point. This level of social knowledge then could be compared with the individual's actual deployment of social skills when constructing the degree of discrepancy in the social domain. In a more pure academic vein, determining the discrepancy between listening comprehension (i.e., ability) and reading comprehension (i.e., achievement) might be a better application in reading, and using one's understanding of math concepts versus math calculations might be better in arithmetic. These suggested variants of the traditional learning disability discrepancy formula actually may capture the essence of academic and social problems more accurately than using IQ and achievement skills; however, these types of applications will require further study.

Problems with definitional clarity also impact on attempts to understand associated comorbidity in this population. Not surprisingly, there are no prevalence rates to describe the presence of learning disabilities in the population of individuals deemed to have AS. Findings from the current review, however, would suggest that these individuals are vulnerable to selected kinds of learning disabilities, or at least learning differences. The Klin, Volkmar, *et al.* (1995) study did show that one-third to one-half of their sample experienced significant academic deficits across reading, arithmetic, and spelling, a rate more than double that of learning disabilities in the general population. Relatedly, many of the neuropsychological and social–emotional characteristics of this population would suggest their alignment with a particular subtype of learning disabilities — nonverbal learning disabilities — and this should receive further clarification as well.

From an educational perspective, it would seem that the presence of a specific profile of abilities asserts the need for a comprehensive assessment of these individuals, perhaps with interdisciplinary input. This assessment should go beyond the traditional school-based evaluation (i.e., intellectual and achievement tests) to include specific measures of information processing (e.g., motor, memory, language) as well as measures that tap social–emotional status, adaptive behaviors, and processing of social-emotional cues. Klin, Volkmar, *et al.* (1995) even suggested that such an evaluation should mirror the neuropsychological assessment protocol used for individuals suspected of having nonverbal learning disabilities.

With respect to educational treatment, as yet there are no clear psychoeducational assessment–treatment linkages for individuals with AS. Despite the initial finding that they receive less special education services than HFA individuals, the emergent description of these individuals would suggest that they should be considered for supportive special education services. Klin, Sparrow, Volkmar, Cicchetti, and Rourke (1995) noted that many of these individuals have received services under the learning disability classification; however, without knowledge of the specific learning characteristics of AS, specific treatment strategies may be misguided, ineffective, and perhaps a hindrance to an individual's learning. In general, many of the educational interventions employed for HFA (Mesibov, 1992; Van Bourgondien & Woods, 1992) and nonverbal learning disabilities (Rourke, 1995) may prove useful to clinicians and teachers working with this population (e.g., employ a verbal teaching approach; develop verbal capabilities; develop visual-spatial-organizational skills; facilitate structured peer interaction; help the caregivers and teachers to understand the individual's needs). Nonetheless, it will be critical for these intervention approaches to receive validation for this population.

SUMMARY

This chapter provided an overview of the emergent literature describing the learning characteristics of individuals with AS. Definitional issues notwithstanding, it would seem that such individuals are prone to a variety of learning deficits and problems that include not only classroom achievement, but neuropsychological and social–emotional functioning as well. In fact, the available literature has begun to relate AS to a specific subgroup of learning disabilities — the nonverbal learning disabilities — and assessment and treatment implications from this model should prove useful in strengthening assessment–treatment linkages for this population.

Finally, one of our primary tasks was to examine the similarities and differences in the learning characteristics of individuals with AS and HFA. We would suggest that AS is a relatively unique taxon, with many similarities to HFA. With only about 20 published studies to date addressing the various learning characteristics of AS, future research clearly is needed to provide greater clarification on this matter. As descriptions of the specific kinds of learning problems experienced by AS individuals become more clear, so too should the similarities and differences between this diagnosis and HFA.

ACKNOWLEDGMENTS

This chapter was completed with support from grants from the Maternal and Child Health Bureau and the Administration for Developmental Disabilities awarded to the Center for Development and Learning.

REFERENCES

American Psychiatric Association. (1994). *Diagnostic and statistical manual of mental disorders* (4th ed.). Washington, DC: Author.

Asch, S. E. (1951). Effects of group pressure upon the modification and distortion of judgments. In H. Guetzkow (Ed.), *Groups, leadership and men: Research in human relations* (pp. 177–190). Pittsburgh: Carnegie Press.

Asperger, H. (1944). Die "autistischen Psychopathien" im kindesalter. *Archiv für Psychiatrie und Nervenkrankheiten, 117*, 76–136.

Barrows, A. (1988). Asperger's syndrome: A theoretical and clinical account (Doctoral dissertation, The Wright Institute). *Dissertation Abstracts International, 49*, 907.

Bennetto, L., Pennington, B. F., & Rogers, S. J. (1995). Intact and impaired memory functions in autism. *Child Development, 67*, 1816–1835.

Berthier, M. L. (1994). Corticocallosal anomalies in Asperger's syndrome. *American Journal of Roentgenology, 162*, 236–237.

Berthier, M. L., Bayes, A., & Tolosa, E. S. (1993). Magnetic resonance imaging in patients with concurrent Tourette's disorder and Asperger's syndrome. *Journal of the American Academy of Child and Adolescent Psychiatry, 32*, 633–639.

Berthier, M., Starkstein, S. E., & Leiguarda, R. (1990). Developmental cortical anomalies in Asperger's syndrome: Neuroradiological findings in two patients. *Journal of Neuropsychiatry and Clinical Neurosciences, 2*, 197–201.

Bigler, E. D. (1989). On the neuropsychology of suicide. *Journal of Learning Disabilities, 22*, 180–185.

Bishop, D. V. (1989). Autism, Asperger's syndrome and semantic–pragmatic disorder: Where are the boundaries? Special issue: Autism. *British Journal of Disorders of Communication, 24*, 107–121.

Blonder, L. X., Bowers, D., & Heilman, K. M. (1991). The role of the right hemisphere in emotional communication. *Brain, 114*, 1115–1127 (Published erratum appears in *Brain, 115*, 645).

Borod, J. C., Koff, E., & Caron, H. S. (1983). Right hemispheric specialization for the expression and appreciation of emotion: A focus on the fact. In E. Perecman (Ed.), *Cognitive processing in the right hemisphere* (pp. 83–110). New York: Academic Press.

Bowers, D., Bauer, R., Coslett, H., et al. (1985). Dissociation between the processing of affective and nonaffective faces in patients with unilateral brain lesions. *Brain and Cognition, 4*, 258–272.

Bowler, D. (1992). "Theory of mind" in Asperger's syndrome. *Journal of Child Psychology and Psychiatry and Allied Disciplines, 33*, 877–893.

Bowler, D. M., & Worley, K. (1994). Susceptibility to social influence in adults with Asperger's syndrome: A research note. *Journal of Child Psychology and Psychiatry and Allied Disciplines, 35*, 689–697.

David, A. S., Wacharasindhu, A., & Lishman, W. A. (1993). Severe psychiatric disturbance and abnormalities of the corpus callosum: Review and case series. *Journal of Neurological and Neurosurgical Psychiatry, 56*, 85–93.

Davies, S, Bishop, D., Manstead, A. R., & Tantam, D. (1994). Face perception in children with autism and Asperger's syndrome. *Journal of Child Psychology and Psychiatry and Allied Disciplines, 35*, 1033–1057.

Denckla, M. B. (1983). The neuropsychology of social-emotional learning disabilities. *Archives of Neurology, 40*, 461–462.

Eaves, L. C., Ho, H. H., & Eaves, D. M. (1994). Subtypes of autism by cluster analysis. *Journal of Autism and Developmental Disorders, 24*, 3–22.

Fine, J., Bartolucci, G., Ginsberg, G., & Szatmari, P. (1991). The use of intonation to communicate in pervasive developmental disorders. *Journal of Child Psychology and Psychiatry and Allied Disciplines, 32*, 771–782.

Fine, J., Bartolucci, G., Szatmari, P., & Ginsberg, G. (1994). Cohesive discourse in pervasive developmental disorders. *Journal of Autism and Developmental Disorders, 24*, 315–329.

Francis, D. J., Shaywitz, S. E., Stuebing, K. K., Shaywitz, B. A., & Fletcher, J. M. (1996). Developmental lag versus deficit models of reading disability: A longitudinal, growth curves analysis. *Journal of Educational Psychology, 88*, 3–17.

Ghaziuddin, M., Butler, E., Tsai, L., & Ghaziuddin, N. (1994). Is clumsiness a marker for Asperger syndrome? *Journal of Intellectual Disability Research, 38,* 519–527.

Ghaziuddin, M., Tsai, L. Y., & Ghaziuddin, N. (1992). Brief report: A reappraisal of clumsiness as a diagnostic feature of Asperger syndrome. Special issue: Classification and diagnosis. *Journal of Autism and Developmental Disorders, 22,* 651–656.

Gillberg, C. (1989). Asperger syndrome in 23 Swedish children. *Developmental Medicine and Child Neurology, 31,* 520–531.

Gillberg, C. (1991). Clinical and neurobiological aspects of Asperger syndrome in six family studies. In U. Frith (Ed.), *Autism and Asperger syndrome* (pp. 122–146). Cambridge: Cambridge University Press.

Goldberg, E., & Costa, L. D. (1981). Hemisphere differences in the acquisition and use of descriptive systems. *Brain and Language, 14,* 144–173.

Goldstein, G., Minshew, N. J., & Siegel, D. J. (1994). Age differences in academic achievement in high-functioning autistic individuals. *Journal of Clinical and Experimental Neuropsychology, 16,* 671–680.

Goodman, R. (1989). Infantile autism: A syndrome of multiple primary deficits. *Journal of Autism and Developmental Disorders, 19,* 409–424.

Hooper, S. R., & Willis, W. G. (1989). *Learning disability subtyping. Neuropsychological foundations, conceptual models, and issues in clinical differentiation.* Berlin: Springer-Verlag.

Interagency Committee on Learning Disabilities. (1987). *Learning disabilities: A report to the US Congress.* Washington, DC: Author.

Johnson, D. J., & Myklebust, H. R. (1971). *Learning disabilities.* New York: Grune & Stratton.

Jones, P. B., & Kerwin, R. W. (1990). Left temporal lobe damage in Asperger's syndrome. *British Journal of Psychiatry, 156,* 570–572.

Kanner, L. (1943). Autistic disturbances of affective contact. *Nervous Child, 2,* 217–250.

Klin, A., Sparrow, S. S., Volkmar, F. R., Cicchetti, D. V., & Rourke, B. P. (1995). Asperger Syndrome. In B. P. Rourke (Ed.), *Syndrome of nonverbal learning disabilities. Neurodevelopmental manifestations* (pp. 93–118). New York: Guilford Press.

Klin, A., Volkmar, F. R., Sparrow, S. S., Cicchetti, D. V., & Rourke, B. P. (1995). Validity and neuropsychological characterization of Asperger syndrome: Convergence with nonverbal learning disabilities syndrome. *Journal of Child Psychology and Psychiatry and Allied Disciplines, 36,* 1127–1140.

Kracke, I. (1994). Developmental prosopagnosia in Asperger syndrome: Presentation and discussion of an individual case. *Developmental Medicine and Child Neurology, 36,* 873–886.

Lai, Z. (1993). A neuropsychological test of cortical circuitry subserving affective processing in the developing human brain (Doctoral dissertation, University of Minnesota). *Dissertation Abstracts International, 53,* 4399.

Mesibov, G. B. (1992). Treatment issues with high-functioning adolescents and adults with autism. In E. Schopler & G. B. Mesibov (Eds.), *High-functioning individuals with autism* (pp. 143–155). New York: Plenum Press.

Minshew, N. J., & Goldstein, G. (1993). Is autism an amnesic disorder? Evidence from the California Verbal Learning Test. *Neuropsychology, 7,* 209–216.

Minshew, N. J., Goldstein, G., Muenz, L. R., & Payton, J. B. (1992). Neuropsychological functioning in nonmentally retarded autistic individuals. *Journal of Clinical and Experimental Neuropsychology, 14,* 749–761.

Minshew, N. J., Goldstein, G., & Siegel, D. J. (1995). Speech and language in high-functioning autistic individuals. *Neuropsychology, 9,* 255–261.

Minshew, N. J., Goldstein, G., Taylor, H. G., & Siegel, D. J. (1994). Academic achievement in high functioning autistic individuals. *Journal of Clinical and Experimental Neuropsychology, 16,* 261–270.

Mottron, L., & Belleville, S. (1993). A study of perceptual analysis in a high-level autistic subject with exceptional graphic abilities. *Brain and Cognition, 23,* 279–309.

Myklebust, H. R. (1975). Nonverbal learning disabilities: Assessment and intervention. In H. R. Myklebust (Ed.), *Progress in learning disabilities* (Vol. 3, pp. 85–121). New York: Grune & Stratton.

Ozonoff, S., Rogers, S., & Pennington, B. (1991). Asperger's syndrome: Evidence of an empirical distinction from high-functioning autism. *Journal of Child Psychology and Psychiatry and Allied Disciplines, 32,* 1107–1122.

Pennington, B. F. (1991). *Diagnosing learning disorders. A neuropsychological framework.* New York: Guilford Press.

Ross, E. D., & Mesulam, M.-M. (1979). Dominant language functions of the right hemisphere? *Archives of Neurology, 36,* 144–149.

Rourke, B. P. (Ed.). (1985). *Neuropsychology of learning disabilities: Essentials of subtype analysis.* New York: Guilford Press.

Rourke, B. P. (1988). Socio-emotional disturbances of learning-disabled children. *Journal of Consulting and Clinical Psychology, 56,* 801–810.

Rourke, B. P. (1989). *Nonverbal learning disabilities: The syndrome and the model.* New York: Guilford Press.

Rourke, B. P. (Ed.). (1995). *Syndrome of nonverbal learning disabilities. Neurodevelopmental manifestations.* New York: Guilford Press.

Rourke, B. P., Young, G. C., & Leenaars, A. A. (1989). A childhood learning disability that predisposes those afflicted to adolescent and adult depression and suicide risk. *Journal of Learning Disabilities, 22,* 169–185.

Semrud-Clikeman, M., & Hynd, G. W. (1990). Right hemisphere dysfunction in nonverbal learning disabilities: Social, academic, and adaptive functioning in adults and children. *Psychological Bulletin, 107,* 196–209.

Shea, V., & Mesibov, G. B. (1985). The relationship of learning disabilities and higher-level autism. *Journal of Autism and Developmental Disorders, 15,* 425–435.

Shields, J. R. (1991). Semantic–pragmatic disorder: A right hemisphere syndrome? *British Journal of Disorders of Communication, 26,* 383–392.

Siegel, D. J., Minshew, N. J., & Goldstein, G. (1996). Wechsler IQ profiles in diagnosis of high-functioning autism. *Journal of Autism and Developmental Disorders, 26,* 389–405.

Steffenburg, S. (1991). Neuropsychiatric assessment of children with autism: A population-based study. *Developmental Medicine and Child Neurology, 33,* 495–511.

Szatmari, P., Bartolucci, G., & Bremner, R. (1989). Asperger's syndrome and autism: Comparisons on early history and outcome. *Developmental Medicine and Child Neurology, 31,* 709–720.

Szatmari, P., Bremner, R., & Nagy, J. (1989). Asperger's syndrome: A review of clinical features. *Canadian Journal of Psychiatry, 34,* 554–560.

Szatmari, P., Tuff, L., Finlayson, A., & Bartolucci, G. (1990). Asperger's syndrome and autism: Neurocognitive aspects. *Journal of the American Academy of Child and Adolescent Psychiatry, 29,* 130–136.

Tantam, D., Evered, C., & Hersov, L. (1990). Asperger's syndrome and ligamentous laxity. *Journal of the American Academy of Child and Adolescent Psychiatry, 29,* 892–896.

Tantum, D., Holmes, P., & Cordess, C. (1993). Nonverbal expression in autism of Asperger type. *Journal of Autism and Developmental Disorders, 23,* 111–113.

Van Bourgondien, M. E., & Woods, A. V. (1992). Vocational possibilities for high-functioning adults with autism. In E. Schopler & G. B. Mesibov (Eds.), *High-functioning individuals with autism* (pp. 227–239). New York: Plenum Press.

Voeller, K. K. S. (1986). Right-hemisphere deficit syndrome in children. *American Journal of Psychiatry, 143,* 1004–1009.

Voeller, K. K. S., Hanson, J. A., & Wendt, R. N. (1988). Facial affect recognition in children: A comparison of the performance of children with right and left hemisphere lesions. *Neurology*, *38*, 1744–1748.

Volkmar, F. R., Klin, A., Siegel, B., Szatmari, P., Lord, C., Campbell, M., Freeman, B. J., Cicchetti, D. V., Rutter, M., Kline, W., Buitelaar, J., Hattab, Y., Fombonne, E., Fuentes, J., Werry, J., Stone, W., Kerbeshian, J., Hoshino, Y., Bregman, J., Loveland, K., Szymanski, L, & Towbin, K. (1994). DSM-IV autism/pervasive developmental disorder field trial. *American Journal of Psychiatry*, *151*, 1361–1367.

Weintraub, S., & Mesulam, M.-M. (1983). Developmental learning disabilities of the right hemisphere: Emotional, interpersonal, and cognitive components. *Archives of Neurology*, *40*, 463–468.

Wing, L. (1981). Asperger's syndrome: A clinical account. *Psychological Medicine*, *11*, 115–129.

Wing, L. (1991). Mental retardation and the autistic continuum. In P. E. Bebbington (Ed.), *Social psychiatry: Theory, methodology, and practice* (pp. 113–138). New Brunswick, NJ: Transaction.

World Health Organization. (1990, May). *International classification of diseases: Tenth revision.* Chapter V. Mental and behavioral disorders (including disorders of psychological development): Diagnostic criteria for research. Geneva: Author.

VI

Personal Essays

15

A Personal Account of Autism

THOMAS A. McKEAN

INTRODUCTION

In preparing for writing this essay, I looked over the contributions in the sister book to this one, *High-Functioning Individuals with Autism*. Needless to say, I was impressed by the quality of writing that went into that book, and I was (as always) particularly impressed by the extreme honesty and candor of my colleagues. I feel honored now to be asked to make a contribution to this fine series.

I was born in mid 1965 at the Ohio State University. Everything was fine until I was about 6 months old. My parents took me in for glasses. I put them on, saw the world for the first time, and I didn't like what I saw. That's the way the story goes as I hear it, I can't really say that I recall being 6 months old. What I do know is that 32 years later, I still don't like what I see.

Growing up, I thought that what was happening to me was also happening to everyone else. I thought they just handled it better. I really had no idea what was going on, though it was painfully obvious to me by kindergarten that something was. I kept a volley from one doctor to the next, but because I could talk (though I never really said much, and if I did, it never really mattered) they refused to give me the diagnosis.

Because no one would confirm the diagnosis, acting "autistic" in any way was the wrong thing to do. I was often punished for reasons I didn't understand, simply because what I was doing was being myself. It has been suggested to me

THOMAS A. McKEAN • Columbus, Ohio 43229.

Asperger Syndrome or High-Functioning Autism?, edited by Schopler *et al.* Plenum Press, New York, 1998.

that maybe this is a reason I turned out as well as I did, and that may be true. But it doesn't make the memories any easier to live with.

For this reason, I very strongly advocate telling your children. Because I didn't know, I was under the impression that what I did wrong was my fault and that I was basically an all-around bad person. If you don't tell them what is wrong, their own imaginations will make something up and things will only get worse from there. Just as I knew something was wrong at a very young age, I suspect most people with autism are the same in this respect. I am sure many professionals will shake their heads and tell me (or you) that I am crazy for even suggesting you tell your children the truth. Let them. They haven't been there. They haven't felt the pain.

School was pretty much a nightmare. I was held back a year before kindergarten, stayed in regular classrooms until halfway through third grade. Then I spent every year (sometimes even half years) in a different school and in a different special-ed class. (Part of this was because I was among the first unfortunate victims of the now defunct and now admittedly wrong "desegregation" experiments of the 1970s, not to mention one of the first affected by P. L. 94–142.) If my parents or the professionals wondered why I never made any friends, it may have simply been because they never gave me a chance before moving me again. Sixth grade came along and I was placed back in the regular classroom. That's when I dabbled with writing for the first time.

Junior high proved to be a mixture of the previous experiences. Half of the day I was in regular classes, half of the day I was in with a special-ed teacher, who, like many before her, had next to no compassion and really didn't understand her job or the students in the class. Nor did she have any desire to. Now, many years later, I am always happy when a teacher shows up at conferences. It is too late for me, but it is not too late for them. If there are any teachers reading this and you see my name on a conference ad, come to the conference and tell me you came because you believe this essay in the sense that teachers need more education. *Doing so will make me one very happy Thomas.*

I was never very popular in school. Being in the "special classroom," as the other students called it, I was an easy target and I dreaded things like gym and recess. I would usually just walk around on the playground by myself and watch the other kids play. By this time, drugs had become a problem in schools and thus they did away with the private stalls. This was a problem for me back then. I have since outgrown it.

In the seventh grade, I had a mainstreamed math class (nowadays it would be an "included" math class) immediately following the lunch hour. All of the kids, being that they were indeed kids, seemed to be rather pumped after lunch and the teacher, "Mr. Dekker," never could keep control of things. One day he just gave up. Walked out on us in the middle of class, went into the office, announced that he quit, and marched triumphantly out the door of the school. I never saw him again after that. Too bad, really. He was one of my favorite teachers and he was also one of the few who could really connect with the students when he chose to do so. An important attribute for any educator.

Eighth grade came along and just before finals, it was announced to me that I was going into a psychiatric facility. I had gone to see yet another doctor and she labeled me with PDD-(NOS). I was also, in her opinion, "in severe danger of becoming schizophrenic." (That is a direct quote from personal medical records of the 1970s.) Why in the world they placed me in a mental institution is beyond me. *Autism is* not *a mental illness. It is a neurological disorder.* Nevertheless, I was rather pleased to be going as it meant no study for finals. I was told that I would be there for 3 weeks and that I would be "automatically passed" into the next grade. Unethical, yes. But I was young then and didn't care. Now I am older and feel a little guilty about it. (Because of a clerical error, I was also illegally graduated from high school without ever attending. I passed the GED test, but legally it was too soon for me to graduate. I graduated anyway, beating everyone else in my class. Unlike the previous promotion, I have no guilt feelings about this whatsoever. I proved I knew the material that was required for the diploma. This is all that matters as far as I am concerned.)

I decided to look at the 3 weeks as a vacation. That vacation lasted all of 3 years. If I was helped at all during those 3 years, it was more the result of random day-to-day events than it was by the doctors or any of the therapy. I think that my values and my personality were somewhat ultimately molded in a positive way by what I experienced while I was there. You simply cannot watch people die and not be affected by it. I saw people in pain, heard people screaming, noticed the end results of drug overdose, helplessly observed many suicide attempts and a few successes. Not to mention God only knows how much bloodshed (quite literally, pools and pools of blood) I was there from age 14 to age 17. And even now, looking back, I still feel as though I have never had a chance to grow up, like my adolescence was stolen from me. Yet while I was there I learned something very important that would later help me in my conference speaking, on the board of directors of ASA, in my various writings, and in other advocacy. And that is that there is suffering in the world, and that once in a while, if you happen to be in the right place at the right time with the right attitude, maybe you can do something about it.

It was not all bad. Sometimes there was love. Usually a strong bond of friendship between the patients. We used to pass notes back and forth after hours with a remote control racer I had stashed in my drawer. Sometimes the staff caught us. Usually they didn't. When they did, we were usually punished. They seemed to not approve of us supporting each other. But with all of the bad things that were happening in there, that support sure went a long way with all of us.

There was one living area that was coed, that's where I was fortunate enough to spend most of my time. The boys and girls held secret meetings in the ladies room. The reason we were there was because we needed to talk to each other. Horrors beyond imagination faced us every morning we woke up. We never knew what would happen, or when. But we were always on guard. You were on guard or you were dead. That simple. For those curious, the reason we chose the ladies room was because the room was located in one of the very few areas not visible from the staff booth. We could sneak in and out of there without ever being seen, and both males and females did that frequently during the night. Sometimes prearranged, sometimes not. After the first few times you get "caught" by the opposite sex, it doesn't bother you anymore. There are far more important things to worry about. Like staying alive, or trying to find sanity when you walk only among insanity. Some of the staff even eventually found out that they'd have made better patients than staff. It is unfortunate that by the time this happened, the girls had already been abused and the damage had already been done.

When I was finally released, it was against the better judgment of the doctors. The earth had aged 3 years without me. Thus, I was in an alien world. (Historical reference note: As I write this essay, the *Sojourner* probe is mucking · about on the landscape of Mars. This cute little fellow is pretty much biding his time and every now and again, when the mood strikes him, he can be found taking pictures of big rocks. He takes pictures of big rocks wherever he can find them. Sometimes I wonder if even with MTV and VH-1, he doesn't seem to enjoy his collection of rock videos. But in all seriousness, I think I have a pretty good idea of how that little earth speed buggy is feeling right about now. He is all alone and he is certainly feeling that loneliness. He is fascinated and frightened by what he sees. Both of these emotions he is feeling in the extreme and at the same time. He is confused by this and he wants to be home in his own bed, but his strength and determination drive him forward. Forward to even bigger rocks. Go back in time and remember the television coverage or find a video somewhere. Imagine that it is you all alone out there so many miles from home with nothing but rocks and a video camera. Do this, and you may have some small idea of what autism is truly like.)

Just after I got out, I worked for a veterinarian for a short time. Then I left Ohio for Urbana, Illinois. I lived there for a while, attending a small, community college and studying computer science. No high school diploma was necessary to attend, so long as you studied to get your GED while you were there. And although I failed all of the college courses (except the one that was nontransferable), I did pass the aforementioned GED test the first time I took it. I attribute this now to divine intervention. I never studied for the test. It's also possible that I am smarter than I think I am.

The school had a strong Christian fellowship. And it was here that I met the person who would eventually go on to "bring me out of it." She seemed to *want* to be around me. This was very hard at first because I couldn't figure out why such an attractive and intelligent girl would want to be my friend. But she did, and I owe her a lot for that. She was the first person to ever really bother to look inside. And then she taught me how to look inside. She showed me that I was not really the bad person I thought I was all of those years. Princess Gwendolyn remains a close friend and a close friend she will remain until death does us part. Of this I am certain. I count myself fortunate to be befriended by Royalty. I let her know this on a regular basis. At least I try to.

She has taught me many things in the years that I have known her. For example, she taught me that I (and later I would come to see that this applied to most others with autism) had three things in abundance. These are inner strength, courage, and the capacity and ability to be at peace with myself. She showed me that I had these traits so many years ago. But it took my more recent martial arts training to open my eyes as to just how important and valuable these traits are. The irony of this is that if you look for these things in a person with autism, you will, with only very rare exception, easily find them. Everybody who knows the person knows that he or she has these qualities except the very person who has them. Something must be done to change this.

I returned to Columbus to attend another community college, this time studying mental health. I didn't fare too well academically, but I did learn a lot. Probably more about social interaction than about mental health.

After leaving school a second time, I took a job at Medicare. I processed claims for Ohio and West Virginia from 1986 to 1989. (That means I got Ruth Sullivan's people.) My supervisor, Brigadier Weidner, is to this day one of the most compassionate men I have ever met. I still see him frequently and we do things together even though I no longer work for him. I was proud to serve under the brigadier in the 1980s. Now, in the 1990s, I am a colonel and I am even more proud to be able just to call him my friend.

In 1989, I left Medicare behind me to go back to college. This time to study journalism. And I got passing grades. One quarter I even got all A's. I also met someone on the side. After three or four full-time quarters, I became burned out on college. Melanie and I continued to pursue our friendship and eventually we became engaged. Picture it: Columbus, Ohio, July 4th, 1989, 12:25 AM. Melanie and I are both enjoying a skinny dip in my father's backyard Jacuzzi. The sky is clear and stars are shining. The full moon smiles down on us like a beautiful Willendorf goddess. I take her hand in mine and I look longingly into her eyes. I say to her (and these are the *exact* words; well rehearsed, well remembered, and classic autism) "Melanie, you fabulous babe, would you do me the honor of becoming my wife?" Melanie looks longingly back at me. "Thomas," she replies, "you fabulous babe, I would be honored to be your wife." I gently slide a diamond on her finger and she melts into the water.

At this moment, I find peace. For the first time in my life, I know happiness. I decide at this point that it would be from the 25th year that I would date my life. But the peace and the happiness were not to last.

Friction mounted when it became obvious we had different needs. Her need for intercourse and my need for celibacy was a constant source of uneasiness between us. When she was raped several months after the engagement, she broke it off with me and eventually pursued a relationship with someone who was more able to fulfill her needs. Last I heard, she remains married.

Convinced that I was somehow the reason for the collapse, I began to search my past. It was there that I found the diagnosis. No one had bothered to tell me. This was kept from me for 11 years because of an obscure Ohio law. I had to stumble onto it on my own. Desperate to learn more about what autism was and how to treat it, and even more desperate to learn who this odd person named Thomas A. McKean really was, I put my name on the ballot of the board of directors of the Autism Society of America. I was surprised to be elected. That was in 1992. I have heard from a reliable source that I got the highest number of votes that year, even though at the time I was totally unknown. My thanks to ASA for opening the door for me. (My deeper thanks to Dr. Temple Grandin, for opening another door not only for me but for a few fortunate others to come through.)

SENSORY SENSITIVITIES

As I have spoken to many others in the field of autism, I have come to see how very vital it is that we who are able to talk about how we are affected by autism do so, especially in this area. I believe sensory anomalies may be at the root of many if not all behaviors that seem inappropriate or bizarre compared with the impossibly high standards set by the contemporary general population. (Dr. Gary Mesibov has told me he believes there are cognitive anomalies as well. He and I continue to debate this. I enjoy the debates.)

For me personally, the most annoying problems would have to be in the auditory and tactile/proprioceptive areas. My ears are extremely sensitive. Kind of like someone turned the volume on the universe all the way to high. It is very difficult for me to sleep unless it is absolutely quiet. (I used to leave my window open, then I discovered the birds woke me up with the sun to face the harsh reality that comes with daylight. Now I leave it closed.) This is not at all uncommon in autism. Estimates are that as many as 40% of all people affected by autism have auditory sensitivities. I believe the number is in reality much higher than that. I also believe, based on personal experience and many conversations with parents, professionals, and individuals with autism themselves, that there is in many of these cases a direct link between auditory sensitivities and violent behavior. More recently, I have discovered that a "sound machine" is very calming when trying to get to sleep.

And if you have ever explored the metaphysical side of the universe, there may be some help there, too. Don't jump the gun and think I am going to tell you to call a 900 psychic line. That won't help. Tarot cards and runes won't help you, either. There is the ogham, which has more scientific proof behind it, but that also won't help.

Some say there is love in the earth. Mother Earth, Father Time. Time and space, different yet synonymous and even synergistic. If the earth itself is alive, all that is within the earth is alive. Native Americans were the first to believe this. I think I may believe it, too. My recent research into this area surprisingly pointed me right to autism in the forms of jade, hematite, and gold.

Jade is, to put it one way, "the stone that dreams are made of." Legend has it that jade enables easier sleep, more pleasant dreams, easier dream interpretation, and a relief from nightmares. It is suggested that jade be placed under the pillow before going to bed for this reason.

Hematite is a beautiful crystal. The metallic look is incredible. The belief here is that hematite balances the mental, physical, spiritual, and emotional into one cohesive and healthy person.

Gold is another matter entirely. First there is the price. For metaphysical purposes, only the purest gold will do. Very few people know that gold is singled out as an instrument in the recovery of autism. (See Melody, 1995, *Love Is in the Earth*, Earth-Love Publishing, Wheat Ridge, CO, p. 299.)

Let's get real. Can rocks really help someone with autism? I have a ring carved out of pure jade. It was hard to find. I also found a ring carved out of pure hematite. Both fit me perfectly. I can't sit here and tell you that sliding a ring on your child's finger will help, but I know that it has helped me. The question then is, do the rings really help me because of metaphysics, do they help me simply because I *believe* they will help me (placebo effect), or do they help me as a way of providing a channel for my own energy to do me some good? The truth is I don't know. What I do know is what every parent out there knows. When it comes to autism, you do what works for you and your child. I am just tossing this out as yet another possible way to help amid the various other crackpot ideas.

Like others with autism, I too have noticed a craving for pressure. However, unlike those others, I find that I feel even better when that pressure is applied by the gentle touch of a friend. In fact, I believe that I need the touch more than the pressure. This causes some obvious problems. Contemporary American society is very clear on what is "proper" and what is not. Most touching is not proper. There seem to be unwritten rules and laws and boundaries about this that are somewhat universal in our society. I find I am constantly breaking these rules and laws at the conferences where I am speaking. (It would be interesting to note an observation at this point. That is that the parents often allow some invasion while the professionals usually make it very clear to me that I am doing something wrong. This fascinates me. Why are the parents of other people with autism more understanding and compassionate than the professionals who are said to be the best in the field?)

This "invasion" on my part is not done out of any conscious desire or attraction to that individual person. Rather, it is done out of a very strong platonic need to be close to someone. A friend of mine once observed that the needs for pressure and physical contact are very strong in newborns. One reason babies are wrapped in blankets is because of the drastic change in environments. That infant is used to the pressure of the mother's womb. Wrapping him or her in a blanket will simulate that pressure while acclimating the infant to the pressure-less world we all now live in. The tactile and touch needs are also there for obvious reasons. As we grow, we are supposed to develop and "grow out of" the cravings for these things. Perhaps in my case, that particular development just didn't occur. It would also explain why I sleep with bears and teethers and have a few bottles lying around.

Visually, I am very light sensitive. I have on occasion gotten physically sick from walking outside into the sunlight. Now I wear the darkest sunglasses I can find to avoid that happening. Going from light to dark also hurts my eyes. It is hard on me when I am in a room and someone turns off the lights.

One of the things I do to help me with this problem is wear the Irlen Filters. These are lenses with therapeutic colored filters in them that have been used successfully by people with dyslexia for many years. Donna Williams discovered they were also beneficial for people with autism. Research is currently being done to understand how these filters can best aid the autism community. I also have prisms in my lenses; this helps me with eye teaming, a visual problem common in autism.

I want to go on record as stating that there should be a law prohibiting the fluorescent lights in public and private schools. As the cost would be enormous, this will never happen. Yet if it did, think of how much more intelligent and comfortable our children would be. Having experienced these lights in the schools and in the board rooms, I know firsthand just how painful they truly are.

SOCIAL INTERACTION

Society is very strange. It does things I don't think I will ever understand. For instance, why are sex and violence so popular in the media? Why are children bringing loaded weapons to school? Where are they getting those weapons? Why is tobacco still legal? Why can't the government operate within its budget? What can Thomas do to better fit into mainstream society? And someone, anyone, *please* tell me what eventually happened to Barabbas!

There are no easy ways to answer these questions. Yet I have always wanted (perhaps even *needed*) answers. I knew what was going on around me. I knew *who* was doing *what* and *when* and *where* they were doing it. Usually (though not always), I even knew *how* it was being done. What I could never understand, what I still do not understand, is the *whys*. This is what people with autism have problems with.

I have developed one way to deal with this problem. When I want to know a why, I ask someone who knows and understands me (and who understands autism) well enough to answer my questions in a way I can relate to. There are very few people in this category and I am always looking to make friends of those few who do. I have discovered that a lot of questions simply have no answers. Although I know this is true, it is a truth that is very hard for me to accept. (The answer to Barabbas is out there somewhere.)

I am very dependent on my friends. I know they understand the world much better than I do, and thus there are times when I am forced to rely on their judgment. For this reason, I am also very careful about whom I choose as friends. I want people who are intelligent, compassionate, and trustworthy. People who are savvy to the ways of society in a fashion such that I never will be, and people who have a good heart. These people are very hard to find, but they are out there.

ADVICE FOR NEW PARENTS

Over the past several years, I have had many ask me for advice for new parents. Here is what I believe to be very important at this stage.

1. Go to the library. I can't stress this enough. You cannot appropriately deal with autism until you know what autism is. There is one important thing you need to know before you begin your early research. If you are checking a book written by a professional (or even the book you hold in your hands right now), check the copyright date. If it is over 5 years old, be aware that you may be getting outdated information. We are learning more and more about autism every day. Try to get the most current book(s) available. Doing otherwise may harm your child.

Yet we must also keep in mind that the older books are as important as the newer ones as they show us where we have been. We can know where we are going without knowing where we have been. But we really do need to know where we have been to actually get to where we are going.

If you are curious about where we have been, you may want to read, with great caution, *The Empty Fortress*. After reading this book, it is worth a moment of silence to individually (and collectively) pray we never go down that wrong road again. To see where we are going, read *Thinking in Pictures*, or *A Parents Guide to Autism*. (Not to be confused with *Autism: A Parents' Guide*. Leave that one alone. That is another "where we have been" book best left in the dark until you know where we are going.) Another good book would be the *Autism Treatment Guide*. As a parent, you must know the latest research and therapies, especially regarding sensory integration dysfunction, if you are to help your child. You must know what autism is, not what it was. After you know what it is, you can further help your child (and yourself) by learning what autism was. The history of autism is as fascinating as the disorder itself.

Many people find reading the history of mental or neurological disorders to be somewhat dry and boring. My guess is few can disagree that autism is an exception. Bernard Rimland's research of the 1960s disproving the "cold parent" theory can never be denied by anyone as being the best discovery ever to happen in the field of autism. Occupational therapist A. Jean Ayres and her discovery in the 1970s of sensory integration would go on to further vastly improve the lives of many children and adults with autism.

Look at Temple Grandin in the 1980s, speaking out for the first time only to find she has boldly gone where none with autism have gone before. Even to this day she remains the *Enterprise*. Certainly other starships have come along, myself included, but none of us can ever take the Captain's chair away from her. Oh, we may see the occasional navigator or engineer, maybe even a science officer or two, but the all-important command center seat belongs to Temple. It always will.

Guy Berard and his experiments with auditory training, originally designed to cure his own deteriorating hearing loss, have helped untold people with autism. My own sensory experiments in the early 1990s led to the modified telephones and pressure bracelets that are now being used around the world. Helen Irlen found that a simple thing like color can do wonders toward recovery, and what is probably one of the more significant pieces of history is Doug Biklin bringing back Rosemary Crossley's facilitated communication technique from Australia. Of all things mentioned, none has caused more fanfare, more hype, more media attention, or more controversy.

All of these things, and many more, somehow fit seamlessly together in a simplistically complex tapestry to give us a fascinating glimpse into the curiously almost mystical realm of those with autism and to an extent it provides our society with a private view of the rest of us who love them.

But I digress.

2. Have your child evaluated by an occupational therapist. With all of the sensory issues that are so evident in autism, early intervention is crucial. Ask around for the name of a reputable occupational therapist and have your child evaluated and treated. If there are sensory issues, the earlier you start to work on them, the better off your child will be. You may also want to consider speech therapy.

3. Find a support group. There are several support groups out there for parents of children with disabilities, and for parents of children with autism in particular. Several national organizations have local chapters, including the Autism Society of America and the Autism National Committee. Ask around for a group and then attend. Find a state or national conference and pay the registration fee. Remember that you are looking for answers, and this is one good place with lots of useful information.

After you have done these three things, you will know in your heart what you need to do next. Have no fear; what your heart tells you will be the right thing to do.

ADVICE FOR PROFESSIONALS

Some may say I have the audacity to want to be giving advice to professionals in the autism field. Yet outside of those who specialize in autism (and many times even then), it is common for professionals to make the same mistakes. Here are a few things to keep in mind.

1. Parents know what they are talking about. So often I hear complaints from parents that the professionals didn't believe there was a problem. (This happened in my own case.) You need to keep in mind that no one knows the child better than the parents. If they believe there is a problem, check it out. Give the parents the benefit of the doubt. They deserve it.

2. Be honest with the parents and speak to them in plain English. Many times I have heard parents tell me that the professionals danced around the diagnosis. If the child has autism, tell the parents the child has autism. If the child has PDD-NOS or Asperger syndrome, explain to the parents that this is a form of autism. Proper home treatment cannot begin until the parents know what is wrong. Also, do not use the term *autistic-like behavior*. Either the child has autism or the child does not have autism. For all of your schooling and training, it really boils down to something that is just that simple. As the professional, it is your job to make that determination. I am so aggravated to see so many who claim to be professionals still riding the fence on this one. If the child has autism, *tell the parents the child has autism*. If you determine the child does not have autism, look for other problems. But whatever the diagnosis, be straight and be honest with the parents. As much as it may hurt them to hear the truth, it is the child who will suffer (and suffer greatly) if the truth is not told. Don't be afraid as there is nothing to fear in the truth. (For 11 years, my own parents were told I was "developmentally delayed." Anyone know what the therapies are for someone who is "developmentally delayed"? There are none, because such a condition does not exist.)

3. Keep up to date on the research. Nothing bothers me more than talking to professionals at a conference and discovering that I know more about autism than they do. This happens far more often than I would like it to. It is vital that those working in the autism community, be they doctors, advocates, teachers, or therapists, understand where research (and theories) are going. Views, opinions, research, and therapies are constantly changing in the field. If these children are to be treated appropriately, we need to know the current lines of thinking. We don't need to agree on them (though that would certainly help), but we need to know them.

4. Don't make it look hopeless. Time and time again I have heard parents tell me that when the child was first diagnosed, the doctor said that he or she would never talk and would need to be placed in an institution for life. Then the parents go on to tell me how the child is communicating well and is included in a regular classroom and even has some friends. These people making the diagnoses are condemning the children to hell. You are doctors, you are not gods. You have the right to diagnose but you have no right to condemn. *Give the child a chance.* He or she may surprise you.

CONCLUSION

Now, more than ever, there is hope. With radical therapies and a slow (but definite) international change in attitude, more children will begin to recover and to recover more thoroughly. Although I don't believe there will be a cure for autism anytime soon, I do believe there may someday be a prevention. I believe there are valid treatments that can improve the lives of these worthy individuals. We owe it to them to try anything we can and anything we need to in order to make those lives more fulfilling and beneficial to society. We simply cannot even begin to imagine the benefits society will receive in return.

16

An Essay of Faith, Perserverance, and Hard Work

JEFFREY B. PIGOTT

I will start at the beginning. I was born on Saturday, September 11, 1971, at Rex Hospital in Raleigh, North Carolina. My parents noticed that I was not developing as quickly as they expected. They also noticed that I was not getting over certain fears that other normally developing children usually get over by age 2 or 3. Some of those fears were toilets flushing, fireworks (although today some people tell me that this is a legitimate concern as opposed to a fear and it may be both), race cars, and the like. As a result, I was taken to the Developmental Evaluation Center in early 1973 where my parents were told that I was moderately retarded which really did not fit me at all. They also had been told that I needed to be placed in a special school for children with mental retardation. In early 1974, I was sent to Frankie Lemmon School to receive the best help possible with my "diagnosis" of moderate retardation. I went there for 3 years and I improved to the point where I was able to go to public school. When my parents and teachers told me about this, I was Ecstatic! Now, some of you out there must be thinking: "Great! No more problems! He's living happily ever after!" I am sorry to dash that thought, but that was not the case.

From the time I began public school in August 1977, my academic and social problems continued. Let me give two examples of some of those problems. I remember that math was a real academic problem in my middle and high school years during the 1980s because math is such an abstract field of study. When a

JEFFREY B. PIGOTT • Raleigh, North Carolina 27607.

Asperger Syndrome or High-Functioning Autism?, edited by Schopler *et al.* Plenum Press, New York, 1998.

person with autism works with forms of math like algebra, there is a lot of information coming in to be processed by the brain. Most "normal" people who are really good with forms of math like algebra and trigonometry are able to "take it all at once" as the saying goes because their thinking processes are faster. A person who has autism must filter the information and therefore works at a slower pace. This was pretty much the case with me because there I was asking questions about things that the teacher had gone over already. Others asked also, but I asked the most often. Next is an example of a social problem that I had and this deals with the anger and frustration that I experienced because of my peers making fun of the fact that I was different.

One day in the eighth grade, while I was standing on the sidewalk during my lunch period in the winter of 1986, a student walked up to me and started pounding on my back. I did my best to contain my anger for as long as I could but finally I turned around and started to fight with him. Thankfully, my P.E. teacher intervened and resolved that crisis.

Next I will describe the kinds of classes that I took. I was in regular classes for the most part. At the beginning of sixth grade, I was placed in Curriculum Assistance, which was a special one-hour study hall for students with learning disabilities. Thus, in 1984 my diagnosis of moderate retardation had been upgraded to learning disabled. This upgrade occurred as the result of an individual evaluation program (IEP) by the Wake County Public School System.

I was in Curriculum Assistance until I graduated from Needham B. Broughton High School in Raleigh, North Carolina, on June 6, 1990. One thing (or actually two) about Curriculum Assistance is that while I was in this class I was able to get help for my homework as well as for the social problems I was having, even though my class was not designed for students with autism. During my junior year at Broughton there was a highlight that my family and I will remember for years. I was in danger of failing the 11th grade near the end of the third quarter of the final semester. With that in mind, my dad told me to give him my class ring until things improved. Thankfully, things did get better as a result of a last-minute effort during the final quarter to pass. It worked, but I was not sure of that until my mother called the school one day in May 1989 for positive confirmation that I would be a senior during the 1989–1990 school year at Broughton. That same night I was called to supper and I received a delightful surprise. At my place was a chocolate ice cream cake that said, "Congratulations, Jeffrey! You made it!" and my class ring that I worked so hard for was in the middle of that cake! We had turned near tragedy into triumph. We laughed so hard that we all cried. My senior year, by the way, was really good. I maintained a consistent grade point average of 3.0.

When late 1990 rolled around, events in my life changed quite drastically. I got a job as a bagger at Phar-Mor, Inc. in July and began attending Wake Technical Community College in September. It was there that an academic/personal crisis occurred that would precipitate something very major in my life. This major event began when my English instructor went to the Disabilities Counselor at Wake Tech in very early 1991. She told my counselor that I would drink my entire water thermos before class and then ask to use the restroom, and this really irritated her. With that in mind, the counselor talked with my parents about a referral to Division TEACCH in Chapel Hill, North Carolina. We went there to find out more about the problem that had been affecting me for nearly 20 years. On March 14, 1991, the diagnosis of mild autism was established. Now, you might be asking yourselves, "How did you and your family deal with this and what effect, if any, did the new diagnosis have on your Christian faith?" I was very angry both about the diagnosis and about the way in which it was disclosed to me. Another thing that bothered me was finding out at such a late age (I was 19½ years old when I was diagnosed).

My family was wonderful in helping me to get through those first 8 months of integrating the new diagnosis into my life. I will give two important examples of this. On the day of my diagnosis, my dad told me: "You see, basically nothing has changed!" Now, if you interpret that as meaning that I am still Jeff Pigott, then that's right. Another example concerns my paternal grandmother, Violet L. Pigott. One Saturday afternoon a couple of weeks after the diagnosis, we drove to her house in Clayton, North Carolina, and we talked about the anger that I was experiencing and she told me: "You can help someone in a Christian way and a professional way. The person who diagnosed you is trying to help you in a professional way."

I agree that I was being labeled in a professional way because a trained party from Division TEACCH finally made the correct diagnosis of high-functioning autism. Second is my paternal grandmother's point that a person can be helped in a Christian way. The evangelical conservative Christian values on which I have built my life have played a very important role. Without these beliefs I could have become very depressed about my condition. Because of my beliefs, however, I am excited about my life as a whole, my experiences with TEACCH, writing this chapter, having fun at TEACCH In-Service programs, and so forth.

Division TEACCH really helped me by introducing me to the Social Skills Group (now simply called Social Group) in September 1991. Although it has taken some time, I have really come to enjoy this group. We go to Camp Dogwood in Sheralls Ford, North Carolina, each September, and have done so quite successfully for several years. In addition to enjoying the boating, cook-outs, games, and other activities of Camp Dogwood, I enjoy the Durham Bulls baseball games, individual outings for dinner at restaurants, and the special summer outings to Jordan Lake, North Carolina. Another activity that I really enjoyed when I first went to Social Group in September 1991 was the making of a video entitled *Autism in Review*.

Another way that TEACCH has helped me has been through their superb job coaching program. This progam helped me to locate a job at the North

Carolina Department of Agriculture's Agronomics Services Division as a temporary full-time lab assistant from November 1991 to April 1992. They provided on-site training and continued support. It was really fun and I enjoyed it. The TEACCH job coaching program assisted me again in the early spring of 1992 by referring me to a job fair for people with disabilities at the Raleigh Civic and Convention Center. At the fair, I met with Underwriters Laboratories and a few weeks later, on May 4, 1992, I got a job as a sample room attendant at Underwriters Laboratories, Inc. I am still happily employed there. I continue to participate in the Division TEACCH job coaching program and I would like to thank David Laxton for doing such a wonderful job in training me. I would also like to thank Dr. Lee Marcus, Clinical Director of Chapel Hill TEACCH, for referring me to the job coaching program.

Let me now discuss my living arrangements and conference speaking opportunities. I lived with my parents all of my life until March 1994, when I moved into Meredith Village Apatments with the help of Residential Support Services of Wake County, Inc. as well as my dear family. That day was so special because it began this latest chapter in my adult life. Living in my apartment has really taught me a lot about what it means to be independent and also how to communicate in a calm, clear manner.

I have had some problems along the way, but my family and friends have been there to help and that's very comforting and important. One problem was with my first roommate, who lived with me from March until July 1994. I had a problem with his stepfather coming over to the apartment and deciding what the thermostat should be set at, as opposed to letting my roommate and I make that decision ourselves, as we should have been allowed to do. This problem was only one of many that I had with my roommate. I have learned to be very thankful for my good independent living skills because I saw what can happen when a person with a developmental disorder such as my first roommate is so overly protected to the point that he is not properly prepared for independent life.

On the conference trail, I gave my first presentation in February 1994, at a Winter In-Service for Division TEACCH. I really enjoyed that because it was a great opportunity to meet professionals from across the state, country, and world who work with autistic people and I am glad that I was able to meet David Moser, a fine young man with high-functioning autism. I was glad to meet David because he has successfully dealt with his autism. As I spoke at the conference, he stood in the back of the room and told Dr. Gary Mesibov that he really wanted to meet me because he had noticed similarities between the two of us.

A friend of mine from Division TEACCH said that David and I make a fine team and she is right. However, David and I would not make a fine team if we did not have the same moral convictions and beliefs. I spoke at the Division TEACCH Winter In-Service on February 23, 1995, in Durham, North Carolina. That was really neat because it is always good to be able to talk to new audiences as well as those you have addressed before. Another really exciting aspect about all of this is that the people who come to these In-Services benefit from hearing me speak.

At my third consecutive successful (as well as enjoyable) TEACCH Winter In-Service talk in Durham on February 22, 1996, I had a great turnout. We laughed and enjoyed ourselves as I not only informed my audience but also entertained them with my sense of humor and an unexpected blooper that had everybody laughing! I will not mention that blooper, however, because I was very embarrassed.

I was invited to speak at the annual conference of the Autism Society of America in 1995 by Dr. Julie A. Donnelly. Regarding this, she had contacted Dr. Gary Mesibov, who, in turn, called and asked me if I would give him permission to pass on my name and address to her. Subsequently, I was invited to the conference held in Greensboro, North Carolina, on July 12–15, 1995. It was really great to be able to share with a national audience my experiences with autism, my faith in Christ Jesus, and my TEACCH experiences. Being on the panel was also neat because I was able to listen to three other high-functioning individuals with autism.

I have written this chapter to let my readers know that I will make it! I have been to more doctors than I can count and at one point saw a psychologist for over 2 years. After everything that I have gone through in the past 25 years, I can honestly say that I am very thankful for everyone and everything that has played a major role in my success. I close by extending an invitation. For those who want to write me, my address is: Jeffrey B. Pigott, 2429-D Wesvill Court, Raleigh, NC 27607. Also, if you are parents of autistic children, keep the faith! To all my dear readers, hang in there, and remember the late North Carolina State University basketball coach Jim Valvano: "Whatever you do, don't you ever, ever give up!"

17

How Fate Taught Me the Violin

DARIEN BROOKS

Have you ever wondered how many of us got interested in playing a musical instrument at an early age?

Although our parents and grandparents were the first people to teach us our musical talents after we heard them play the piano, guitar, violin, brass or woodwinds, they were only but among our first influences.

Some youngsters learned how to play the guitar after becoming inspired by a George Harrison solo on their first Beatles song, either on record or on radio.

Others first learned how to play the piano after becoming inspired by the greatness of Vladimir Horowitz or Elton John, although they never needed to wear flashy glasses or stage costumes while playing Chopin's "Minute Waltz" to imitate the latter in their first recital.

They might begin the clarinet to emulate Benny Goodman's swing, the trumpet for Louis Armstrong's New Orleans jazz, or the flute after hearing James Galway perform another soul-stirring performance before an enthralled audience.

But for me, my first involvement with the violin involved not hearing a great artist, but with fate playing the piece for me.

I remember when I was 11 years old, in fifth grade in Wilmington, North Carolina, that fate played a part in inspiring me to take up my first musical instrument, and the subsequent involvement of my parents and teachers to help me develop that talent.

It was in 1977 (I can't remember the exact date) that I first heard an announcement over the PA system in my fifth-grade class. It said that any

DARIEN BROOKS • Wilmington, North Carolina 28412.

Asperger Syndrome or High-Functioning Autism?, edited by Schopler *et al.* Plenum Press, New York, 1998.

interested student who wanted to play the band or orchestral instrument of their choice should go to the auditorium and sign up for that chosen instrument.

This got me curious, so being the interested student who was eager to try anything new, I joined up with my fellow schoolkids outside the auditorium in two separate lines — one for band instruments, the other for orchestral instruments.

I joined the line that was for the latter. When it came my turn to sign up, I casually put my name down on the list, along with the name of the instrument I wanted to play, the violin.

A few evenings later, as my family and I were having dinner, my mother received what would become the phone call that changed our lives forever.

"Your son put his name down on the list of interested orchestra students a few days ago, and if he wants to take part in the program, you may have to buy a violin for him."

My mother didn't know the person on the other end of the phone, but what she heard prompted her to put down the receiver and give me the biggest look of concern on her face that she ever sported.

What was this all about, she wanted to know, about me signing up to play a violin.

I had to let the truth out the best I could — anything to escape a possible whipping — and told her everything that had happened just a few days before: the PA announcement, the long lines at the auditorium, my signing up to play the violin, and my interest in joining the school orchestra.

She believed my story, but told me that if I was going to take part in such a program, we would have to cough up as much as $300 to buy it.

I bravely accepted her offer, but my mother added I would have to spend my after-school hours practicing as hard as possible to master the instrument.

I did, and soon learned to play scales, individual notes, and at times the different pieces in my first method book. This process had been so fast that my first teacher — the same teacher whose voice my mother had heard over the phone — placed me in the first violin section in the hope of helping me to learn how to read music.

That didn't work out at first. I could not even try to read one chord of either Beethoven, Bach, or Mozart along with the rest of the students while we were rehearsing, let alone try to emulate the partner playing next to me — and performing better than me.

It soon became frustrating and exhausting at times, trying to practice and sacrifice all of my TV time simply to master a piece of music on an instrument I knew nothing about when I first signed up, and I wondered if all of this was just an exercise in curiosity gone haywire.

But I kept trying and trying to master first violin with each school day — and still I was not able to read the right notes and play along with my partner and the rest of the students.

This continued into sixth grade and junior high, until my second teacher decided on a solution to my problem, when she noticed I didn't know how to sight-read.

She put me in the second violin section hoping that my frustrations would be exorcised and I would learn how to play better and without further difficulty.

To hers and my mother's surprise, it worked. I was able to read enough notes and copy my partner's playing as a second section player with no trouble at all.

I was to continue in the second section in high school, all the way to my first audition with the Wilmington Symphony, where I have been a community volunteer since 1985.

At the audition to become a WSO member, you have to bring a piece of music of your choice, and prepare to sight-read a symphonic work the conductor has made ready, in front of a small committee.

Remembering my experiences as a frustrated first violinist, I tried hard not to be nervous as I prepared for my audition — and to the committee's surprise, I passed it with no trouble at all, sight-reading and playing every note like a true professional.

In the 11 years since that audition, I have enjoyed getting to perform, and create friendships, with other members of the community who play not just violin, viola, and cello, but woodwind and brass instruments such as trumpet and clarinet.

I have had the honor and privilege of performing with world-renowned singers and musicians who have guest-performed with us, from sopranos to violinists, or simply with individuals from area high schools, who showcase their abilities with us each year, helping to ensure another sold-out season for our audiences and giving Wilmington its own cultural identity, all for sheer enjoyment.

Looking back at what I have just written, I am struck by how all of this came into being — how a simple announcement had launched my avocation as a musician — and how fate had inspires so many other young people who have a developmental or physical disability to pick up their first musical instrument, inject some positive thinking into their practicing, and say to themselves, "I can learn how to play this instrument all by myself just by believing in myself."

Fate can touch us in so many ways, including over a PA system in a classroom on a school afternoon.

18

How the Diagnosis of Asperger's Has Influenced My Life

VAN BRUCE MacDONALD

I was born in Evanston, Illinois, on January 24, 1938, the first child of a family no member of which had previously had developmental problems or mental illness. At that time, developmental problems and mental illnesses were in general poorly understood. At the ages of 2 and 3, in nursery school, I developed "theoretical skills," such as understanding letters and numbers, spelling words, following adults' commands, and even simple arithmetic skills, but did not develop "play skills," or the ability to interact socially with other children my age at all! For example, when the other children moved their hands to "imitate" a bird, I just exclaimed "I don't want to be a bird!" in a very loud and angry-sounding voice.

In Edmonton, in 1943 and 1944, where father was stationed on military duty, I again had great trouble interacting with other children in nursery school, often not attending it when scheduled because I was too busy daydreaming about things that were interesting to me. I read the longest and most complicated words in my neighbors' dictionary and even father's college math books. Once I wandered out into the country without knowing where I was going, and the police took me back home.

At grandpa's home in Seattle later during the war, I climbed the cherry tree in his backyard in order to "be a giant, with head at the actual position of my head up in the tree and feet on the ground," as that was a symbol of superiority.

VAN BRUCE MACDONALD • Denver, Colorado 80210

Asperger Syndrome or High-Functioning Autism?, edited by Schopler *et al.* Plenum Press, New York, 1998.

But when I tried to attend first grade, my developmental problems really revealed themselves as "something very serious, but no one knew just what," because I played in the toilets, screamed and sang and talked to myself in class so that other children couldn't study, used vile language, and had to be pulled out of school after 6 weeks. Mother and I had weekly meetings with a psychologist, Miss French, but she could do nothing to help us. However, she suggested that I completely lacked understanding of the "nebulous" rules of good social interaction with other people, both children and adults. During this time, Leo Kanner in the United States and Hans Asperger in Austria first characterized "autism" and "Asperger syndrome," the latter of which would eventually turn out to be exactly my diagnosis.

In Chicago after the war, I had to go to a tutor for an education. I "was even more superior," as I climbed much taller trees than I had climbed in Seattle, looking down from my perches up high in the trees on the electric wires and insulators "so as to be superior to an electrician." I rode my bike around nearby suburbs of Chicago so as to "be an explorer." I balanced very difficult designs with wood blocks, with one block at the bottom and several rows of eight blocks above, held together just by friction, not corrugations, so as to "be a circus performer" when the designs did not fall down. I threw several dice repeatedly and noted how frequently all or all but one showed the same number on top, so as to "be a probability-theory mathematician." (The frequencies actually agree with what I later calculated in algebra.)

At this time I was evaluated by the great Dr. Bruno Bettelheim, but he said that I was "too far gone to retrieve." At the office of another psychiatrist, Adrian Vandervere, I did nothing but lie on the floor and read the medical dictionary!

After moving to Denver in 1948, I satisfied my desires for "uniqueness" and "superiority" by excelling in school, getting all A's and B's except for a very few C's in such uninteresting subjects as "social science" (in which children study how people interact socially in this country or in the world so as to create a good life for everyone). I also took such subjects as algebra and Latin at an earlier age than most children take them, but still got high grades in them.

In Latin I became very fascinated with the letter V, five verbs (*valeo*, I am well; *venio*, I come; *video*, I see; *vinco*, I conquer; and *vivo*, I live) that begin with it, and their derivatives. I also became very fascinated with Dutch "van" (which resembles some of these Latin verbs, meaning "of" or "from," and is the most common word in that language!), as used as a man's first name in the United States. (That is why, on October 12, 1995, I changed my legal name, by court action, from Donald Bruce MacDonald to Van Bruce MacDonald.)

Since then, I have been deriving "unspeakably tremendous fun, pleasure, thrills, and gratifications to my emotions" out of being enclosed, completely alone, by the closed doors to my house, the closed door to my bathroom, and the curtain which did not enclose any of my property but did enclose me, while showering to maintain good hygiene. I have obtained some of my greatest thrills out of associating Van as a man's first name (now my favorite word in the English language) with showering, thinking of my own name while showering myself, and visualizing Van Cliburn (my favorite living real-life personage today) or myself taking showers.

At that time I had weekly meetings with a psychiatrist, Dr. Young, and mother met with a psychologist, Mr. Mandelbaum, both of the University of Colorado Medical Center. But for several years they did neither of us any real good. I had to take my first 2 years of high-school education from tutors, just as I had taken elementary education from them in Chicago. But in early April 1954, Mr. Mandelbaum moved to Topeka, Kansas, to work for the famed Menningers' Foundation. Just before he moved, he suggested to my parents and me that we all have a very thorough evaluation at Menningers.' In the middle 2 weeks of April, we did have such an evaluation. Most of the psychiatrists there gave us the gloomy prognosis that "I was destined to be a ward of the state or, at best, a patient 'put away' in the State Hospital, for the rest of my life," and told my parents to "pay us, walk away, and forget you had this son." But one psychiatrist, who did have hope, and who diagnosed me as having "severe, chronic, hebephrenic-type schizophrenia," suggested that shock treatment might help. Two forms of shock treatment, insulin and electric, were then in vogue for the seriously mentally ill, the latter being somewhat safer and more promising.

From May 1, 1954, to June 15, 1955 (at ages 16 and 17), I was locked up in Woodcroft, a private hospital in Pueblo, Colorado (totally unrelated to the State Hospital in the same city). There I received 32 electric shock treatments, all administered in the most frightening way possible. As my ability to reason and remember improved, the extremely sudden loss of consciousness became more frightening than ever. In 1955, I considered these treatments as consequences of my inappropriate or antisocial behavior, just as spanking would have been had I been mentally well, but much more severe (from my point of view). This status, of absolutely having to behave as appropriately as possible in order not to be extremely frightened by more treatments, absolutely forced me to develop the drive to free myself from my mental, emotional, behavioral, and social disabilities as completely and as soon as possible! This stay at Woodcroft was the most "negative" and frightening, but most important and momentous, chapter in my life! As a result of struggling as hard as possible all of the time to behave appropriately and to get mentally well, both before and after my release from Woodcroft, I would receive absolutely no more electric shock treatments after release. This made the summer of 1955 the happiest time in my life so far.

I took my senior year of high-school education at Mullen, a small Catholic parochial high school, and got all A's and B's there. By far the most interesting of my subjects there was physics, the study of the matter and energy of which our universe is composed. This has turned out to be my special savantlike skill, as it is still the one subject that I get the greatest fun and enjoyment out of devoting all of my attention to. Most of my college education (at the University of Colorado) has been in physics. Just before I started getting a college education, I was already daydreaming about minimizing the cost of energy produced by controlled earthbound nuclear fusion (now it would be cold, or muon-catalyzed, fusion) and freeing the world from chronic and serious mental illnesses and from violent and heinous crimes.

As long as I lived with my parents after release from Woodcroft, I got high grades (all A's and B's except for a very few C's in the most difficult or least interesting subjects at CU, grade point average 3.51), "had blowups," or did inappropriate things jeopardizing my right to go to school, only about once in 6 months on the average, became a member of Sigma Pi Sigma physics honor society, and worked for pay in physics in the summers of 1960 and 1961. But in the autumn of 1958, I tried living alone in Boulder while my parents were still in a suburb of Denver, "went berserk," and did only about half of my schoolwork (with A- and B-grade study traits). I got so much fun, pleasure, and thrills from my "dreamworld" (daydreaming about things, some realistic and some pure figments of my own imagination, for my very own fun) that I couldn't stop daydreaming to do the other half of my schoolwork, that I displayed exceedingly strange and bizarre behavior, with very little awareness of it, and that I felt absolutely no such unpleasant emotions as "feeling guilty," "being ashamed of myself," "hurts to my conscience," or "wishing I had done otherwise," no matter how much I was criticized, punished, or confronted by the police. After 2¼ months of living alone in Boulder, I had to be pulled out of school and returned to live with my parents.

In June 1959, I returned to school, living with my parents until October 24, 1961, when United Air Lines transferred father's job from Denver to Chicago. On that day my parents moved to Chicago and left me living with friends named Delia and Woody in Denver. Again I "went berserk" and did all of the things I did in the autumn of 1958, but now for 7 months, and across the country from my parents. Both times I just wasn't able to live without the care of either my parents or a mental institution. These things pointed out that I would need long-term, intensive treatment and support before I could get by on my own.

On May 1, 1962, CU put me under the care of its Colorado Psychiatric Hospital for a 6-week evaluation of my developmental problems, again pulling me out of school. At that time autism and Asperger syndrome were rarely talked about in the United States, and the only mental-health treatment then available was intended for quite different mental illnesses. The best that could be done then was to put me on Thorazine and Cogentin, intended for severe chronic schizophrenia, and to have me undergo 8 months of highly unpleasant discipline, in which the staff dictated everything I would do, in the form of a regular weekly schedule of therapeutic-community activities, at the Fort Logan Mental Health Center. After that I spent 2¾ years living in family-care homes with too few activities available to me, resulting in a very upsetting "vacuum," just waiting for psychiatry to become a better-developed branch of medical science.

(Despite the almost complete lack of understanding of my true developmental problem, Asperger syndrome, the treatments that were then available for quite different mental illnesses helped me struggle to improve my behavior and to overcome my abnormalities, so that, starting in 1970, I would stay out of mental hospitals for good, and would eventually live in my own apartment and then in my own duplex. I would also support myself with my income from my job at Bayaud Industries and my rental income from my tenants, completely on my own.)

On November 5, 1965, I became a worker at Fort Logan's industrial therapy shop. From then on I worked on decreasingly "sheltered" jobs, first there, then at Goodwill Industries of Denver, and finally for a year as a secretary and typist on "semicompetitive" jobs. These work experiences resulted in my getting the treatment needed eventually to live completely on my own. The skills needed to live and work more responsibly without others' help or guidance, and to practice very appropriate social behavior and very good social skills and work and study traits, came more and more "automatically."

By June 15, 1969, at the end of my year of semicompetitive work, I was sufficiently rehabilitated to realize my long-time prime goal, namely, returning to school and to the field of physics. Under the relatively emotionally unchallenging situation of studying the very topic that I get the greatest amount of fun and enjoyment out of devoting all of my attention to, I was destined for very good social behavior and high grades in physics. After my last semester of undergraduate study, I became a postgraduate student of modern quantum physics at CU in Boulder on August 18, 1969. For the next 3 years, I was to get all A's and B's except for one C in plasma physics in the final semester (grade point average 3.29), finally receiving a "special" or "honorary" degree of Master of Science in Engineering Nuclear Physics from CU on August 11, 1972 The reason I couldn't get a regular degree is that I had a very strong and irresistible temptation and urge to devote two thirds of my time in any laboratories to which I might be admitted to performing unauthorized experiments of my very own, just to get the extreme thrill of seeing the principles of physics and chemistry at work, and only the other one-third of my time to the assigned experiments, and that any further graduate work leading to a doctorate or employment in physics would entail extensive laboratory experimentation with intricate and expensive equipment.

My behavior at home and on the busses to and from Boulder was usually very appropriate, as long as I lived in family-care homes and even after I moved into a boarding home on October 8, 1970 (at the boarding home I really was successfully living under the care of neither my parents nor a mental institution). But in late January 1971, my housekeeper sold the boarding home to an extremely strict man who had high blood pressure, was overweight and overworked, and had had many traumatic experiences earlier in life. His being "absolutely too difficult to live under the authority of at home" precipitated very much inappropriate behavior at home, although everywhere else my behavior was usually very appropriate. (I can say that at school I still enjoyed a "good emotional utopia," getting my extreme fun, pleasure, and thrills from the real world, not from the dreamworld.)

On October 8, 1972, I began 24 years of work at a rehabilitation program, called Bayaud Industries (because it is on Bayaud Ave.), with the purpose of developing the ability to meet, successfully and with very appropriate social behavior and excellent social skills and work and study traits, all of the emotional and other challenges that will be entailed with my actually conferring my hoped-for future benefits, in physics and so on, on the world. For the first year my work there demanded little of my attention, and I enjoyed it very much while daydreaming about my favorite topics or socializing about appropriate topics with co-workers while working. My behavior at the workshop was always very appropriate. But early in my second year of work at Bayaud I was assigned to packaging fishhooks, in which I had to devote 100% of my attention just to being absolutely sure that I put exactly ten hooks in every little box, all the time I was at the workshop. Extremely frequent work-related variances between the way things were and the way I wanted them to be, by provoking unreasonably intense anger in me, elicited tremendous amounts of antisocial behavior at the workshop, in addition to my inappropriate behavior at home. This antisocial behavior provoked by unreasonably intense anger at little variances, and my getting just as angry at purely trivial, dreamworldly variances, having absolutely nothing to do with reality, as I got at genuine, real-life variances and frustrations, testified even more explicitly to my very serious, improperly treated developmental disability than excessive daydreaming and the strange and bizarre behavior resulting from the daydreaming had before.

But on June 1, 1975, I moved out of my boarding home into my very own private apartment, where I lived all by myself. On exactly the same day, I reverted to working on jobs demanding little of my attention and giving me great freedom to daydream and socialize while working. The resulting emotional unchallenged-nesses resulted in my best social behavior and work quality in my life save for the time since April 17, 1996. However, at the beginning of 1976, I reverted to packaging fishhooks all the time I was at the workshop, and from November 5, 1976, to March 3, 1978, I was transferred, one step at a time, to far more responsible and demanding work as a staff assistant (chiefly a timecard-calcu-lating accountant, calculating all of the financial transactions of Bayaud employ-ees, using their timecards). This very emotionally challenging and attention-demanding work precipitated blowups (violent displays of anger-pro-voked antisocial behavior) caused by work-related variances. Their frequency decreased from once in 5 days at the beginning of 1976 to once a month by June 1987, thereafter remaining at once a month until February 1992. For the next 3 years I had blowups only once in 4 months — but when I had them, my behavior was so much more antisocial and challenging to my employer's and tenants' authority than before that several times I came frighteningly close to losing, permanently and for the rest of my life, both of my sources of income (my job and my tenants' rental). With the gradual transfer of authority over me, as I perceived it, from my parents (who passed away during this period) in part to my employer and my tenants and in part to me myself, I was prone to "test others' limits" by behaving in any way I thought I newly had the right to behave, regardless of all other people's rights and freedoms. (It is natural for anyone, but was especially so for me, to "take advantage of" the removal of parental authority and to overindulge in such newly found freedom.)

Then came, on March 10, 1995, my correct diagnosis of Asperger syndrome! With my switchover from psychotropic drugs intended to treat schizophrenia, to abate anger, and to make me want to struggle harder to control my temper during anger—such as Thorazine, Stelazine, Tranxene, Haldol, Cogentin, and Benadryl—to a more appropriate kind (amitriptyline, a low-dose tricyclic antidepressant intended to counteract anxiety induced by Asperger syndrome, the main cause of all of my past antisocial behavior), with the realization that anxiety, not anger, was the most significant symptom, and with the acknowledgment of the tremendous differences between my previously assumed and my actual developmental disorders, my behavior improved more sharply than at any previous time in my life! Since my rediagnosis, I have "punished myself with an imperfect day" only once, on October 2, 1995, when a purely trivial, dreamworldly variance (something by which I have absolutely never been challenged since January 24, 1996), resulting from three "extremely negative" memories then haunting my mind, made me verbally threaten a Bayaud staff member's life (without any use of physical force). In January 1996, I stopped taking Haldol (the last of the old type of medications I had been on since 1962) and for several weeks took only amitriptyline. But several very physically violent and loud blowups at home at my duplex (although practically none anywhere else) forced me to resume taking Haldol. On March 14, my brother Clay showed me that using "common sense," "using everyday life as a physics laboratory," and not daydreaming too much would eliminate most of the variances that previously elicited inappropriate behavior. I have made full use of these suggestions ever since, and have also overcome all of my previously unrecognized stubbornnesses. However, the Haldol caused symptoms of "tardive dyskinesia," such as my tongue's flicking in and out of my mouth, my knees, elbows, and hands shaking a little, and my unknowingly having silly expressions on my face. For these reasons, on April 17, 1996, I was transferred from Haldol to Risperdal, and my tardive dyskinesia symptoms have vanished. It also does not require Cogentin (as Haldol did) to counteract side effects. Rating my behavior during anger on a scale of 0 to 10, with 0 being behaving so antisocially as to come very close to permanently losing my sources of income and 10 being displaying no inappropriate behavior at all during anger, I have gone below 10 only once during the more than 8 months since April 17. That one time was on May 22, when I went down to 6 by having a very loud and violent blowup in the middle of the night when my lights burned out and it took 10 minutes to put in new bulbs, thus waking everyone in the house.

My next social goals are to eliminate from my behavior such "very little inappropriatenesses" as whispering to myself, gritting my teeth, moving my fingers as though I were playing a piano or writing, and "appearing excited and in my dreamworld"; to exercise automatically the "little social graces" that people who have never been mentally disabled exercise around others, such as letting ladies on the bus or through doors first, being polite to waitresses in restaurants when they do not give me exactly what I want, saying "excuse me," and so on; to develop normal nonverbal communication; and to feel true social emotions such as love, sympathy, empathy, and repentance for past misdeeds "with my heart." Because of my medications I now semiautomatically do exercise some graces, such as picking up papers that others have dropped on the ground, letting old or disabled people through doors first and helping them by holding the doors open, saying "please" and "thank you," writing letters about twice a year to those who have really helped me, and getting out my bus pass before the bus comes so as to have it ready to show to the driver from the outset. People have observed that I am much calmer in general, and that when I talk, there is much less "high-pitched rapid-fire" affect in my voice. After another couple of years I hope to impress everyone around me "very positively," as though I had never been developmentally disabled. My social groups, led by well-trained mental-health workers, are greatly helping me become more aware of such graces all the time.

My medications have made it much easier for me to leave my dreamworld when that is important, to limit my daydreaming so as not to overindulge in it, to appear calm, relaxed, and "in the real world" when I approach other people with whom I have business, and to remain at all times well aware of all of my responsibilities to control myself and to put as much of my free time as possible to constructive use. Recently, when I "appear to have daydreamed about and analyzed exhaustively all there is to daydream about in all parts of my dream-world," short of my future professional work in the same fields, and "it is not my scheduled time to be in the machine room" (see below), I have been using my spare time considering other people's maintaining good hygiene, their studentship, job-seekership, workership, or none of these, their mental illnesses, and my own history in all of these respects, and so on. At first I did this about 3 hours a day, while listening to the radio; but now, with more constructive preparations for my future to occupy myself with, I do it only about half an hour a day. I spend this half hour analyzing the memories that spontaneously come to my mind each day as I think, observe, perceive, and experience both the real world and my dreamworld, memorizing my dreams during my sleep each night (all of which I can and do now memorize, as the result of my medications), and being enabled by my medications to feel a greater range of emotions than before.

My dreamworld is now divided into seven "rooms": the "Beethoven room" (music), the "cosine room" (mathematics), the "potassium room" (chemistry), the "Valentine room" (physics), the "customs room" (current national and international affairs, the news, economics, law, and so on), the "autobiography room" (my own extremely unusual, interesting, and remarkable life history and mental-health success story), and the "machine room" (not daydreaming at all in order to do my Bayaud Industries work, listen to the news, socialize with other people I know, or pay attention to others when it is particularly important). In particular, I now very much like "living on a schedule," which dictates what I am to do at each time of the week or when I have spare time to do as I please, such that when it's time to be in the machine room, that room has foremost prominence. This is because I have to do certain things, which demand all of my attention, at preset times of the week, in order to succeed in life. I am now enjoying every aspect of life more and more every day. My enjoyment of nuclear physics is increasing most rapidly (as my greatest hoped-for future benefit to the world is to maximize as far as is theoretically possible the number of fusions catalyzed by each muon in cold, or muon-catalyzed, fusion before it decays into an electron and neutrinos so as to minimize the cost of energy produced by controlled earthbound nuclear fusion); solid-state physics is becoming second most rapidly more "fun"; followed by molecular biophysics and psychophysics, "mesoscopic physics" (using the recently discovered Bose–Einstein condensate and "quantum dots"), elementary-particle physics, the autobiography room, and the machine room. (The first five of these seven are all in the Valentine room.) Nowadays the Beethoven, cosine, and potassium rooms are quite completely and permanently "saturated," meaning that there is nothing new in them that I have not already exhaustively analyzed in my daydreams before, and I now spend almost no time in these rooms; but I spend lots of time in the customs, Valentine, autobiography, and machine rooms.

On December 14, 1996, I took the Graduate Record Examination advanced test in physics, a test that I scored in the 98th percentile on in April 1971 (the new test, unlike the old, treats the many advances made in modern physics during the last 25 years). My scores were 78th percentile this time, and were reported to the University of Colorado at Boulder and at Denver, the CU Health Sciences Center, and me on January 11, 1997. About February 7, I hope to submit my final, fine-tuned and computer-written doctoral thesis (on explaining why light travels more slowly through material media than through a vacuum, why it undergoes reflection and refraction, and various of its other properties, including the new nonlinear optics, solely by quantum-mechanical, not classical, concepts) to Dr. John P. Cumalat, the new chairman of the CU Department of Physics. I hope on January 17 to become a tuition-paying student of physics (probably taking mostly lab courses) once again, remaining a Bayaud Industries worker at least until September 2, 1997, then, hopefully, to become a true, professional physicist, a paid worker in physics. Starting then, I hope actually to confer my hoped-for future benefits on the world. I have written a 200-page autobiography, *From Darkness to Light*, which I hope to publish and popularize around May 30, 1997. I hope to use it to "teach by example" that seriously developmentally disabled people throughout the world can overcome their abnormalities as I have nearly overcome mine, to enable them to benefit the world with their special savantlike skills, to advocate for the creation of paid jobs for them, to help identify and correct the various circumstances and factors that really do predispose a very small fraction of the people throughout the world to violent and heinous crimes, and to make several other, somewhat less major, advances in physics, such as using modern quantum theory to explain the elusive phenomenon of consciousness.

I am already preparing for such a future by studying my back issues of *Scientific American* and *Physics Today* back to January 1972, by learning how to connect with the Internet and World Wide Web, by reading and sending my e-mail every day, by attending social psychotherapeutic groups (mainly at the University of Colorado Health Sciences Center) as a means of socially greatly improving myself, by participating in research projects in which scientists at the Health Sciences Center study the abnormalities in the brains of those afflicted with what ranges from autism to Asperger syndrome (such as me), which will pinpoint the parts of the brain that have abnormalities, which will eventually lead to their being cured and ultimately using their special savantlike skills to benefit the world (for which I have already been paid for participation in one, based on magnetoencephalography), by having my brother Bill fine-tune and computer-print my doctoral thesis, by seeking help from you, Dr. Gary B. Mesibov, in publishing my autobiography, by having my brother Clay fine-tune it, reading it from a layman reader's point of view and not my own, and by reading your previous essays for inclusion in your book.

I hope in the future to be "one of the most unusual Americans, one of the greatest benefactors to the world, one of the most complete men in all history." In particular, I look forward to being the first person in history, at least whom I know of, to become great in physics despite chronic, very serious developmental disabilities. With my autobiography, *From Darkness to Light*, I hope to follow such American writers as Clifford W. Beers (*A Mind That Found Itself*), Joan Greenberg (*I Never Promised You a Rose Garden*), Donna Williams (*Nobody Nowhere* and *Somebody Somewhere*), and Temple Grandin (*Emergence Labeled Autistic*), to become famous in this manner.

19

Autistic and Undiagnosed

My Cautionary Tale

DAVE SPICER

OVERVIEW

Living with undiagnosed autism for many years has a profound effect on one's life. As someone who has done this, I felt it would be useful to others for me to describe some aspects of my experience. In particular, three groups may benefit most: professionals who work with autistic people diagnosed later in life, those autistic people who were identified only in recent years, and those people who are autistic and still do not know it. My hope is that what I say here will be useful to you, and to the present and future clients you will work with. The body of this essay is divided into three sections: internal mechanisms that I developed in childhood, the results of these mechanisms and other influences, and suggestions for other folks like me and those who work with them.

INTERNAL MECHANISMS

Somewhere fairly early in childhood, I realized that something was different about me. My reaction to situations and events was not what my family expected. This resulted in puzzlement, then frustration, as it became increasingly clear that what had worked well for my older sister and brother was not working

DAVE SPICER • Asheville, North Carolina 28805.

Asperger Syndrome or High-Functioning Autism?, edited by Schopler *et al.* Plenum Press, New York, 1998.

nearly as well for me. The most expressive thing I could do was to burst into tears over and over, but this did not communicate what was wrong, and despite a large and precise vocabulary I had no words for it.

Over time, I came to develop several coping mechanisms, in an effort to minimize the stress in those around me, and therefore my own stress.

One of these was to internalize others' expectations and criticism. This was necessary because I was extremely sensitive to feelings of disappointment or disapproval in others. These would overwhelm me, and I saw that if I could control myself tightly enough, this would not happen as often. Although this mode of learning might be expected of a toddler, it was all that I had for many years. If I could do a good enough job of conforming to others' expectations of me, and avoid doing things that would result in criticism, then I could "fit in better" with those around me, and attract less awful-feeling attention.

The worst problem with this strategy is that it can be carried too far. Overconforming can ultimately lead to loss of identity, and I went quite far in that direction. As it was safer not to express strong emotion, I learned to suppress it. People who are neurologically atypical can be especially sensitive to medication, and autistic people are often extra-sensitive to sensory input. Looking at these together, I feel that I was — and still am — especially sensitive to my own emotions, and have to control them tightly to keep from being incapacitated by them. Adrenaline, especially, is very powerful and disruptive to me.

Spontaneity was a problem for me as well, because it could produce a wide range of reactions in others, some of which felt awful to me. So again, it was safer to suppress it than to suffer the possible consequences.

What this left me was to appear adultlike, or what I thought was adultlike, and hope for the best. Using precise language was the best way I could see to have a chance of being understood, so I was precise. This wasn't the best solution, as it accentuated the difference between how I often sounded and how I acted when my internal controls failed. But it was all I had.

Suppressing my feelings did not eliminate them, though. A kind of underground reservoir developed inside me, containing frustration, resentment, jealousy, fear — and each instance of social ineptness or rejection added to it.

Over time, I internalized others' beliefs about me — that "there was nothing wrong with me," that I only needed to try harder, that if I really wanted to do things differently I could. In order to deal with each of these premises, I had to develop an interpretation of them, to translate them into something I could (at least partly) understand, and then turn into my beliefs about myself.

So "there was nothing wrong with me" became: "don't ask for help, because I'm not supposed to need any. Besides, if anyone looked really closely and still didn't find anything wrong, all of this really *would* be my fault. It's better just to have a small hope than to risk actually finding out."

And "all I needed to do was try harder" became "the other people around me are succeeding while I am not, and it must be as hard for them as it is for me.

So I am never to complain about difficulty or physical discomfort. If anything is physically at all possible to bear, it should be borne in silence."

Finally, "if I really wanted to change, I could" evolved into "I am deliberately resisting having my life, and the lives of those around me, be any better. I don't know why this is. But everyone feels this way, and they can't be wrong because look who they are and how many of them are saying it." In other words, I was deliberately making the people around me upset and angry.

Trying to function under these self-imposed guidelines was difficult. It was like trying to build a house on swampy ground that could not support any weight despite looking all right at first glance, or like trying to ice-skate on a pond that in many spots was barely frozen over. In each of these cases, the surface impression does not at all reflect what lies beneath, or the fragility of what is seen. And those around me built their houses, or skated on their ponds, and could not understand why I was having so much trouble. And neither could I. My self-esteem was very low, and more than anything else, I was ashamed of myself. Of my being. Of my entire life.

What came from all of this was a state resembling posttraumatic stress. Tendencies toward isolation and passivity, not uncommon in autism anyway, were reinforced. My understanding of what was happening around me had to be faulty, because so many things kept going wrong. I lived with a great deal of uncertainty about what was true and what was not. Unable to rely on my perceptions, I instead constructed a model of what I thought the world was, then lived in constant fear that someone would rush in and tell me that it was wrong.

[There is a phenomenon known as *learned helplessness*, which has been described by Peterson, Maier, and Seligman in a book bearing that title (Oxford University Press, 1993). It was observed that laboratory rats, after being subjected to random, inescapable electric shocks over time, would not try to avoid them when it later became possible to. When I read of this recently, I saw numerous parallels to my own life — in the pervasive stress, passivity, and even in the experiments themselves. The experience of thinking things were going along all right, and suddenly being informed that they were not, because of something I had done hours or days earlier — emotionally, this was close enough to an electric shock. I could definitely relate. What's more, the "learned helplessness" response seems to reinforce some characteristics of autism, making change/growth all the more difficult.]

In hindsight, it seems pretty clear to me that many of the mechanisms I had developed worked actively against my being helped, had effective help been available in the mid-1950s. Effectively, I was locked into an experience of living that looked as good as possible on the outside while barely functioning on the inside. This pattern continued for decades.

It is very important for me to point out that this happened despite the best of intentions on everyone's part. None of what I am relating is meant to assign blame to anyone.

RESULTS

Academically, elementary and junior high school were not difficult, except for "penmanship" at which I was awful. What I remember most clearly is how emotionally fragile I was, often bursting into tears to the dismay of my teachers. By high school, I had managed to become bland enough to not attract very much attention, except when a teacher would notice the difference between my very high performance on standardized aptitude tests and my very average grades. "Unrecognized potential," they called it.

College was a different story. In the fall of 1965, I found myself hundreds of miles from home, at a school where I knew no one, facing demands for self-reliance, initiative, and organization far beyond what I could manage. Also, as the subject material became more and more abstract, I found myself no longer able to understand it. The best I could do was to "survive as long as possible," as I had learned to do years earlier, with grades falling each semester. Toward the end, I stayed away from classes for weeks, afraid and alone. Finally, after three-plus years, it was over, except in my memory — thirty years later, I still have unpleasant dreams about being there.

Along with some of the basics of engineering, I came away from college with a great deal of experience with alcohol. From almost the very beginning, I found myself unable to drink in moderation. The combination of social isolation and academic stress, coupled with the "internal mechanisms" I described earlier, led me to seek relief. I kept seeking it in this manner for many years to come.

The courses I had taken in my first few semesters qualified me for engineering work in the local telephone company, which later led into computer programming. As time went on, my passivity and lack of self-direction interfered seriously with my productivity. Changing employers, which I did twice, would help for a while but the underlying problems were still there. At my last job, I became involved in a huge and very complex project that I was unable to handle my assigned portion of. A couple of years later, I went on long-term disability for anxiety-related issues.

In the midst of my time at college, I had become engaged, and married soon after starting my first full-time job. Between my lack of social development and my drinking, the marriage lasted just a few years. I remarried in 1976, and found that I still did not know how to have a successful intimate relationship. We stayed together to keep from being completely alone.

The first hope for change in my life came in the summer of 1983, when I entered recovery from alcoholism. Many issues still remained, but we had enough hope to have a child. Our son was born early in 1985. We separated in 1986 and divorced 2 years later.

I should add that, during these years, I began to see mental health professionals, in an effort to understand what was going on with me. Several years (and a lot of money) were spent pursuing various possibilities, including codependency, ADD, and nonexistent childhood sexual abuse. In each of these cases, *some* of my affect and experiences matched *some* of the profile for the condition. In a couple of cases, the professionals involved either ignored a clear sign such as my overloading during an exercise and banging my head on the floor, or wanted to continue pursuing a path that was clearly not leading anywhere. So along with everything else, I was seeing professionals during this time, trying to find out why my life had gone as it had.

Parenting is said to be a very demanding occupation. As a "shared-custody single parent," I found the stresses of parenthood barely manageable. My son, too, was having increasing difficulty in preschool, then in school and after-school programs. Finally, in the fall of 1993, we were referred to the Asheville TEACCH Center. My son was evaluated and diagnosed HFA/Asperger. At my request, I was also evaluated, and was diagnosed HFA/AS in April 1994. By this time, I was on disability leave, which ultimately became long-term disability for anxiety-related issues. My son was placed into therapeutic foster care in the spring of 1995, and remains there.

It's not really possible to condense 30 years of experiences into one presentation, but I hope several themes have come through this brief history: I was still having major difficulties with socialization, became unable to work, and was barely able to cope with the stress of parenthood. Without any understanding of why my life was as it was, without any effective support, and with the added complication of years of active alcoholism, at times I'm surprised that I survived it all. Although my experience was not as destructive as it could have been, it serves to illustrate what can happen when an autistic person does not receive the help he or she needs. This is why it's called a "cautionary tale."

SUGGESTIONS

A newly identified autistic adult needs support, and needs understanding. It may not be at all apparent to the person that his or her life could be any different than it has always been. If the reasons for difficulties in different areas can be explained, matter-of-factly, this information can be processed much more easily than profuse expressions of emotion. As one's life experience begins to make more sense, then much of what happened can be reframed in ways that no longer involve guilt or shame or self-hatred. This process may take quite a while, because of the amount of trauma involved.

It seems important that a person in this position be able to meet others who will listen, and who will understand. Being able to tell one's own story, and have it listened to, can be a major step in gaining back — or gaining for the first time — one's self-respect. I have been fortunate to be in the company of many other autistic folks, both in person and via the Internet. Together we are doing what we could probably never do alone.

Even those who have suffered for many years can find hope, and can experience a much higher quality of life. Perhaps it is this process of awakening, rather than the achievement of specific goals, that deserves the greatest attention. This is what has worked so far for me.

VII

Conclusion

20

Premature Popularization of Asperger Syndrome

ERIC SCHOPLER

Asperger (1944) described a disorder showing amazing overlap with autism first introduced by Kanner (1943) during the same time period. Since then, some clinicians and researchers have emphasized what they considered important differences between the two sets of descriptions, whereas others believed that Asperger syndrome (AS)[*] was the same as Kanner's autism when confined to children with high-functioning autism (HFA). Yet, paradoxically, AS appears in the title of an ever-increasing number of professional publications, including this volume, and AS is increasingly being used as a clinical designation, thus adding to the unresolved confusion.

CONTEXT THEORIES

This controversy has spanned over half a century, a period long enough to provide a backdrop of shifts in four major psychological theories, guiding and shaping mental health research and practice. First was psychodynamic theory, prevalent in post-World War II United States and Europe. Based on theory

---

[*] Some refer to AS as Asperger syndrome, whereas others call it Asperger's disorder (AD) as used in DSM-IV. In this discussion I will only use the broader terms AS and HFA in referring to the two groups.

ERIC SCHOPLER • Division TEACCH, Department of Psychiatry, University of North Carolina at Chapel Hill, Chapel Hill, North Carolina 27599-7180.

Asperger Syndrome or High-Functioning Autism?, edited by Schopler et al. Plenum Press, New York, 1998.

unrelated to empirical evidence, such Freudian theories produced considerable misunderstanding of "mental illness" and treatment, especially when applied to autism and related developmental disorders (Schopler, 1971). Autism as defined by Kanner (1943) was rescued from the untested assumptions of psychodynamic speculation by a growing emphasis on behavior theory, the second major psychological theory. Behaviorism saw its heyday during the 1960s and 1970s, when behaviors were quantified in research, and normal psychological processes were deduced from rat running experiments, repetitions of nonsense syllables, and measurements of galvanic skin reflexes. With its computational emphasis, behaviorism helped to rescue families from the misunderstanding of psychodynamic fancy, and it also produced concerns with missing the child in behavioral reductionism.

This led to the third theoretical orientation, sometimes called the "cognitive revolution" (Gardner, 1985), bringing renewed interest in the "mind," including the work of psycholinguists, brain modelers, and computer scientists. For this group of researchers, primary interest in stimulus strength and response patterns was replaced by mental actions such as thinking, attending, understanding, imagining, remembering, feeling, knowing the minds of others, and executive function.

The parallel trends of information processing and neurological specificity have also been linked with risks of reductionism, prompting Bruner (1996) to promote as a fourth new direction, "cultural psychology." He sees culture as being conveyed by oral history, composed of selected information and shared values. He considers the art of narrative the way in which we organize our experience and knowledge. In this chapter I will trace evidence from the work in these various theoretical frameworks, and show the lack of support for distinguishing AS from HFA from the history of Asperger's publications, from empirical research evidence, and the negative indicators from cultural psychology. I will also review medical and cultural bases for diagnostic classification, and the consequences of using AS as a meaningful category before the supporting evidence has been established.

HISTORY OF CONTROVERSY

It is to Asperger's credit that during the era when freewheeling psychodynamic theories were in prominent use, his own clinical papers refrained from such speculations. Nevertheless, the seeds for our current syndrome confusion were sown in the rich soil of his few publications. In his first paper, Asperger (1944) chose the label *autistic psychopathy*. The term *psychopathy* has been objectionable to many professionals familiar with children diagnosed by Kanner's autism criteria. Such children sometimes engage in aggressive, self-injurious, and destructive behaviors, but even when high functioning they do not usually engage in antisocial behaviors, such as manipulative lying, intentional cruelty, and behavior generally regarded as psychopathic. Wing, in Chapter 2, interprets Asperger's psychopathy as an "abnormality of personality." However, Asperger's own case descriptions (1944) leave little doubt that he referred to psychopathic characteristics in the currently accepted sense of the word. On p. 124, he refers to masturbation and sexual behavior engaged in public and rebellious fashion. "Even when treated affectionately they respond with malice and cruelty. They delight in malice, bordering on actual sadism, directed either physically or psychologically" (p. 126).

For Asperger, such psychopathy was not the idiosyncratic characteristics seen in a few of his clinic cases. He regarded such behavior sufficiently important to have it appear in the title of his seminal paper (Asperger, 1944). In the same paper he also referred to autistic characteristics, the same as in Kanner's autism. The main distinguishing feature between Kanner and Asperger could then be defined by the presence of psychopathy.

However, such a diagnostic distinction could also be the product of a sampling error rooted in Austrian culture. In a 1979 lecture, Asperger told his audience "of my rich childhood. My mental development owes much to the German youth movement, the noblest manifestation of the German spirit" (p. 45). As a precursor to the Hitler Youth Movement, with its intense nationalism and related psychopathies, Asperger could easily have drawn many of his subjects from that Youth Group, quite different from Kanner's American sample.

Characteristics without Priority

Another major source of diagnostic confusion originated in Asperger's (1944) paper. Instead of developing diagnostic criteria, he cited a host of different characteristics. A noble attempt to identify his eight most important points can be found in Wing's chapter. These include attributes like socially odd, egocentric, poor communication, circumscribed interests, clumsiness, lack of common sense, and extensive vocabulary with normal or better intelligence, all characteristics often associated with HFA. Her list does not include characteristics given equal weight by Asperger such as sadism, antisocial behavior, tendency to homesickness, and so on (Asperger, 1979, p. 50).

In other words, Asperger's publications include many different characteristics many of which are found in Kanner's definition of childhood autism. Asperger, primarily a clinician and educationalist, described his cases according to his experience. These characteristics had only the loosest connection to the summarizing label attached to the children. This was similar to the writing of U.S. clinicians in the immediate post-World War II era. Many different diagnostic labels were assigned then to severely disturbed children. These labels were attached to psychodynamic explanatory theories, most of which were not supported by either empirical or replicated clinical evidence. For example, Mahler (1952) postulated symbiotic psychosis as the development of psychosis and schizophrenia from excessive mother–infant attachment. Rank (1949) in Boston identified them as atypical. Bender (1953) used childhood schizophrenia, Ekstein and Wallerstein (1954) on the West Coast preferred borderline psychosis, and Bettelheim (1950) in Chicago sometimes used primary disorder of childhood. There was no agreement as to how these labels distinguished children. A child's diagnosis most predictably reflected the region or clinic offering the diagnosis. There was a great deal of overlap between the descriptions of Asperger and Kanner. Nevertheless, the difference between the work of Asperger and his American psychiatric contemporaries, on the one hand, and the work of Leo Kanner, on the other, was quite striking.

Kanner's writing was different from most of his colleagues. His case descriptions were not only clinically lucid, they were also behaviorally observable. Children with Kanner's autism were immediately diagnosed in other countries. The syndrome could be conceptualized into defining features, still used in diagnostic manuals today, more than 50 years later. During that period, Kanner founded the *Journal of Autism and Childhood Schizophrenia,* the only international journal devoted to autism-related research. His robust diagnostic category has arguably inspired more empirical research and scientific understanding of a mental disorder than any other psychiatric label. It is fair to say that prior to Kanner's contribution, the field of child psychiatry was dominated by idiosyncratic and theory-based classification. Kanner's contribution to the field emphasized behavioral observation, empirical research, and rational intervention strategies.

AS, on the other hand, had a very different effect on the field. Prior to 1980, it was mostly ignored in the United States. In Chapter 5, Gillberg and Ehlers were only able to identify four papers specifically referring to "autistic psychopathy." These four were written by European scientists. Following Wing's (1981) paper, Gillberg and Ehlers found more than 140 articles written in English through 1995. The distinction between AS-related papers before and after 1981 shows that the impact of AS on the field was far less than the impact of Kanner's work. Most likely the renewed interest in Asperger's publication rolled in on the wave of Kanner-inspired research and on his primary interest in HFA. Asperger's own publications did not inspire research, replication, or scientific interest prior to 1980. Instead, he laid the fertile groundwork for the diagnostic confusion that has grown since 1980 and is still blooming in this volume.

CORRECTIVE EFFORTS TO ESTABLISH AS DIAGNOSTIC CRITERIA

Because Asperger had not succeeded in identifying a replicable psychiatric syndrome, several investigators have formulated their own view of the essential features. The resulting ambiguities were translated into "research criteria" in ICD-10, research criteria not found in the most important reference book based on diagnostic consensus namely, DSM-IV (APA, 1994).

However, before reviewing individual research efforts to ameliorate the diagnostic confusion produced by Asperger's undifferentiated array of descriptive characteristics, it is worth reviewing the five requirements for defining a specific syndrome, cited by Wing in Chapter 2. They are: (1) if the cause is known as different from other conditions, (2) if the condition has a specific neuropathology, (3) if a consistent and unique pattern of psychological dysfunction is present, (4) if a condition shows the same course over time, and (5) if there is a specific response to a unique intervention. She concluded that none of these conditions served to distinguish AS from HFA.

However, before employing these general classification criteria, Wing (1981) tried to formulate AS diagnostic criteria from the available clinical information. She cited seven problem areas identified from Asperger's own account, namely, difficulties in (1) speech, (2) nonverbal communication, (3) social interaction, (4) repetitive activities, (5) motor coordination, (6) special skills, and (7) school difficulties. However, she added a number of additional items, observed in some of her own cases, but not recorded by Asperger. These are: (1) lack of human interest the first year of life, (2) limited babbling, (3) limited imaginative play, (4) speech before walking, but slow to walk, (5) rote language with long obscure words, (6) unlike Asperger, she reported no sign of creativity, only narrow literal reasoning, (7) poor comprehension, (8) careers in special interests like math and science, and (9) anxiety, depression, and suicide attempts. These observations broadened the definition and served to suggest a spectrum and broadened the AS definition without reducing the diagnostic confusion.

Szatmari, Bartolucci, and Brenner (1989) tried to improve the situation by setting forth their own diagnostic criteria (see Chapter 5, this volume). Their fifth criterion recommends that the individual does not meet DSM-III-R criteria for autistic disorder, a most difficult requirement considering the overlap prescribed in both DSM-III-R and DSM-IV.

Gillberg (1991) published his own criteria, an elaboration of his previously published criteria (Gillberg & Gillberg, 1989). There is considerable overlap with Szatmari and colleagues' (1989), but Gillberg recommended six criteria instead of five, and emphasized extreme egocentricity among the social impairments, and that some individuals may have an autism diagnosis at one point and AS at another, presumably with either the same or different diagnosticans. Obviously, it becomes increasingly difficult to arrive at a usable classification system as increasing numbers of authors introduce their own variations in criteria.

Perhaps a step toward the resolution of the diagnostic confusion was taken through the consensus approach employed by the publishers of DSM-IV and ICD-10 (WHO, 1993). Diagnostic criteria were formulated by committee consensus, but an effort was also made to give special weight to empirical evidence. The DSM-IV criteria were based, in part, on multicenter field trials (Volkmar *et al.*, 1994). Both of these diagnostic systems describe great overlap with the autism definition. The ICD-10 criteria are distinguished from DSM-IV as research criteria. Apparently this was done to accommodate finer distinctions than seemed clinically meaningful to the authors of the DSM-IV definitions. This distinction helps to confuse diagnostic hypotheses about specific functions with validated diagnostic clusters. The classification criteria for a clinical condition should probably not be distinguished from research criteria for projected research. Under ICD-10, specific diagnostic requirements are given, such as single words should have developed by 2 years of age or earlier, or communicative phrases be used by 3 years or earlier. These represent important research issues. But surely they do not have to be studied under the AS label, one already compromised by too many overlapping yet different diagnostic requirements.

Both ICD-10 and DSM-IV posit that there be no signs of early language retardation or abnormality. Unfortunately, this distinguishing feature has not been shown to differentiate AS from HFA. Moreover, it broadens the likelihood of producing false positives, and over inclusively encompassing contributing professors of math and science with an undesired AS label. Partly inspired by the apparent definition consensus published in DSM-IV and ICD-10, several important empirical studies were launched in the search for identifying syndrome features.

EMPIRICAL RESEARCH EVIDENCE

During the era sometimes called the *cognitive revolution* (Gardner, 1985), a number of research concepts became popular, concepts that distinguished specific facets of cognitive development, useful for operationalizing specific steps in socialization and communication. They included motor development, visuospatial components, executive function, and theory of mind. Other communication characteristics have been suggested as unique to Asperger disorder, such as pedantic speech, and early language development, but these have also been observed in HFA.

Motor Functions

Several studies investigated the possibility that AS could be distinguished from HFA by the criterion of clumsiness (Gillberg & Gillberg, 1989; Tantam, 1988). No distinction in clumsiness between Asperger disorder and HFA was found by Ghaziuddin, Tsai, and Ghaziuddin (1994), a finding replicated by Marjiviona and Prior (1995). Klin, Volkmar, Sparrow, Cicchetti, and Rourke

(1995) and Volkmar and Klin (Chapter 6, this volume) reported more clumsiness for AS than for HFA, but this result is consistent with their subject selection, for which clumsiness helped to define their AS sample.

Visuospatial Function

If clumsiness does not uniformly differentiate AS from HFA, perhaps differences in intellectual strengths and weakness can be documented. That individuals with autism have lower scores on verbal subtests and higher scores on performance tests was reported by Lincoln, Allen, and Kilman (1995) and Green, Fein, Joy, and Waterhouse (1995). Klin et al. (1995) found the reverse—higher verbal IQ and lower performance IQ for AS. However, no verbal–performance IQ discrepancy was found by Szatmari, Tuff, Finlayson, and Bartolucci (1990), Ozonoff, Roger, and Pennington(1991), and Marjiviona and Prior (1995).

Theory of Mind and Executive Function

The possibility that AS individuals performed better on theory of mind tests than individuals with HFA was examined by Prior, Dahlstrom, and Squires (1990) and Ozonoff et al. (1991), but this was not found. Another possibility was that individuals with Asperger disorder showed more impairment in executive functioning than did individuals with HFA. Szatmari et al. (1990) found that their Asperger disorder group did somewhat better than their autistic group, but this study did not control for IQ differences. Ozonoff et al. (1991) reported no differences in executive function between Asperger disorder and HFA.

These studies have been inconclusive for several considerations: (1) The distinguishing AS feature reported in the results of the study was part of the definition by which the sample was selected. (2) AS characteristics published in clinical studies were also present in some HFA cases. (3) The AS characteristic reported in one study was not replicated or not found in replication. We have here the interesting phenomenon that there is no agreement on the defining features or on the validity of the syndrome from one sample to the next. Yet there appears to be an ever-increasing number of studies and clinical referrals using the AS designation. The question has arisen whether new insight or clinical practice has resulted from studies conducted with the controversial AS designation.

Probably the most intriguing possibilities have been reported from the neuropsychological direction suggesting neural correlates for certain cognitive functions, and intervention implications. Only two of the possible examples discussed in this volume are cited here.

Executive function impairment has been found for both AS and HFA. The impairments have been reported both clinically and in research (see Ozonoff, Chapter 12) with probable frontal lobe involvement. Among innovative interventions, Ozonoff suggests the inclusion of the individualized educational program (IEP) recommendation of teacher support for impaired executive function. This leads toward a new direction in knowledge and intervention. In this research, a distinction between HFA and AS was not found. However, one is not needed to support the importance of their study.

Another innovative direction has been identified in connection with nonverbal learning disabilities (NLD). NLD characteristics were reported to include: lower performance IQ relative to verbal IQ, worse on visuospatial tasks than on auditory linguistic tasks, better memory for verbal than nonverbal information. Such individuals are also described as clumsy and have poor handwriting, are impaired in math, and show interpersonal difficulties (Rourke, 1989). Similarities between NLD and AS were also noted by Denckla (1983), and are discussed in Chapter 6 of this volume, where Volkmar and Klin report similarities in the neuropsychological profiles for AS and NLD. They also found distinctions in such profiles for AS and HFA. Because their sample was preselected for related AS characteristics (Klin & Volkmar, 1995), it is unlikely that their fine profile distinctions between AS and HFA described in Chapter 6 will be validated. The functions compared may refer to a distinction between left and right brain deficits with rather different intervention implications. As with the previous example, the significance of the new directions in this admirable line of research is not dependent on whether a distinction between AS and HFA is found.

Controversy Resolution with Survey Data

In an attempt to have this volume resolve the controversy of whether HFA and AS are the same or different disorders, we asked the authors of the first 14 chapters to give their own opinion on this question. However, not all of the authors complied with a direct response. It was therefore necessary for me to surmise their views. The impression is that my ratings in Table 20-1 are highly accurate. However, if there is any doubt, the reader may want to check with the author directly.

Twelve of the fourteen chapters regard the distinction between HFA and AS to be nonexistent or ambiguous. It is of special interest that Lorna Wing, whose 1981 publication was instrumental in generating this discussion, now does not believe in the distinction. Likewise, Sally Ozonoff, who reported a distinction between AS and HFA some years ago (Ozonoff *et al.*, 1991), now believes that no valid distinctions exist. It is also noteworthy that none of the four chapters in Part IV (Treatment Issues) report a distinction between AS and HFA. The

Table 20-1. Author Survey: Is High-Functioning Autism Distinct
from Asperger's Disorder?

Author	Chapter	Not distinct	Ambiguous	Distinct
Wing	2	X		
Pomeroy	3			X
Szatmari	4		X	
Gillberg & Ehlers	5	X		
Volkmar & Klin	6			X
Wolff	7		X	
Lincoln et al.	8		X	
Gray	9	X		
Twachtman-Cullen	10	X		
Kunce & Mesibov	11		X	
Ozonoff	12	X		
McDougle	13		X	
Hooper & Bundy	14		X	
Schopler	20	X		
		6	6	2

discussion of the two categories as distinct or ambiguous seems to relate to the use of the ICD-10 research definition, not easily used in a clinical diagnosis.

Only two chapters endorsed a clear distinction between AS and HFA. Pomeroy's (Chapter 3) differentiation is based on a previously unpublished factor analysis, a statistical procedure recognized for generating factors, not often reflected in the real world. Volkmar and Klin (Chapter 6), on the other hand, drew their AS sample from the DSM-IV field trial data. Although this was a multicenter study important to the DSM-IV classification, it is unlikely that all centers selected their AS sample according to the same criteria.

Earlier in this chapter, I reviewed the historical basis for the classification confusion produced by the interaction between Asperger's diffuse case reporting style and the mental health field's use of idiosyncratic and dynamic theory-based diagnostic labels. This was followed by a review of the eruptions of AS publications over the past 15 years. During this period a number of characteristics published by Asperger were investigated in terms of a clinically meaningful distinction between AS and HFA. So far none have been established with validity.

This raises the question of whether a reliable distinction between AS and HFA could be made. No doubt a consensus could be reached that all individuals with the autism syndrome are called AS if they are clumsy, use pedantic speech, show impaired executive function, have higher full-scale IQ, and so on. The closest consensus to this was the DSM-IV definition, positing no significant delay in language, but even this important language development feature represents only the consensus of a small DSM-IV study committee. Even if a consensus differentiating AS from HFA could be reached, should such a distinction be made? What are the advantages and disadvantages, the cost–benefit ratio? Is it worth doing?

CULTURAL PSYCHOLOGY FACTORS

The answers to such questions are found in the context of a new banner of cultural psychology, raised by Bruner (1996) in divergence from what he regarded as the excesses of reductionisms that he associated with the cognitive revolution. For Bruner, what brings the mind to focus is culture — "the way of life and thought that we construct, negotiate, institutionalize, and finally (after it's all settled) end up calling 'reality' to comfort ourselves" (Bruner, 1996). It is from this perspective that we examine both the development and the probable consequences of institutionalizing as a syndrome "Asperger disorder."

Cultural Influences on Diagnostic Classification

When Wing's (1981) paper stimulated the resurgence of AS for clinical application and research publications, I was among those who thought it counterproductive to introduce a psychiatric syndrome prior to the establishment of its clinical validity (Schopler, 1985, 1996). It is noteworthy that, throughout her illustrious career, Dr. Wing had made important contributions to our understanding of autism through her empirical research and astute behavioral observations. Yet her rationale for reintroducing AS was drawn from the informal perspective of cultural psychology. Although she acknowledged that HFA and AS could not be differentiated clearly (Wing, 1986), she offered the following two major reasons (Wing, 1991):

The first reason was that the diagnosis of autism in the minds of many lay people is synonymous with total absence of speech, social isolation, and absorption in bodily stereotypes. Parents of a relatively high-functioning child will not accept the diagnosis of autism but find AS much more acceptable. However, this observation may represent a cultural difference between England and the United States. Where in England the popular understanding of autism may be based on the severe end of the continuum, characterized by bodily stereotypes and self-aggressive behavior, in the United States a more positive stereotype is prevalent. It is based on the upbeat film portrayal, by Dustin Hoffman in *Rain Man,* of an appealing young man with special memory skills. Therefore, most parents tend to prefer the diagnosis of HFA, especially when it is explained in the context of potential skill development.

The second reason given (Wing, 1991) was that too many professional workers including psychiatrists working with adults, have a narrow view of autism as a condition of childhood, not of adulthood. The publications on AS have had the effect of alerting nonspecialist professionals that an autistic person of normal intelligence can be undiagnosed in childhood and develop AS later in life.

Although this kind of assessment may have a positive component, there is no reason to think the same awareness could not also have been produced with the designation of HFA. Moreover, this awareness has brought with it a great increase in referrals, more of which are false positive than was the case in the past. An increase in referrals appears to be a phenomenon seen in virtually all countries. Possible reasons usually cited for this include: greater public awareness, more at-risk births surviving, and increase in environmental toxins. But the emphasis is frequently placed on the ever-increasing use of the AS diagnosis.

CONSEQUENCES OF THE AS LABEL

In order to obtain broader understanding of the label, and issues for people directly involved, I led a discussion of about 400 individuals at a conference for More Able Autistic People (MAAP) (Schopler, 1995). The conference participants were individuals given a diagnosis of HFA or AS, their parents or relatives, and professionals. During our discussion of the consequences for the newly popularized AS designation, it frequently appeared that advantages from a professional perspective were disadvantages from the client/parent perspective.

Increased Professional Interest and Knowledge

Wing (1991) mentioned that adult psychiatrists and others not immediately working with developmental problems showed better interest and understanding of the new AS label and social-communication problems shared by individuals with AS or HFA. They learned that a child undiagnosed during childhood can receive an AS diagnosis as an adult. It is said to give them a better understanding of the wide developmental spectrum involved and it helps policemen understand some of the special social-communication problems so often misunderstood with such individuals.

From the client/parent perspective, professional pursuit of a new label is not necessarily consistent with sounder professional practice. It is more akin to the pursuit of new treatment fads with their unanticipated negative side effects and misunderstanding. That the undiagnosed child can be labeled AS as an adult has also produced more false positives, and as mentioned before has included productive professors of science and mathematics who are not seeking professional help.

Rather than broadening public understanding of the broad autism spectrum, the AS label draws attention primarily to the narrow high-functioning end of the continuum. Moreover, all such "new" insight can be disseminated more easily with the HFA designation. For example, police in San Sebastian, Spain, had been alerted to autism problems by Dr. Fuentes's autism program for the past two decades. They have been able to mediate any number of misunderstandings in social interactions, coming to their attention from adults with autism in their community.

New Research Initiated and Funded with the AS Label

The increasing number of publications in the English language using the AS label since 1981 has already been noted, and is represented in this volume. They present some new knowledge, especially in neuropsychology where cognitive functions have been correlated with specific neural patterns, and intervention procedures (see various chapters in this book). The "new" AS label has, no doubt, also generated new research funding. Moreover, the additional referrals requiring diagnostic evaluation and consultations provide new job opportunities for increasing numbers of graduating professionals.

From the consumer's perspective, this increase is not necessarily advantageous. The new research knowledge could have been achieved more efficiently had HFA been used without the confounding AS characteristics. The research funds would have reached further, had the focus on central cognitive functions investigated not been diffused by unclear label distinctions. In Chapter 7, Wolff provides ample examples for the scope of the label confusion. She mentions that AS has possible overlap or bordering with a number of diagnostic categories including: schizoid personality, schizotypal, Type A personality disorder, schizophrenic spectrum disorder, elective mutism, autistic psychopathy, developmental language disorder, school refusal, conduct disorder, personality disorder, benign psychosis, borderline status, multiplex developmental disorder, right hemisphere deficits, autistic spectrum, dyslalia, and language disorder. Such profusion of labels almost ensures the likelihood for a regression to the diagnostic confusion of the psychodynamic period discussed above. The availability of many related diagnostic labels may provide professional stimulation, but it will also increase the cost to affected individuals, their families, and communities for diagnostic service and consultation. In some regions, AS organizations have been formed requiring interested parents to join both AS and autism societies, increasing family cost for finding information and support.

Access to Services

Considerable discussion occurred at the MAAP conference on the question of whether better service access was available for the label of AS or for HFA. Although some reported improvement in service availability when AS was used, the large majority of individuals reported better service with the more familiar HFA label. The difference was regional, depending on where autism was known and what special services were available under the more familiar label. A number of professionals thought that the consensus represented by the DSM-IV definition would be clinically compelling and provide better support for those fitting AS, but clients and their relatives thought that reeducation to a "new" label produced additional obstacles.

Unfortunately, in the United States there is more experience with the benefits of reducing than adding controversial labels. For example, homosexuality was considered a form of mental illness until the mid-1970s. At that time, by a simple majority vote, APA decreed that homosexuality was no longer a mental illness. Few would argue that removal from that category was less than a positive experience for the individuals involved.

It is unlikely that the inclusion of a diagnostic category like AS in the DSM, before its clinical validity has been established, will be particularly helpful. Instead it will support followers of Szasz (1974) who claim that mental illness is a myth. When no specific and measurable neurobiological or biochemical process can be demonstrated for a given symptom or symptom cluster, the latter claim to be dealing with a behavioral disorder and not a psychiatric illness.

CONCLUSION

In this chapter I have traced the history of the AS, a condition overlapping with autism and normal language development plus a set of diffuse characteristics lodged in German and European culture. I have reviewed how the differentiation between HFA and AS has been attempted through clinical formulation, empirical research using cognitive and neuropsychological procedures, and cultural psychology factors. None of these have to date identified or replicated a valid clinical subgroup. AS appears to be a product of culture, with a life independent of empirical evidence.

In the final analysis, if a valid distinction is found between HFA and AS, it may be unimportant which term is used for overlapping phenomena. In the meantime, the premature use of the AS label serves as a seriously flawed model for how psychiatric diagnostic categories are formed. It should have been left in the investigative state until a valid subgroup had been established. It appears to me that premature use of the AS label has had far more negative consequences than positive, slowing down what progress in understanding and treatment of autism has been accomplished to date.

REFERENCES

American Psychiatric Association. (1994). *Diagnostic and statistical manual of mental disorders* (4th ed.). Washington, DC: Athor.

Asperger, H. (1944). Die 'autistischen Psychopathen' im Kindesalter. *Archiv für Psychiatrie und Nervenkrankheiten, 117*, 76–136. Translated by U. Frith (Ed.), *Autism and Asperger syndrome* (1991, pp. 37–92). Cambridge: Cambridge University Press.

Asperger, H. (1979). Problems of infantile autism. *Communication, 13*, 45–52.

Bender, L. (1953). Childhood schizophrenia. *Psychiatric Quarterly, 27*, 663–681.

Bettelheim, B. (1950). *Love is not enough.* New York: Free Press.

Bruner, J. (1996). *The culture of education.* Cambridge, MA: Harvard University Press.

Denckla, M. (1983). The neuropsychology of social-emotional learning disabilities. *Archives of Neurology, 40*, 461–462.

Ekstein, R., & Wallerstein, J. (1954). Observations on the psychology of borderline and psychotic children. *Psychoanalytic Study of the Child* (Vol. 9). New York: International Press.

Gardner, H. (1985). *The mind's new science: A history of the cognitive revolution.* New York: Basic Books.

Ghaziuddin, M., Tsai, L. Y., & Ghaziuddin, N. (1994). Is clumsiness a marker for Asperger Syndrome? *Journal of Intellectual Disability Research, 38*, 519–527.

Gillberg, C. (1991). Clinical and neurobiological aspects of Asperger syndrome in six family studies. In U. Frith (Ed.), *Autism and Asperger syndrome* (pp. 122–146). Cambridge: Cambridge University Press.

Gillberg, I. C., & Gillberg, C. (1989). Asperger syndrome — some epidemiological considerations: A research note. *Journal of Child Psychology and Psychiatry, 30*, 631–638.

Green, L., Fein, D., Joy, S., & Waterhouse, L. (1995). Cognitive functioning in autism: An overview. In E. Schopler & G. B. Mesibov (Eds.), *Learning and cognition in autism* (pp. 13–31). New York: Plenum Press.

Kanner, L. (1943). Autistic disturbance of affective contact. *Nervous Child, 2*, 217–250.

Klin, A., & Volkmar, F. R. (1995). *Asperger syndrome: Some guidelines for assessment, diagnosis and intervention* (pp. 2–14). Learning Disability Association of America.

Klin, A., Volkmar, F. R., Sparrow, S. S., Cicchetti, D. V., & Rourke, B. P. (1995). Validity and neuropsychological characterization of Asperger syndrome. *Journal of Child Psychology and Psychiatry, 36*, 1127–1140.

Lincoln, A. J., Allen, M. H., & Kilman, A. (1995). The assessment and interpretation of intellectual abilities in people with autism. In E. Schopler & G. B. Mesibov (Eds.), *Learning and cognition in autism.* (pp. 89–114). New York; Plenum Press.

Mahler, M. (1952). On child psychosis and schizophrenia. Autistic and psychotic infantile psychoses. *Psychoanalytic Study of the Child* (Vol. 7). New York: International Press.

Marjiviona, J., & Prior, M. (1995). Comparison of Asperger syndrome and high-functioning autistic children on a test of motor impairment. *Journal of Autism and Developmental Disorders, 25*, 23–39.

Ozonoff, S., Rogers, S., & Pennington, B. (1991). Asperger's syndrome: Evidence of an empirical distinction from high-functioning autism. *Journal of Child Psychology and Psychiatry, 32*, 1107–1122.

Prior, M., Dahlstrom, B., & Squires, T. L. (1990). Autistic children's knowledge of thinking and feeling states in other people. *Journal of Child Psychology and Psychiatry, 31*, 587–601.

Rank, B. (1949). Adaptation of the psychoanalytic technique for the treatment of young children with atypical development. *American Journal of Orthopsychiatry, 19*, 130.

Rourke, B. P. (1989). *Nonverbal learning disabilities: The syndrome and the model.* New York: Guilford Press.

Schopler, E. (1971). Parents of psychotic children as scapegoats. *Journal of Contemporary Psychotherapy, 4*, 17–22.

Schopler, E. (1985). Convergence of learning disability, higher level autism, and Asperger syndrome [Editorial]. *Journal of Autism and Developmental Disorders, 15*, 359.

Schopler, E. (1995, September 15). *Is AS different from HFA?* Presented at the Conference for More Able Autistic People (MAAP), Indianapolis, IN.

Schopler, E. (1996). Are autism and Asperger syndrome different labels or different disabilities? *Journal of Autism and Developmental Disorders, 26,* 109–110.

Szasz, T. S. (1974). *The myth of mental illness* (rev. ed.). New York: Harper & Row.

Szatmari, P., Bartolucci, G., & Bremner, R. (1989). Asperger's syndrome and autism: Comparisons on early history and outcome. *Developmental Medicine and Child Neurology, 31,* 709–720.

Szatmari, P., Tuff, L., Finlayson, M. A. J., & Bartolucci, G. (1990). Asperger's syndrome and autism: Neurocognitive aspects. *Journal of the American Academy of Child and Adolescent Psychiatry, 29,* 130–136.

Tantam, D. (1988). Lifelong eccentricity and social isolation II. Asperger's syndrome or schizoid personality disorder? *British Journal of Psychiatry, 153,* 783–791.

Volkmar, F., Klin, A., Siegel, B., Szatmari, P., Lord, C., Campbell, M., Freeman, B. J., Cicchetti, D. V., Rutter, M., Kline, W., Buitelaar, J., Hattab, Y., Fombonne, E., Fuentes, J., Werry, J., Stone, W., Kerbeshian, J., Hoshino, Y., Bregman, J., Loveland, K., Szymanski, L., & Towbin, K. (1994). DSM-IV autism/pervasive developmental disorder field trial. *American Journal of Psychiatry, 151,* 1361–1367.

Wing, L. (1981). Asperger's syndrome: A clinical account. *Psychological Medicine, 11,* 115–130.

Wing, L. (1986). Clarification on Asperger's syndrome [Letter to the editor]. *Journal of Autism and Developmental Disorders, 16,* 513–515.

Wing, L. (1991). The relationship between Asperger's syndrome and Kanner's autism. In U. Frith (Ed.), *Autism and Asperger syndrome* (pp. 93–119). Cambridge: Cambridge University Press.

World Health Organization. (1993). *International classification of diseases: Tenth revision* Chapter V. Mental and behavioral disorders (including disorders of psychological development): Diagnostic criteria for research. Geneva: Author.

Index